TRENDS IN GENOME RESEARCH

TRENDS IN GENOME RESEARCH

CLYDE R. WILLIAMS
EDITOR

Nova Biomedical Books
New York

Library of Congress Cataloging-in-Publication Data
Available upon request

ISBN 1-60021-027-9

Published by Nova Science Publishers, Inc. ✢New York

Contents

Preface

The genomic approach of technology development and large-scale generation of community resource data sets has introduced an important new dimension in biological and biomedical research. Interwoven advances in genetics, comparative genomics, high throughput biochemistry and bioinformatics are combining to attack basic understanding of human life and disease and to develop strategies to combat disease. Genomic Research began with The Human Genome Project (HGP), the international research effort that determined the DNA sequence of the entire human genome, completed in April 2003. The HGP also included efforts to characterize and sequence the entire genomes of several other organisms, many of which are used extensively in biological research. Identification of the sequence or function of genes in a model organism is an important approach to finding and elucidating the function of human genes. Integral to the HGP are similar efforts to understand the genomes of various organisms commonly used in biomedical research, such as mice, fruit flies and roundworms. Such organisms are called "model organisms," because they can often serve as research models for how the human organism behaves. This new book brings together leading research from throughout the world in this cutting-edge field.

Sophisticated new molecular scanning technologies have the ability to rapidly identify the underlying bases of complex genetic disorders, which allows early diagnostics and targeted therapeutics to be implemented in the clinic rapidly. Additionally, current technology now provides the ability to comprehensively monitor surrogate molecular markers, which will revolutionize how clinical trials will be implemented. The authors discuss in Chapter 1 the evolution of genomic technologies and how these technological advances will affect the strategies used to diagnose and, ultimately, to cure complex and common human diseases.

As explained in Chapter 2, a great number of aerobic endospore-forming Gram-positive *Bacillus* species have been isolated on a number of occasions from a variety of terrestrial and deep-sea environments, including the Mariana Trench which has a depth of 10,897 m. Some of these *Bacullus* species are known to have various capabilities for adapting to extreme environments. In fact, *Bacillus*-related species can grow in a wide range of environments— at pH 2-12, at temperatures between 5 and 78°C, in salinity from 0 to 30% NaCl, and under pressures from 0.1 Mpa to at least 30 Mpa. The authors are now exploring how these adaptive capabilities, as reflected in their genomes, were acquired and what intrinsic genomic structures are present in *Bacillus*-related species that have allowed them to adapt to such a wide range of environments. To answer these questions, they initiated a genome sequencing project in early 1998 and have to present determined the entire genomic sequences of three extremophilic bacilli: alkaliphilic *Bacillus halodurans*, extremely halotolerant and alkaliphilic *Oceanobacillus iheyensis*, and thermophilic *Geobacillus kaustophilus*. We provide the first comparative analysis of the extremophilic bacillar genomes with those of three other phylogenetically related mesophilic and neutrophilic bacilli, *B. subtilis*, *B. anthracis* and *B. cereus*, in order to highlight the commonality and diversity of the bacillar genome.

The stable and site-specific modification of mammalian genomes has a variety of applications in biomedicine and biotechnology. In Chapter 3 the authors outline two alternative approaches that can be employed to achieve this goal: homologous recombination or site-specific recombination. Homologous recombination relies on sequence similarity (or rather identity) of a piece of DNA that is introduced into a host cell and the host genome. The frequency of homologous recombination is generally markedly lower than the process of random integration. Especially in somatic cells homologous recombination is an extremely rare event. However, strategies involving the introduction of double-strand breaks can increase the frequency of homologous recombination.

Site-specific recombination makes use of enzymes (recombinases, transposases, integrases), which catalyse DNA strand exchange between DNA molecules that have only limited sequence homology. The recognition sites of site-specific recombinases (e.g. Cre or ΦC31) are usually 30 - 40bp. Retroviral integrases only require a specific dinucleotide sequence to insert the viral cDNA into the host genome. Depending on the individual enzyme, there are either innumerable or very few potential target sites for a particular integrase/recombinase in a mammalian genome. A number of strategies have been utilized successfully to alter the site-specificity of recombinases. Therefore site-specific recombinases provide an attractive tool for the targeted modification of mammalian genomes.

As presented in Chapter 4, large-scale compilation of the 5'-end data of human full-length cDNAs enabled us for the first time to identify the precise locations of the transcriptional start sites (TSSs) on a genome-wide scale. The information obtained on the TSSs was further utilized to retrieve the adjacent promoter regions from the recently completed human genomic sequence. Now, with the massively compiled information about the TSSs and promoters, analyses are underway to obtain a comprehensive view of the regulatory mechanisms of the transcriptional regulation. Detailed analysis of the positional information of the TSSs revealed that the TSS(s) of a gene are generally scattered over a 50-bp region on average and the patterns of the distribution of the TSSs differ significantly depending on the promoter, possibly reflecting the dynamics of the interaction between the promoters and the transcriptional machineries. A catalogue of representative promoter sequences was generated and provides a database that will serve as a foundation for further network-level studies of human transcriptional regulation. Moreover, recent advances in genome sequencing in other organisms, such as mouse, rat and dog, made it possible to study the molecular evolution of the promoters. Interestingly, intensive comparative studies of the human and mouse promoters suggested that quite a few promoter motifs seemed not to be conserved between human and mouse. Constant evolutional generation and loss of transcriptional regulatory modules may help to explain the molecular basis of speciation.

Array-based comparative genomic hybridization (array CGH) enables simultaneous genome-wide screening for regions of genomic alterations in a test genomic sample relative to a reference sample. Genomic alterations may be identified by regionspecific copy number gains or losses. Identification of these specific regions of copy number change may aid identification of genomic alterations associated with specific diseases, such as tumorigenisis.

The detection of genomic alterations using array CGH requires careful statistical analysis to account for many sources of variation, such as spatial correlation along each chromosome, and heterogeneity of variances. The hybrid adaptive spline (HAS) method has been previously applied to array CGH data to deal with spatial inhomogeneity, by modeling copy numbers in terms of an adaptively selected set of basis functions. The traditional HAS procedure uses a fixed inflated degrees of freedom (IDF) to account for the increased cost of adaptive basis function selection. However, the authors demonstrate in Chapter 5 that a fixed selection cost may lead to HAS selecting too many basis functions in the final model. To overcome this problem, they propose a data-driven measure of the IDF based on the concept of the generalized degrees of freedom (GDF). Our extended hybrid adaptive spline procedure based on this estimated IDF is more adaptive to different data sets and basis functions. The authors use a bootstrap method to compute p-values, which does not require a Gaussian assumption. They also use the False Discovery Rate (FDR) to circumvent the problem of multiple comparisons. They use a well known BAC array data set to illustrate our methods.

Common fragile sites of the human genome are suggested to be potentially involved in cancer development; *FRA6E* (6q26), one of the most frequently expressed common fragile sites in humans, is located in a region frequently found rearranged in cancer. We have mapped *FRA6E* by FISH analysis with YAC, BAC and PAC genomic clones, and have characterized the fragility of the region by sequence analysis. Recent published data indicated that the location of *FRA6E* is about 2.5 Mb beyond the telomeric side of the region considered in the present study. Taken together, the data and previously reported data indicate that *FRA6E* spans approximately 9 Mb, corresponding to a chromosomal region located at 6q25.3-6q26. It has been recently suggested that unusual structural features, detected as high flexibility motives by sequence analysis, are overrepresented within fragile sites, and that this organization can be relevant for the intrinsic fragility of these regions. We have carried out a search for fragility motives within the genomic sequence corresponding to *FRA6E,* confirming the significance of unusual structural organization of chromosome sequences with respect to the location of common fragile sites. A number of expressed genes map at *FRA6E,* which can be relevant for cancer. RT-PCR analysis revealed that some of them are down-regulated in melanoma tumors. The results outlined in Chapter 6 underline the need for a deep investigation of the fragility regions of the human genome, which are probably wider than previously thought.

As outlined in Chapter 7, The National Institute of Standards and Technology (NIST), formerly called the National Bureau of Standards (NBS), has developed over 1300 Standard Reference Materials (SRMs). The Office of Standard Reference Materials defines and describes a SRM as a: "well-characterized material produced in quantity to improve measurement science. It is certified for specific chemical or physical properties, and is issued by NIST with a certificate that reports the results of the characterization and indicates the intended use of the material. A SRM is prepared and used for the following three purposes: 1.To help develop accurate methods of analysis; 2. To calibrate measurement systems used to facilitate exchange of goods, institute quality control, determine performance characteristics, or measure a property at the state-of-the-art limit; and 3. To assure the long-term adequacy and integrity of measurement quality assurance programs" (http://patapsco.nist.gov /srmcatalog/about/ Definitions.htm).

To provide quality assurance in the analysis of human DNA, five Standard Reference Materials - SRM 2390, SRM 2391b, SRM 2392, SRM 2392-I, and SRM 2395 have been developed by NIST and are currently available. Two additional DNA SRMs (# 2394 and # 2399[1]) have been developed and released since the writing of this chapter. Three of these SRMs - the DNA Profiling Standard 2390, the Polymerase Chain Reaction (PCR)-based DNA Profiling Standard 2391b, and the Human Y-Chromosome DNA Profiling Standard 2395 - are intended for use in forensic and paternity identifications, for instructional law enforcement, or non-clinical research purposes. They are not intended for any human/animal clinical diagnostic use. The DNA SRMs, 2392 and 2392-I, are for standardization and quality control when amplifying and sequencing the entire or any segment of human mitochondrial DNA (16,569 base pairs) for forensic identification, disease diagnosis or mutation detection. SRM 2394 is called the Heteroplasmy mtDNA Standard and will permit investigators to determine the limit of their heteroplasmic mutation detection techniques and hopefully, will be useful in promoting the development of new and more sensitive mutation detection methods.

As explained in Chapter 8, the completion of numerous genome projects is changing the focus of research to the gene products, most often proteins. Proteomics approaches can be divided into four clearly distinct classes based on studied systems and produced data. Proteomics and other data intensive techniques rely on bioinformatics to organize, analyze, store and distribute large data sets. The major trends and bioinformatics services of the four subcategories of proteomics, i.e. expression proteomics, interaction proteomics, functional proteomics, and structural proteomics are discussed. Numerous references and links are provided to validated proteomics databases and programs. Since many of the bioinformatics routines in proteomics can be run in Internet mainly Internet-based systems are described, especially those that are freely available.

[1]SRM 2399 provides quality control to clinical laboratories that test human samples for Fragile X and that need to determine the accurate number of CGG trinucleotide repeats.

In: Trends in Genome Research
Editor: Clyde R. Williams, pp. 1-24
ISBN 1-60021-027-9

Chapter 1

Evolution of Translational Genomic Research Strategies

Travis Dunckley, Winnie S. Liang, and Dietrich A. Stephan*
The Translational Genomics Research Institute, Phoenix, Arizona

Abstract

Sophisticated new molecular scanning technologies have the ability to rapidly identify the underlying bases of complex genetic disorders, which allows early diagnostics and targeted therapeutics to be implemented in the clinic rapidly. Additionally, current technology now provides the ability to comprehensively monitor surrogate molecular markers, which will revolutionize how clinical trials will be implemented. We discuss in this chapter the evolution of genomic technologies and how these technological advances will affect the strategies used to diagnose and, ultimately, to cure complex and common human diseases.

Genomics Holds the Key to Human Disease

All human disease has a genetic component. Since the initial findings that human traits are determined by inheritance of discrete genetic units, the study of human disease has undergone profound and unforeseen changes. Initial genetic studies of human disease focused on identifying single-gene mutations with strong effect that drive the disease process, such as in cystic fibrosis and muscular dystrophy. However, diseases that satisfy these criteria affect a relatively limited number of individuals compared to complex, multigenic disorders. The recent complete sequencing of the entire human genome, and the significant technological advances that have been developed to study it, have placed the genetic study of human diseases at a critical point. The opportunity now exists to understand these more common complex human diseases that result from the functional interplay of multiple genetic

---

* E-mail address: dstephan@tgen.org, Phone: 602-343-8727, FAX: 602-343-8844 (To whom correspondence should be addressed: Dietrich A. Stephan, PhD Director, Neurogenomics Division, The Translational Genomics Research Institute, 445 N. 5th Street, Fifth Floor, Phoenix, Arizona 85004)

determinants superimposed on environmental influences. These diseases, which include many forms of cancer, diabetes, cardiovascular disease, and numerous neurodegenerative disorders, account for millions of deaths and billions of dollars in healthcare expenses annually. This represents a large human tragedy and economic burden that genomic technologies have the potential to alleviate.

Sophisticated new molecular scanning technologies have the ability to rapidly identify the underlying bases of complex genetic disorders, which allows early diagnostics and targeted therapeutics to be implemented in the clinic rapidly. Additionally, current technology now provides the ability to comprehensively monitor surrogate molecular markers, which will revolutionize how clinical trials will be implemented. We discuss in this chapter the evolution of genomic technologies and how these technological advances will affect the strategies used to diagnose and, ultimately, to cure complex and common human diseases.

DNA Variants Underlying Disease: from Mendelian to Complex Trait Dissection

Positional cloning has been widely successful in identifying disease-causing mutations. This strategy works because humans are all products of their ancestors. Every disease-causing genetic variant present within our cells can be traced through our family pedigrees (Figure 1). During meiosis homologous recombination events can shuffle DNA sequences between pairs of chromosomes, such that resulting children will have a slightly modified combination of chromosome parts that are originally inherited from the parents. These recombined chromosomes are likewise shuffled to subsequent progeny. When there is a disease causing genetic mutation segregating in a family, multiple generations of meiotic recombination will reduce the region of shared DNA sequence between affected individuals that contains the disease-causing mutation of interest to a relatively limited region of the genome, thereby facilitating identification of the relevant chromosomal region. That region can then be scanned to identify the mutated nucleotide of DNA. This process, whereby successive generations of related individuals are screened to identify regions of the genome that coinherit with the disease phenotype, is referred to as linkage analysis.

Historically, performing a linkage scan requires genotyping polymorphic DNA sequence markers spaced throughout the genome in families of affected and unaffected individuals (Figure 2). The essential premise is that some DNA markers will be genetically linked with the disease mutation and will cosegregate with the trait through the pedigree. Prior to sequencing of the human genome, this was a labor intensive process, restricted by limited knowledge of the genomic DNA sequence from which these markers could be selected. As a result, markers were often spaced 10cM or more apart. This allowed identification of large genetic intervals, often spanning multiple chromosomal bands, that co-segregate with the disease. These intervals contain hundreds of genes and millions of bases of DNA that must then be further characterized, often by direct DNA sequencing, to identify the specific genetic mutation that causes disease. This step has traditionally been the bottleneck for disease gene identification. Bacterial or yeast artificial chromosome libraries of overlapping genomic DNA sequence that spanned the genetic interval of interest needed to be constructed. Time-consuming high resolution physical mapping of these genomic contigs through chromosome walking using additional DNA markers that were often generated by end sequencing of each clone was then performed. This physical mapping enabled the identification of candidate genes by direct selection, exon trapping, or cDNA selection, followed by mutation screening using single-strand conformational polymorphism (SSCP) or direct sequencing of gene/exon candidates in affected individuals and controls to isolate and clone the gene of interest. Despite the significant input of time and labor, this approach has led to the identification of hundreds of disease causing mutations, providing valuable information about the mechanisms of a multitude of diseases. For example, trinucleotide expansions in the huntingtin protein, which cause Huntington's disease, were identified with this approach[1].

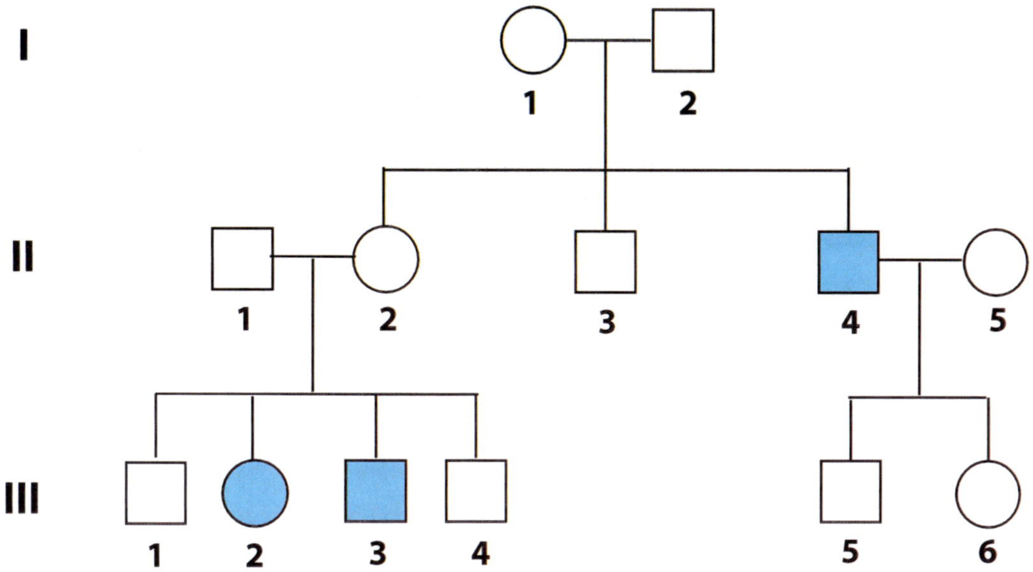

Figure 1. Pedigrees are commonly used to illustrate inheritance of disease through multiple family generations. Illustrated here is transmission of a disease showing a classic Mendelian recessive inheritance pattern. Affected individuals are shaded in blue. Males are represented by squares and females by circles. Accurate pedigrees are essential for genetic linkage studies to identify the underlying causative disease gene (see text).

The approach to linkage analysis described above is most successful with Mendelian inherited diseases of high penetrance. Penetrance refers to the percentage of individuals carrying a disease-causing mutation that will actually display the disease phenotype. In the most extreme scenario, a penetrance of 100% indicates that all of the individuals who have the given mutation will develop the disease, regardless of any other genetic or environmental influences. Thus the disorder would be completely monogenic. A penetrance of 50% means that half of those with the disease-causing mutation will be expected to develop the disease and that additional genetic or environmental influences are necessary to manifest disease. For whole genome linkage scans, followed by positional cloning, high penetrance is critical to ensure that only the affected individuals and none of the control individuals carry the disease gene so that co-segregation analysis can be performed effectively. Erroneous classification of disease classes risks the possibility of reducing the effective power to detect the disease causing alleles.

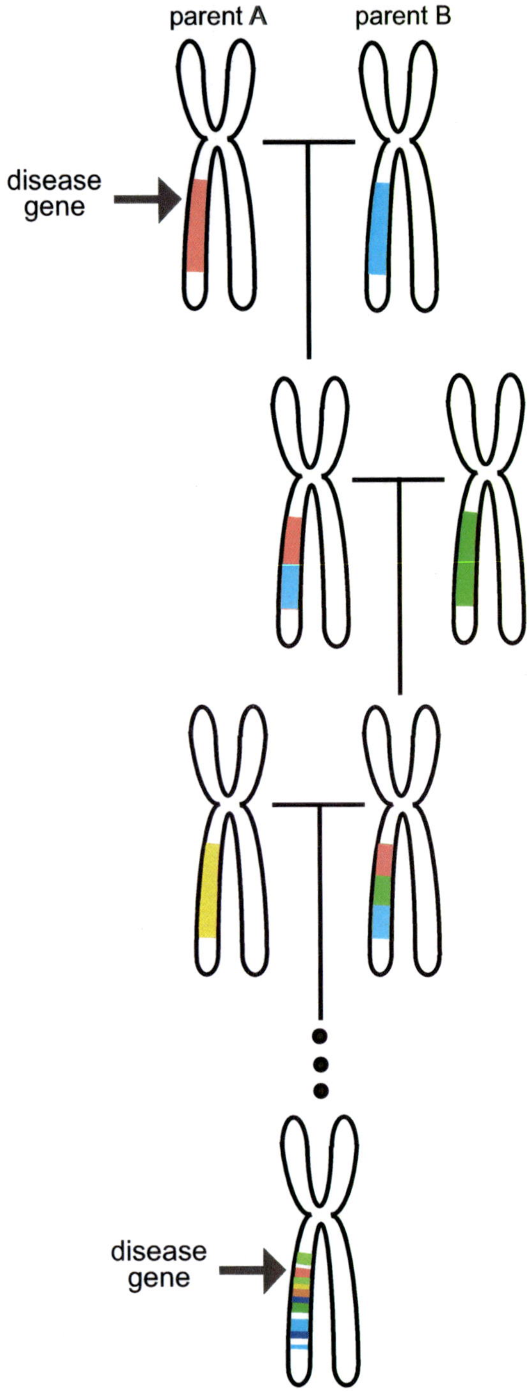

Figure 2. Linkage scans have been extremely successful for the identification of disease-causing genetic mutations. To perform a linkage scan, DNA markers are genotyped throughout the genome and those markers that are always associated with the disease phenotype define the critical genomic region that harbors the relevant genetic mutation. Subsequent high resolution mapping and direct DNA sequencing are then necessary to clone the relevant gene.

Though traditional linkage analyses and positional cloning approaches have yielded significant insights into studies of Mendelian diseases, it has been difficult thus far to study complex human diseases using these traditional approaches. Complex diseases result from the coordinate function of multiple genetic determinants in conjunction with environmental influences. The low resolution of linkage analyses will fail to identify these genetic determinants, even in very large populations. The completion of the human genome project affords, for the first time, the opportunity to address the genetic underpinnings of complex human diseases by enabling the development of high-throughput technologies to hasten the pace and increase the resolution at which the human genome can be analyzed. Additionally, current genomic technologies, such as gene expression profiling, allow one to elucidate molecular and cellular mechanisms of disease, something which has heretofore often necessitated cloning the relevant disease-causing mutation.

Significant advances in our understanding of complex human diseases have thus far come from the study of rare, familial forms of these complex disorders. For example the identification of mutations in the amyloid precursor protein gene, as well as mutations in the presenilin 1 and presenilin 2 genes, which uniformly cause early onset familial Alzheimer's disease (AD) have led to the development of numerous molecular models of AD pathogenesis and to the pursuit of multiple treatment strategies that may be effective on both sporadic and familial forms of AD[2]. Additionally, literally dozens of predisposing mutations and familial mutations of cancer predisposing genes have been identified through traditional positional cloning strategies, including p53, the retinoblastoma protein, the Ras oncogene, and BRCA2 among many others. Each of these examples illustrate how the study of Mendelian inherited, rare forms of common sporadic diseases has provided valuable information about the development and progression of human diseases. However, current genomic advances will obviate the need for this single gene approach to the study of complex disorders and will allow the direct investigation of the functional interplay of multiple genes that underlies sporadic and common human disease.

Post-human Genome Genomics: Uncovering the Genetics of Complex Human Disease

The human genome provides a wealth of biological information and its complete sequencing signals a key transition in the approach to understanding human diseases. The challenge since the sequencing of the genome was completed has been to access and analyze that information efficiently and to translate any findings into clinically relevant applications of disease diagnosis and therapy. Complete knowledge of the entire genomic sequence allows intelligent design of assays to interrogate disease states. To that end, multiple high-throughput assays have been developed to capture relevant genetic information across the entire genome. For example, ever improving technology now allows one to determine the expression levels of every mRNA expressed in the cell on a single standard expression profiling array and allows over 500,000 single nucleotide polymorphisms (SNPs) to be genotyped on high density oligonucleotide arrays to determine nearly the total genetic variability between individuals. Both expression arrays and SNP arrays, as well as comparative genome hybridization (CGH) arrays, DNA sequencing arrays, exon arrays, and siRNAs have very powerful and synergistic uses for understanding disease mechanisms, identifying disease genes, and for developing rapid, reliable diagnostics and effective therapeutics in common and complex genetic disease.

Single Nucleotide Polymorphisms: Enabling Rapid Disease Gene Identification and Diagnostics

Any two humans are 99.9% identical at the DNA sequence level. This ~1 nucleotide in 1,000 variation defines our uniqueness as well as our differential susceptibility to disease. SNPs represent single base pair differences between individuals at a specific location in the genome. There are an estimated 10 million single nucleotide polymorphisms (SNPs) that differ between individuals in the population[3-5]. A comprehensive cataloguing effort of these variable positions through efforts such as the SNP consortium (TSC), the Celera sequencing effort, and the HapMap project now allows the utilization of these SNPs to interrogate the combinations of SNPs that, when inherited, predispose to any human trait. Locked within these SNPs are the keys to identifying the genetic differences that function in concert to increase susceptibility of certain members of the population to one complex genetic disorder and not to another, susceptibility to heart disease versus Parkinson's disease for example. Only recently have genomic advances matured to the point that genotyping large numbers of SNPs to address the genetics of complex disease is becoming possible. SNP analysis also provides a rapid and informative alternative to traditional microsatellite genotyping for familial linkage analyses of Mendelian inherited traits.

SNPs are currently categorized according to their predicted functional effects (Figure 3). For example, a single SNP occurring in the coding region of a gene that alters the protein sequence of the gene product can have a strong functional effect. These are the classically defined Mendelian inherited single base-pair mutations, and have historically been identified through classic PCR-based microsatellite positional cloning strategies or on a candidate gene basis using information from the study of model systems, such as the mouse. A second class of SNPs, referred to as functional SNPs, encompass those that have subtle effects, contributing to disease only when occurring in the context of additional genetic variants or environmental influences. The final category is nonfunctional SNPs that are functionally completely silent, but may nevertheless be genetically linked to a nearby functional sequence variant.

With respect to common and complex genetic disorders, functional SNPs are of particular interest since they are thought to occur at high frequencies in the general population and, only when occurring in specific combinations, to result in disease. Complex diseases that are thought to arise primarily through this genetic paradigm of synergistic interplay between multiple low penetrance functional DNA sequence variants include diabetes, cancer, cardiovascular disease, and numerous neurodegenerative diseases. Until only very recently, identifying these highly common genetic variants has been an insurmountable task. However, recent advances in high-throughput SNP genotyping technologies provide an opportunity to identify these SNPs in large case-control association studies. SNP analysis also enables more rapid identification of Mendelian inherited diseases through linkage analyses, in some cases condensing the previous time-frame for disease gene identification from several years for traditional approaches to less than a week for high-throughput SNP based assays[6].

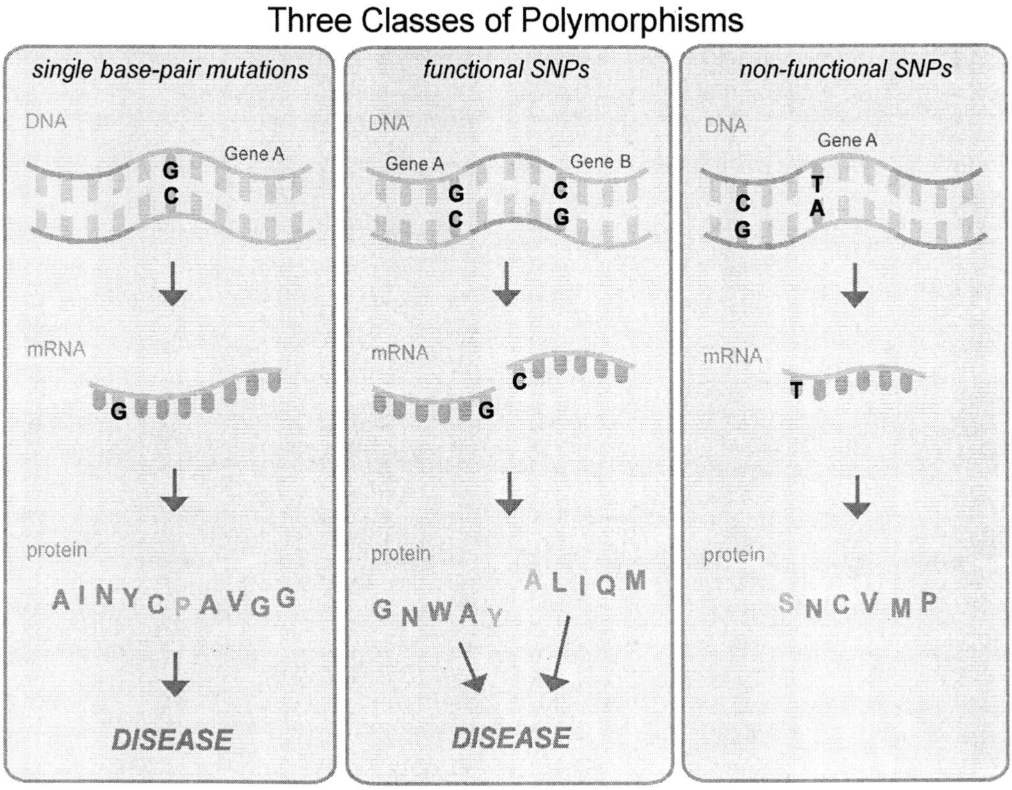

Figure 3. There are currently three broad categories of single nucleotide polymorphisms (SNPs). Single base-pair mutations are SNPs that alter the function of the encoded protein and are sufficient to cause disease. Functional SNPs are those that have subtle effects on either protein function or expression and are phenotypically silent on their own but can cause disease when combined with additional functional SNPs. Non-functional SNPs have no apparent function, either alone or in combination with other SNPs or environmental factors. However, they can be very useful in genetic analyses as they may be linked to nearby functional SNPs. Thus they can provide an anchor in the genome from which to identify the relevant disease-causing genetic variant.

Detecting Familial, Single Gene Mutations in Days Instead of Years

Traditionally, linkage analyses have been done on a genome-wide scale using PCR-based assays to genotype microsatellite markers at a density of ~10cM (Mb) intervals. This is a tedious methodology. We now have access to a high resolution SNP map of the human genome, as well as new technologies for rapidly genotyping these SNPs. Several technologies are currently available for high-throughput SNP genotyping, including the BeadArray platform from Illumina, the MassArray system from Sequenom, and the GeneChip mapping arrays from Affymetrix. For the Affymetrix and Illumina platforms, SNP allele detection is based on hybridization to a complementary oligonucleotide probe. The Sequenom system uses matrix-assisted laser desorption/ionization time-of-flight mass spectrometry (MALDI-

TOF) for accurate SNP detection. Each of these platforms provides the ability to quickly genotype thousands of SNPs. Both the Illumina and Affymetrix platforms allow the simultaneous genotyping of hundreds of thousands of SNPs and the Sequenom platform has demonstrated advantages for quantifying pooled samples and is more easily amenable to genotyping custom SNPs. These abilities make the MassArray system a useful complement to the Affymetrix and Illumina systems.

Although SNPs are biallelic and thus less informative than multiallelic microsatellites, their large numbers and high density of ~every 3kb (on the new Affymetrix ~1,000,000 SNP array) provides more overall, evenly distributed information[7-9]. Whole genome genotyping of 3,000 to 10,000 SNPs has been demonstrated to be a sufficient density for familial linkage analyses. SNP genotyping also provides a speed advantage relative to microsatellite analysis. For example, using SNP genotyping approaches to linkage analysis, the causative mutation underlying sudden infant death with dysgenesis of the testis (SIDDT) and multiple additional heritable disorders have been identified in less than one week[6](unpublished observations). This represents a dramatic ~100-fold increase in the speed of the positional cloning process that effectively removes the previous crucial bottleneck of gene discovery prior to the development of new therapies. In addition to leveraging recently gained knowledge of specific SNP sequences, the SNP approach to gene discovery also depends on the concurrent advances in annotation of gene databases and in high-throughput DNA sequencing capabilities, each of which has resulted directly from the human genome project[10]. In addition to the SIDDT example, SNP linkage analyses have led to the identification of mutations in the HOXD10 gene in Charcot-Marie-Tooth disease[11], to the identification of multiple linkage peaks in 167 families affected by prostate cancer[12], as well as to studies of rheumatoid arthritis and bipolar disorder[13,14].

SNP analysis also provides the opportunity for rapid diagnostic tests to determine genetic risk for complex diseases. For example, currently genetic testing is done one gene at a time using a candidate gene approach. That is, one has a family history of a particular disease for which a common genetic variant is known, such as cystic fibrosis, and can be tested for the presence of that variant within their genome. This information can then be used to guide life decisions, such as reproductive choices or exercise and eating habits in other instances. However, most human disease is sporadic and multigenic. Risk for these diseases cannot be diagnosed using traditional approaches. SNP analysis can be performed on a genome-wide scale in large case-control association studies of outbred populations to identify all of the genetic variants that contribute simultaneously to a specific disease. These variants can then be packaged into a diagnostic to predict an individual's overall genetic risk for developing a given disease. SNP diagnostics would be most effective when coupled to an effective therapeutic strategy. However, such a diagnostic could have a significant impact on human health, even in the absence of a specific therapy because environmental influences, which are modifiable, also affect the development and course of disease. For example, high cholesterol diets have been shown to increase the risk of some forms of cancer and may also be an important factor in the development of Alzheimer's disease. Knowing that you are at heightened genetic risk for these disorders could motivate significant lifestyle changes. In this way, as the analysis of complex diseases continues to evolve, the ease of use and the versatility of SNP genotyping for identifying relevant genetic variants, such as point mutations, deletions, and amplifications, will lead to significant advances in human health.

Data Analysis

Data analysis of linkage studies has been well established through previous approaches relying on genotyping multiallelic DNA markers. However, SNP genotyping introduces new considerations by virtue of the large number of markers genotyped. As with microsatellite linkage analyses, LOD scores are used to interpret the significance of SNP marker associations. The LOD score represents the likelihood that a disease mutation is genetically linked to the SNP marker. A LOD score greater than 3 is considered significant, indicating a 1,024:1 probability that a disease gene is in close proximity to that marker in the genome. To generate this LOD score, traditional programs for linkage analysis are designed for a few hundred multiallelic microsatellite markers. SNP data consists of thousands of biallelic markers. New software programs are being developed to handle this type of data, including Varia (Silicon Genetics), simwalk2snp (UCLA) and DChipSNP(Harvard University) and have been used to successfully identify linkage peaks that contain disease genes from SNP genotyping data. The concomitant development of bioinformatics tools and genomic technologies illustrates clearly the interdependent and symbiotic relationship of technological advances in genomics to query over 3 billion base-pairs of information with advances in computational biology to sift through the masses of data to extract only the relevant information. For continued advancements in our understanding of human disease, this synergistic relationship and mutual advancement will continue to be critical.

Because of the high numbers of SNPs currently being genotyped, many SNPs are in significant linkage disequilibrium (LD). This means that SNPs are often coinherited at a rate higher than would be predicted by random chance. Thus two adjacent markers in close proximity will cosegregate more frequently than distant markers due to a decreased probability of meiotic recombination occurring between the adjacent proximal markers. Established calculations of multipoint LOD scores assume that each marker is not linked to every other marker. Application of these calculations to SNP analysis, which violate the assumption of independence, will bias LOD score calculations. Therefore, one must note LD between two markers when interpreting the LOD score significance.

Once linkage peaks have been determined, a combination of informatics and DNA sequencing is required to identify the relevant mutation in affected individuals. Essentially one must identify all of the genes under the linkage peak by referencing available databases. Linkage peaks from SNP data are often significantly smaller than microsatellite generated linkage peaks owing to the high density of SNP markers, which narrows the number of candidate genes. Candidate genes must then be selected, where possible by interpreting the known biological function of the gene candidates in light of the clinical presentation of the disease, and then sequenced to identify the causative mutation.

Analyzing Complex, Multigenic Disorders: from Candidate Genes to Whole Genome Screens

SNP genotyping technology has already worked to significant effect to identify novel single gene disease-causing mutations at an unprecedented rate. Perhaps more significantly, this technology holds great potential for discovering multigenic contributions to complex disorders. Indeed, these complex disorders, which are influenced by multiple genetic determinants and environmental factors, affect the most people[15,16]. These disorders are usually not inherited in a Mendelian fashion and, in many cases, may be referred to as "sporadic" cases of disease. Thus, traditional familial linkage studies are not effective[17]. Rather case-control whole genome association studies of outbred populations hold the most promise.

Traditionally, case-control association studies have analyzed single genes using a candidate gene approach. Thus hundreds of individuals would be genotyped for a given gene or single base-pair change. This approach makes analysis and understanding of multigenic diseases extremely difficult and cost prohibitive. The development of SNP technology now allows the simultaneous testing of every gene.

Two key issues must be considered in a case-control association study (reviewed in Craig and Stephan, 2005). First, sufficient numbers of SNPs must be used to ensure that some genotyped SNPs are in significant LD with the disease-causing genetic variant. From a practical standpoint and because the location of the relevant genetic variants are unknown prior to screening, a set of SNPs must be selected that is in LD with the majority of the genome[15,18,19]. A major effort, referred to as the International HapMap Project, is currently ongoing to define this informative set of SNPs[20]. The primary goal of this consortium is to identify the minimal set of "tagSNPs" that define all of the haplotype blocks in the genome[21]. These haplotype blocks represent ancestrally conserved regions of the genome that appear to be largely free of recombination and that are passed from generation to generation intact. Defining these blocks will reduce the number of SNPs required for an association study since few SNPs within these blocks will need to be genotyped. The number of SNPs needed for a whole genome scan is currently estimated at 300,000 to 1 million.

The second issue to be considered is the size of the population analyzed. Case-control association studies on common complex diseases will require hundreds to several thousand case and control individuals[22,23]. The sample size needed will vary for a given study depending on the disease allele frequency in the population, the SNP allele frequency being genotyped, and the allelic odds ratio of the disease gene of interest. Additionally, due to the large number of false positives predicted from this approach, it is critical to validate candidate associations and similarly sized independent patient cohorts of control and affected individuals.

These requirements for genotyping a large number of SNPs in a large sample size of patient cohorts for whole genome association studies, as well as validation genotyping in large independent populations, have thus far limited the application of SNP genotyping to a more straightforward candidate gene approach. The candidate gene approach has successfully identified the apolipoprotein E, ε4 allele as a significant risk factor for Alzheimer's disease[24] and polymorphisms of the lymphotoxin-α gene as a risk factor for myocardial infarction[25]. Though these examples represent an important first step, the future of association studies lies in non-biased queries of whole genome disease associations and will become feasible as SNP genotyping capabilities move beyond 300,000 SNPs. For example, a whole genome association study using the Affymetrix array based platform with 116,204 SNPs successfully identified a SNP within an intron of the complement factor H gene as being associated with age related macular degeneration (AMD)[26]. This study used 96 AMD cases and 50 controls and identified only this one SNP to be significantly associated with AMD. Reconstruction of the haplotype block using additional SNPs from the HapMap project revealed that the associated SNP was within a 41 kb haplotype block. Resequencing of the complement factor H gene revealed an exonic polymorphism 2 kb upstream of this 41 kb haplotype block resulting in an amino acid substitution. There are at least two important implications of these findings. First, genotyping nonfunctional SNPs can be extremely informative, particularly when they are located in haplotype blocks that are linked to functional allelic variants. Second, this study reveals the power of SNP genotyping outbred populations to identify a disease susceptibility locus. However, it is relevant that only a single significant SNP was identified in this study, which was found in all of the AMD cases and in none of the controls. Thus, this example likely does not represent a truly complex, multigenic disorder, although it does provide a valuable paradigm for how those disorders may be approached using this technology.

The utility of identifying genetic variants for complex diseases lies in their use as a predictor of disease risk, as a diagnostic for disease, as a predictor of response to therapy, or for the identification of therapeutic targets. For example, currently genetic testing is done one gene at a time using a candidate gene approach. That is, one has a family history of a particular disease for which a common genetic variant is known, such as cystic fibrosis, and can be tested for the presence of that variant within their genome. This information can then be used to guide life decisions, such as reproductive choices or exercise and eating habits in instances of other disorders. However, most human disease is sporadic and multigenic. Risk for these diseases cannot be diagnosed using traditional approaches. SNP analysis can be performed on a genome-wide scale in large case-control association studies of outbred populations to identify all of the genetic variants that contribute simultaneously to a specific disease. These variants can then be packaged into a diagnostic to predict an individual's overall genetic risk for developing a given disease. These SNP diagnostics would be most effective when coupled to an effective therapeutic strategy. However, such a diagnostic could have a significant impact on human health, even in the absence of a specific therapy because environmental influences, which are modifiable, also affect the development and course of disease. For example, high cholesterol diets or smoking have been shown to increase the risk of some forms of cancer and may also be an important factor in the development of Alzheimer's disease. Knowing that you are at heightened genetic risk for these disorders could motivate significant lifestyle changes. In this way, as the analysis of complex diseases continues to evolve, the ease of use and the versatility of SNP genotyping for identifying relevant genetic variants, such as point mutations, deletions, and amplifications, will lead to significant advances in human health.

Data Analysis

Significant findings in case-control association studies are represented by an odds ratio (OR). The OR is a measure of the likelihood that an individual carrying a given genetic variant will have a particular disease and is influenced by the OR of the actual disease-causing variant, the extent of LD between the genotyped SNP and the disease variant, the SNP marker frequency, and the disease allele frequency. An OR greater than 1 indicates increased risk and an OR less than 1 signals decreased risk for disease. Calculation of an odds ratio works very well for single candidate gene approaches. However, analysis of high-density SNP data across the entire genome presents a substantial complication. High numbers of false positives are expected using standard χ^2 tests[27]. Calculation of the False Discovery Rate (FDR) can be used to reduce the number of false positives[28]. Alternatively, p values can be empirically determined by comparison with large sets of randomized, unassociated data. Permutational statistics are advantageous to approaches that assume standard data distributions since they do not make any assumptions about the distribution of the data, which may be unknowingly altered due to stratified populations or admixed individuals[29].

Calculating all possible combinations of SNP markers associated with a given complex disease is desirable in a whole genome association study of a multigenic disease but is not computationally feasible because of the enormous number of SNPs and SNP combinations that must be tested. Several approaches have been developed to reduce the number of statistical tests to be performed including set-association algorithms that group SNPs based on allelic association and FDR to reduce the set of interesting SNPs[27,29,30]. However, there is no current standard approach to these analyses.

In addition to false associations resulting from multiple testing issues, additional erroneous associations of SNPs with specific diseases can result from population stratification or population admixture. Population stratification occurs when regionally or ethnically distinct populations with different disease risks are unknowingly sampled. This stratification can be detected by genotyping as few as 50 random SNPs, which should show no preferential association with cases versus controls[31]. Population admixture occurs when a population with high proportions of a specific SNP and of disease mixes with a population with low proportions of both. In these instances, SNP association with disease can result from this admixture rather than from physical proximity to the disease-causing genetic variant.

Because of the combined factors leading to high false positive associations, including statistical multiple testing issues, population stratification, population admixture, and the number of predisposing genes for a given disease, validation and replication of any associations in independent populations should be done.

RNA Variants: From Northern Blots to Gene Expression Microarrays

Just a decade ago analysis of gene expression was performed one gene at a time using northern blot and RNase protection assay approaches. In these techniques, the mRNA is anchored in a gel matrix and detected by hybridization to a labeled, homologous oligonucleotide. The development of gene expression microarrays reverses this approach, allowing the simultaneous interrogation of expression of every mRNA. With expression microarrays, oligonucleotide probes homologous to cellular mRNAs are anchored to a solid support and probed with labeled mRNA, rapidly generating an expression profile for every cellular mRNA.

Alterations in cellular metabolism will underlie any disease phenotype. These effects can be seen as altered mRNA expression profiles in diseased cell types. Even members of phosphorylation cascades can be dysregulated at the mRNA level. Thus far, multiple approaches to interrogate global gene expression have been used, including differential display[32], serial analysis of gene expression (SAGE)[33], and suppression subtractive hybridization[34]. However, these approaches are technically difficult, hard to standardize, and allow for the simultaneous study of only a few biological samples. Gene expression microarrays provide a powerful alternative. Gene expression microarrays are used to rapidly assess the gene expression profiles of thousands of genes in a single experiment. In fact, following completion of the human genome, expression profiling technology rapidly expanded such that it is now possible to test the expression levels of all mRNA coding sequences in a single rapid assay. Usually, mRNA from unaffected cells or tissue is compared to mRNA from diseased cells or tissue. Significant differences that are observed in the diseased state can then be used as a diagnostic expression signature of the disease or to inform as to the cellular mechanisms of disease, thereby leading to a potential new therapy.

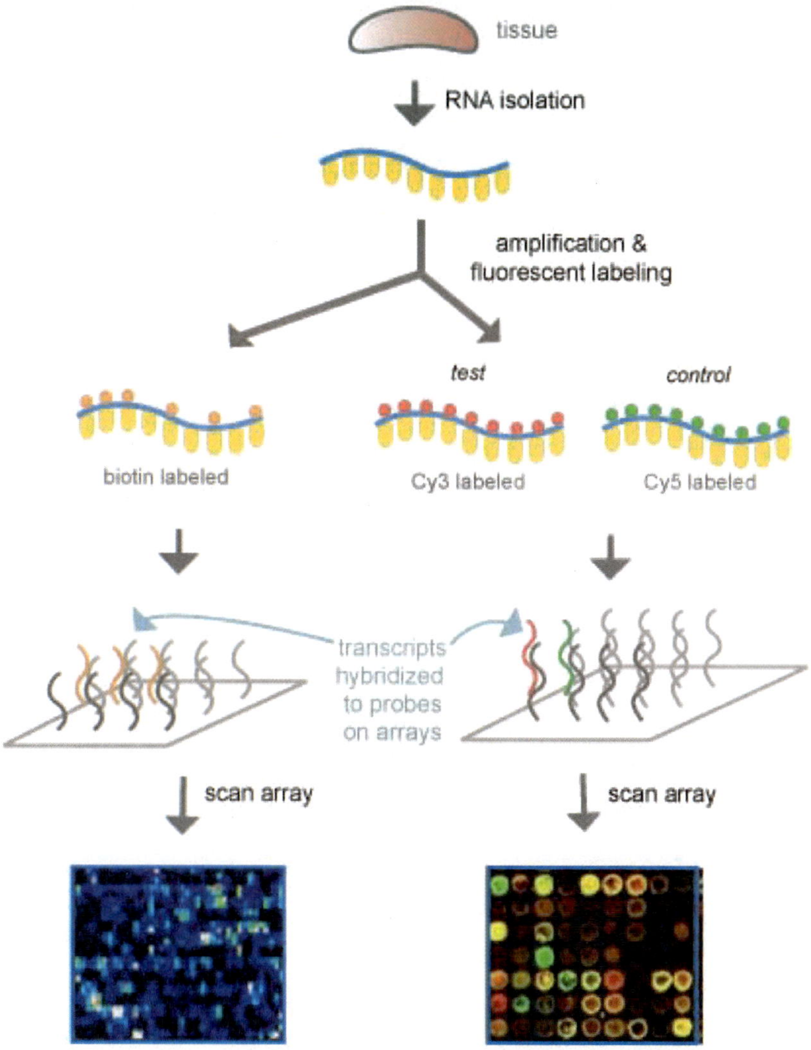

Figure 4. A typical one-color and two-color microarray experiment is shown. RNA from the relevant cells or tissue is amplified and labeled. The labeled sample is then hybridized directly to the DNA probes on the microarray, which can be either oligonucleotides or PCR-generated cDNAs. For two-color arrays, this is a competitive hybridization of labeled RNA from control and test samples, which are each labeled with different fluorophores. As illustrated, genes that are upregulated in the test sample appear red and genes that are downregulated in the test sample appear green. Yellow spots indicate equivalent expression for the given gene in control and test samples.

There are two primary variations of expression arrays currently in use, cDNA and oligonucleotide microarrays (Figure 4). Oligonucleotide arrays provide the benefits of greater specificity since the probes used are of shorter sequence (~25-70 nucleotides) than those used for cDNA arrays (200-2000 nucleotides). cDNA arrays have greater sensitivity but cannot, for example, discriminate between splice variants because the size of DNA probes used often spans splice junctions. For each type of array, sequences of DNA that are homologous to different genes of interest are attached to a solid support at distinct locations. Each probe (or probe set for oligonucleotide arrays) on a slide corresponds to a single gene and each array can hold thousands of probes. One then hybridizes either labeled cRNA or cDNA from the cell type of interest to the microarray, rapidly generating an mRNA expression profile for thousands of genes. Indeed, the large amount of data generated present daunting bioinformatic and data warehousing issues.

Technical Variability

Numerous comparisons of repeated microarray measures within and between different platforms have been reported. The overall theme is that technical variability between replicates using the same platform is very low when performed by skilled technicians using standard protocols. However, comparisons of replicates run on arrays from different manufacturers should not be performed as the concordance rates can be 30% or less[35]. The majority of the inter-platform differences appear to arise from the fact that each platform uses different oligonucleotide probe sequences that have slightly different hybridization specificities, particularly with regard to alternatively spliced gene variants. An ambitious and costly solution would be for all manufacturers to use common probe sets. However, a more realistic approach is to restrict replicate analyses to a single array platform.

Biological Variability

For expression profiling results to be clinically valuable, they must be specific to the disease of interest or to the broader cellular dysfunction that underlies the disease, such as aberrant apoptotic signaling in cancer cells. Working against these goals are multiple sources of variability, including tissue heterogeneity, clinical heterogeneity of the disease itself, and technical variability in the experimental assay. Expression profiling technology and protocols have become routine such that technical variability is now negligible when the assays are performed with standardized protocols by trained personnel. In many cases advances in clinical diagnostics are necessary to achieve more precisely stratified patient sample cohorts to reduce disease heterogeneity. For example, in neurodegenerative diseases in particular, such as multiple sclerosis, Alzheimer's disease, and Parkinsons's disease, clinical diagnostics need further refining[36-39]. In Alzheimer's disease, where diagnostics are arguably the most advanced, the post-mortem neuropathological confirmation rate of a clinical diagnosis of "probable" Alzheimer's disease is as low as 65% in some instances[40]. In fact, a definitive diagnosis can only be made for many neurodegenerative diseases using a combination of clinical and post-mortem neuropathological criteria. For the purposes of gene discovery and the elucidation of pathogenic disease mechanisms, it is imperative to analyze clinically well-stratified cohorts of affected and unaffected individuals. With current limitations of antemortem clinical diagnostics, this often limits the research to working with post-mortem tissue and places a significant emphasis on tissue banking protocols, which have rapidly advanced to standardize tissue procurement and processing procedures, with the goal of obtaining high quality tissue specimens with low post-mortem intervals.

The second issue of tissue heterogeneity is being addressed through microaspiration techniques, automated cell sorting, and, more recently, through the development and maturation of laser capture microdissection technology (LCM). LCM allows the isolation of individual cells from a heterogeneous tissue sample. This technology, coupled with standard RNA amplification protocols, enables the analysis of homogeneous cell populations such that expression profiles are specifically correlated to the cellular dysfunction of interest[41,42].[43,44]. For example, this approach has been used to identify candidate genes involved in colon cancer progression[45], liver cancer progression[46], prostate cancer[47], and oral cancer[48] among many others. Application of LCM to other complex disorders such as Alzheimer's disease, Parkinson's disease, schizophrenia, and vascular disease are also underway[49,50]. These approaches will provide masses of information about the genes that are specifically dysregulated in aberrant cell types in each of these disorders. The main challenge will then be to develop adequate functional assays to determine which dysregulated genes actually contribute to the disease phenotype. This is currently a time-consuming task. However, high-throughput RNA interference-based validation methods are now approaching a whole genome scale and should help to expedite this validation process.

Expression profiling has been used successfully to identify disease diagnostics[51-54], predict the prognosis of specific forms of disease[52,55], predict patient response to current therapies[56], and to identify dysregulated genes and signaling pathways that contribute to cellular dysfunction and disease[57-59]. In the latter examples, these genes can serve as novel targets for the development of new and effective therapeutics. In the future, as nanotechnologies are merged with genomics, these assays will be packaged into rapid, affordable diagnostics that can be used in a clinic setting to provide accurate molecular diagnoses of disease subtypes and to enable the most efficacious treatment options to be initiated for those disease subtypes. This will represent a significant advancement in patient care as nonresponders will no longer be subjected to unnecessary medications and concomitant adverse side-effects.

Data Analysis

A standard whole genome microarray assay now generates over 47,000 individual gene expression data points, presenting a significant analytical challenge. Usually, this large number of data points is assayed in a comparatively small number of biological samples. Extensive texts cover microarray data analysis in great detail[60]. In general, microarray expression data is typically analyzed at three levels:

1) Image analysis where the images for each spot are analyzed in order to assign a confidence value based on the quality of the spot
2) Statistical data analysis where values for expression are examined for normality, bias, signal drift and correlation between replicates.

3) Biological interpretation where data is related back to genes, data reduction/filtering is done, and feature selection and classification, clustering, and prediction of gene regulatory networks is done.

For most commercial arrays (Affymetrix, Agilent, etc) the image analysis is software driven. Data is assigned a confidence value based on parameters such as spot shape, intensity, local and global background, overall signal level, and statistical analysis of the pixels composing a spot. Most experiments done on clinical samples are high throughput, exceeding 20 arrays per experiment, and often exceeding 100 arrays. Thus individual, manual attention to image analysis is done at the data analysis and quality control steps.

Data from array experiments is normalized using loess (for Agilent two-color arrays) or MAS5, dChip, or RMA/GC-RMA (for Affymetrix). All of these programs work well to detect the most significant outliers. Following normalization, the data distributions, scale, standard deviations within and across arrays, and concordance across replicates must be determined. Statistical measures of power (when adequate replicates are available) across replicates and across sample types are also calculated to get the power per probe and the minimum detectable fold change. This is calculated using standard t-test-based power calculations and standard deviations computed from either $\log_2$ ratios or raw values. Although statistical analysis of microarrays (SAM), False Discovery Rate (FDR), Hochberg and Benjamini, can be used to calculate false discovery rates, arrays are usually of such high quality across replicates that the p-value for differentially expressed genes can be set below the level where false positives appear (typically $p<0.00001$ yields no false positives). False negatives are addressed at the validation stage. At this stage specific genes of high biological interest can be analyzed individually via secondary validation measures.

Biological validation of any differentially expressed candidate gene is essential via secondary measures such as RNA interference or overexpression studies and occurs following completion of the initial statistical procedures, quality control procedures, and model building steps. Here, a binomial analysis against the Gene Ontology database can provide clues about the functional bias of a given list of genes. The hypothesis that functional properties of genes occur together at higher-than-random frequencies often provides the investigator with a functional category that guides the researcher toward a cellular process that can be evaluated using other methods.

Additionally the user may run feature selection and classification methods to predict those genes which best predict the phenotype, outcome, or survival prognosis. These methods are combined with an exploration of gene regulatory networks using commercially and publicly available tools (i.e. Ingenuity, GeneGo, BioRag, KeGG, David, GenMAPP, EASE), where expression data is combined with two-hybrid, synthetic lethal, and literature findings to identify patterns of expression that match known functional pathways. Biochemistry or molecular biology approaches are critical to further validate hypotheses generated by data mining of expression profiling results.

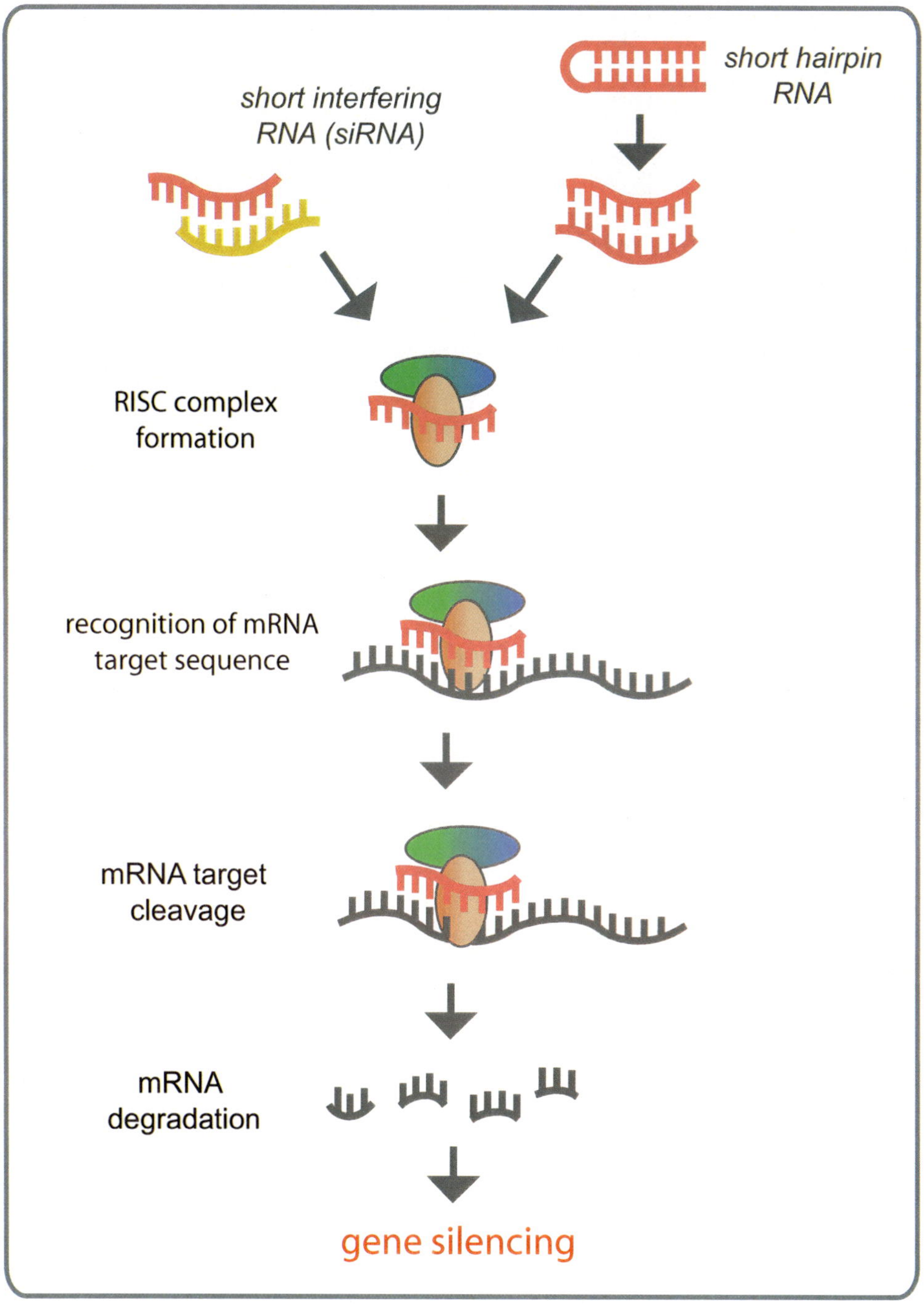

Figure 5. RNA interference can be used to specifically target and degrade most cellular mRNAs. Small interfering RNAs (siRNAs) or short hairpin RNAs, which are processed to siRNAs inside the cell, are bound by the RNA-induced silencing complex (RISC). This complex then binds to the appropriate mRNA based on homology of the siRNA for the target gene of interest. Following mRNA binding, the target mRNA is cleaved and subsequently degraded, thereby achieving targeted knockdown of a single gene of interest. This is a post-transcriptional mechanism of gene silencing that works only when the siRNA is present.

Validation of Gene Candidates: Identifying True Diagnostic and Therapeutic Targets

Whole genome expression profiling and SNP genotyping strategies are generating lists of candidate genes implicated in a multitude of disease processes at an unprecedented rate. A major challenge to continued gene discovery, determining pathogenic disease mechanisms, and developing new and effective treatments lies in the validation of those gene candidates. Validation is essential at both the protein and functional levels. Validation of expression changes at the protein level is most appropriately performed on a set of independent biological samples, those that were not used in the original microarray study. Quantitative western analyses or, when not practical as in the case where LCM isolated cells are the starting material, qualitative differences in gene expression can be observed using immunohistochemical approaches.

Genes that validate at the protein level must then be tested for functional effects. In model systems such as yeast, drosophila, and even mice, more facile genetics enables systematic mechanistic studies of individual gene candidates. However, human cells have historically been genetically intractable in comparison. The recent discovery of a highly conserved post-transcriptional gene silencing mechanism, referred to as RNA interference (RNAi), provides the opportunity to rapidly investigate disease mechanisms in human cells.

RNA interference involves the use of small interfering RNAs (siRNA), which are RNA duplexes of 20-23 nucleotides (nts) in length that base pair with a homologous sequence within mature mRNA products[61,62]. This base-pairing interaction serves as a guide for the RNA-protein complex termed the RNA-induced silencing complex (RISC)[63,64], which directs the cleavage and subsequent degradation of the target mRNA resulting in a reduction of gene expression (Figure 5). These synthetic siRNA duplexes are very useful for studying gene function through transient gene suppression but cannot be used for long-term gene suppression because the RNA duplex is degraded very quickly in mammalian cells. The study of small nucleic RNAs and their transcription led to the discovery of the transcription of short hairpin RNA or shRNA *in vivo* from RNA polymerase III promoters such as those of the H1 RNA, the RNA subunit of RNase P complex and U6 snRNA genes, which have well defined transcription initiation and termination signals. Short hairpin RNAs are processed into siRNAs *in vivo* and induce RNAi gene silencing[65,66].

The use of RNAi for analysis of gene function is advancing rapidly. For example, Brummelkamp and co-workers employed a novel retroviral RNAi vector system to functionally target the oncogenic version of KRAS2 involved in pancreatic cancer progression[67]. Targeted reduction of this gene led to a loss of anchorage independent growth and decreased the tumorigenic capacity of the pancreatic cancer cell line, CAPAN-1, in nude mice, clearly illustrating the utility of RNAi in the identification and validation of potential targets for anticancer therapies. Additionally, RNAi has been used to identify important molecules that function to mediate gemcitabine resistance in pancreatic cancer[68-74].

One of the most important advantages to RNAi technology is that it is amenable to high-throughput analysis. For example, RNAi genomic libraries have been used to screen the entire genome for functional effects with respect to a given phenotype, such as proteasome function and p53-mediated cell cycle arrest[75-77]. This type of assay will facilitate the understanding of the function of a large number of genes with respect to specific disease phenotypes and will greatly advance our understanding of complex biological processes such as cancer and neurodegenerative disorders. Continued and expanded application of RNAi approaches will lead to significant biological insights into these diseases, as well as to the rapid validation of gene candidates emerging from expression profiling and SNP genotyping screens and, subsequently, to the development of new treatment options.

Clinical Applications of Genomic Technologies

Clearly identification of the underlying DNA or RNA defects leading to development of disease will translate directly into effective diagnostics and drug design. For example, SNP analyses provide the potential for early and reasonably noninvasive cancer diagnosis by detecting heritable cancer specific mutations in peripheral tissues, such as blood. As a result, treatments may be commenced earlier than was previously possible[78]. Additionally, SNP analysis could become a routine screening procedure to identify individuals with SNP haplotypes that place them at risk for developing specific forms of cancer. This information could be used to direct at risk individuals to appropriate prevention strategies. As the technology matures and is merged with developing nanotechnologies, diagnosis and screening using this methodology will become economically feasible for general practice. In addition to providing a diagnosis method, SNP analyses will be useful for identifying causative mutations and affected molecular pathways in various cancers. Following validation of these pathways new targets for therapy will emerge.

Gene expression profiling has numerous important clinical applications. Expression profiling data can be used to categorize tumor subtypes according to such factors as chemotherapeutic response or predicted outcome[56,79] In breast cancer susceptibility screening, genetic testing to identify individuals carrying known predisposition alleles has been used to indicate when more extreme prevention strategies, such as surgical resection of at risk tissue, are needed. However, this approach suffers from the limitation that not all individuals carrying susceptibility genes will develop cancer. Expression profiling allows the further subclassification of a person's cancer risk based on additional genetic determinants, restricting such surgical prevention strategies to only a subset of individuals with the highest likelihood of developing particularly aggressive forms of disease. The example of breast cancer illustrates the expectation that, as more tumors are profiled and subcategorized, expression profiling could become a general tool for predicting the course of cancer progression and for guiding prevention strategies in unaffected individuals. For example, the Molecular Profiling Institute now offers the first commercially available microarray cancer diagnostic (MammaPrint®) based on gene expression profiling 70 genes in breast cancer cells that indicate which subset of lymph node negative individuals will have recurrent disease with an accuracy of 96.7%, thereby enabling directed therapy for only those lymph node negative women that will most benefit from treatment. This represents a significant advance in the treatment of breast cancer since less than half of the women with lymph node negative breast cancer currently being treated with chemotherapy will experience recurrence. The rest are unnecessarily experiencing adverse side effects of expensive chemotherapy treatment. In the future, subcategorizing tumors based on their expression profiles will further aid in patient-specific therapies that are designed to be most effective in the clinic on a real-time basis for the treatment of particular forms of cancer and other genetically complex disorders.

Microarrays are also important for identifying dysregulated genes and signaling pathways that are involved in tumor development and progression[57]. Identification of these genes and pathways will have important implications for the development of novel anticancer therapies since they provide novel targets for treatment.

As expression profiling in the study of human diseases moves forward, a critical goal will be to translate the vast amounts of biological data into meaningful clinical advances. This will require large collaborative efforts pooling the combined knowledge and expertise of different institutions to successfully accomplish all of the required goals from sample acquisition, to genomic analysis, to target identification and validation, to drug design and discovery.

Summary

The study of the human genome has seen a dramatic progression from the single gene approach to a more rapid holistic approach to understanding human disease. High-throughput technologies are speeding up identification of core genetic variants underlying human disease through parallel assays that allow immediate application in diagnostic settings and targeted "knowledge-based" therapeutic development. As technology has progressed to allow the study of the human genome on an ever-increasing scale, the focus of research efforts can now be placed squarely on the development of disease prevention strategies, diagnostics, and therapeutics based on resulting novel genetic discoveries. Analysis of SNPs and gene expression profiling are valuable methods for identifying the genetic determinants of disease. However, to fully realize the value of these techniques, it will be critical to translate those findings into practical applications that can benefit affected individuals as well as those who are at risk for developing particular diseases. Knowledge of an individual's innate susceptibility to various diseases gained through SNP genotyping can be used to guide the course of prevention strategies that focus, for example, on lifestyle changes such as diet and exercise. In addition, SNP and expression profiles can be used to both accurately diagnose disease and to subcategorize diseases, such as tumor types based on severity of the malignant phenotype. This information could then be used to target the most aggressive therapies to patients with the most severe or invasive forms of disease. Ultimately, the information gleaned from these powerful genomics techniques will be used to identify novel targets for therapeutic intervention with the eventual endpoint of preventing some of the most devastating diseases that are now unfortunately very common.

References

[1] (1993) *Cell* **72**(6), 971-983.
[2] Tanzi, R. E., Kovacs, D. M., Kim, T. W., Moir, R. D., Guenette, S. Y., and Wasco, W. (1996) *Neurobiol Dis* **3**(3), 159-168.
[3] Ardlie, K. G., Kruglyak, L., and Seielstad, M. (2002) *Nat Rev Genet* **3**(4), 299-309.
[4] Carlson, C. S., Eberle, M. A., Rieder, M. J., Smith, J. D., Kruglyak, L., and Nickerson, D. A. (2003) *Nat Genet* **33**(4), 518-521.

[5] Kruglyak, L., and Nickerson, D. A. (2001) *Nat Genet* **27**(3), 234-236.
[6] Puffenberger, E. G., Hu-Lince, D., Parod, J. M., Craig, D. W., Dobrin, S. E., Conway, A. R., Donarum, E. A., Strauss, K. A., Dunckley, T., Cardenas, J. F., Melmed, K. R., Wright, C. A., Liang, W., Stafford, P., Flynn, C. R., Morton, D. H., and Stephan, D. A. (2004) *Proc Natl Acad Sci U S A* **101**(32), 11689-11694.
[7] Matise, T. C., Sachidanandam, R., Clark, A. G., Kruglyak, L., Wijsman, E., Kakol, J., Buyske, S., Chui, B., Cohen, P., de Toma, C., Ehm, M., Glanowski, S., He, C., Heil, J., Markianos, K., McMullen, I., Pericak-Vance, M. A., Silbergleit, A., Stein, L., Wagner, M., Wilson, A. F., Winick, J. D., Winn-Deen, E. S., Yamashiro, C. T., Cann, H. M., Lai, E., and Holden, A. L. (2003) *Am J Hum Genet* **73**(2), 271-284.
[8] Sawcer, S. J., Maranian, M., Singlehurst, S., Yeo, T., Compston, A., Daly, M. J., De Jager, P. L., Gabriel, S., Hafler, D. A., Ivinson, A. J., Lander, E. S., Rioux, J. D., Walsh, E., Gregory, S. G., Schmidt, S., Pericak-Vance, M. A., Barcellos, L., Hauser, S. L., Oksenberg, J. R., Kenealy, S. J., and Haines, J. L. (2004) *Hum Mol Genet* **13**(17), 1943-1949.
[9] Rosenberg, N. A., Pritchard, J. K., Weber, J. L., Cann, H. M., Kidd, K. K., Zhivotovsky, L. A., and Feldman, M. W. (2002) *Science* **298**(5602), 2381-2385.
[10] Venter, J. C., Levy, S., Stockwell, T., Remington, K., and Halpern, A. (2003) *Nat Genet* **33** Suppl, 219-227.
[11] Shrimpton, A. E., Levinsohn, E. M., Yozawitz, J. M., Packard, D. S., Jr., Cady, R. B., Middleton, F. A., Persico, A. M., and Hootnick, D. R. (2004) *Am J Hum Genet* **75**(1), 92-96.
[12] Schaid, D. J., Guenther, J. C., Christensen, G. B., Hebbring, S., Rosenow, C., Hilker, C. A., McDonnell, S. K., Cunningham, J. M., Slager, S. L., Blute, M. L., and Thibodeau, S. N. (2004) *Am J Hum Genet* **75**(6), 948-965.
[13] John, S., Shephard, N., Liu, G., Zeggini, E., Cao, M., Chen, W., Vasavda, N., Mills, T., Barton, A., Hinks, A., Eyre, S., Jones, K. W., Ollier, W., Silman, A., Gibson, N., Worthington, J., and Kennedy, G. C. (2004) *Am J Hum Genet* **75**(1), 54-64.
[14] Middleton, F. A., Pato, M. T., Gentile, K. L., Morley, C. P., Zhao, X., Eisener, A. F., Brown, A., Petryshen, T. L., Kirby, A. N., Medeiros, H., Carvalho, C., Macedo, A., Dourado, A., Coelho, I., Valente, J., Soares, M. J., Ferreira, C. P., Lei, M., Azevedo, M. H., Kennedy, J. L., Daly, M. J., Sklar, P., and Pato, C. N. (2004) *Am J Hum Genet* **74**(5), 886-897.
[15] Zondervan, K. T., and Cardon, L. R. (2004) *Nat Rev Genet* **5**(2), 89-100.
[16] Carlson, C. S., Eberle, M. A., Kruglyak, L., and Nickerson, D. A. (2004) *Nature* **429**(6990), 446-452.
[17] Botstein, D., and Risch, N. (2003) *Nat Genet* **33** Suppl, 228-237.
[18] Wall, J. D., and Pritchard, J. K. (2003) *Nat Rev Genet* **4**(8), 587-597.
[19] Cardon, L. R., and Bell, J. I. (2001) *Nat Rev Genet* **2**(2), 91-99.
[20] (2004) *Nat Rev Genet* **5**(6), 467-475.
[21] Johnson, G. C., Esposito, L., Barratt, B. J., Smith, A. N., Heward, J., Di Genova, G., Ueda, H., Cordell, H. J., Eaves, I. A., Dudbridge, F., Twells, R. C., Payne, F., Hughes, W., Nutland, S., Stevens, H., Carr, P., Tuomilehto-Wolf, E., Tuomilehto, J., Gough, S. C., Clayton, D. G., and Todd, J. A. (2001) *Nat Genet* **29**(2), 233-237.
[22] Risch, N., and Merikangas, K. (1996) *Science* **273**(5281), 1516-1517.
[23] Kruglyak, L. (1999) *Nat Genet* **22**(2), 139-144.

[24] Strittmatter, W. J., and Roses, A. D. (1996) *Annu Rev Neurosci* **19**, 53-77.
[25] Ozaki, K., Ohnishi, Y., Iida, A., Sekine, A., Yamada, R., Tsunoda, T., Sato, H., Sato, H., Hori, M., Nakamura, Y., and Tanaka, T. (2002) *Nat Genet* **32**(4), 650-654.
[26] Klein, R. J., Zeiss, C., Chew, E. Y., Tsai, J. Y., Sackler, R. S., Haynes, C., Henning, A. K., Sangiovanni, J. P., Mane, S. M., Mayne, S. T., Bracken, M. B., Ferris, F. L., Ott, J., Barnstable, C., and Hoh, J. (2005) *Science* .
[27] Hoh, J., Wille, A., and Ott, J. (2001) *Genome Res* **11**(12), 2115-2119.
[28] Benjamini, Y., Drai, D., Elmer, G., Kafkafi, N., and Golani, I. (2001) *Behav Brain Res* **125**(1-2), 279-284.
[29] Hoh, J., and Ott, J. (2003) *Nat Rev Genet* **4**(9), 701-709.
[30] Hoh, J., Wille, A., Zee, R., Cheng, S., Reynolds, R., Lindpaintner, K., and Ott, J. (2000) *Ann Hum Genet* **64**(Pt 5), 413-417.
[31] Hao, K., Li, C., Rosenow, C., and Wong, W. H. (2004) *Eur J Hum Genet* **12**(12), 1001-1006.
[32] Liang, P., and Pardee, A. B. (1992) *Science* **257**(5072), 967-971.
[33] Velculescu, V. E., Zhang, L., Vogelstein, B., and Kinzler, K. W. (1995) *Science* **270**(5235), 484-487.
[34] Diatchenko, L., Lau, Y. F., Campbell, A. P., Chenchik, A., Moqadam, F., Huang, B., Lukyanov, S., Lukyanov, K., Gurskaya, N., Sverdlov, E. D., and Siebert, P. D. (1996) *Proc Natl Acad Sci U S A* **93**(12), 6025-6030.
[35] Marshall, E. (2004) *Science* **306**(5696), 630-631.
[36] Riaz, S., and Nowack, W. J. (1998) *South Med J* **91**(3), 270-272.
[37] Levin, N., Mor, M., and Ben-Hur, T. (2003) *Isr Med Assoc J* **5**(7), 489-490.
[38] Poewe, W., and Wenning, G. (2002) *Eur J Neurol* **9** Suppl 3, 23-30.
[39] Mangino, M., and Middlemiss, C. (1997) *Nurse Pract* **22**(10), 58-59, 63-58, 70, passim.
[40] Petrovitch, H., White, L. R., Ross, G. W., Steinhorn, S. C., Li, C. Y., Masaki, K. H., Davis, D. G., Nelson, J., Hardman, J., Curb, J. D., Blanchette, P. L., Launer, L. J., Yano, K., and Markesbery, W. R. (2001) *Neurology* **57**(2), 226-234.
[41] Hergenhahn, M., Kenzelmann, M., and Grone, H. J. (2003) *Pathol Res Pract* **199**(6), 419-423.
[42] Gillespie, J. W., Gannot, G., Tangrea, M. A., Ahram, M., Best, C. J., Bichsel, V. E., Petricoin, E. F., Emmert-Buck, M. R., and Chuaqui, R. F. (2004) *Toxicol Pathol* **32** Suppl 1, 67-71.
[43] Cho-Vega, J. H., Troncoso, P., Do, K. A., Rago, C., Wang, X., Tsavachidis, S., Jeffrey Medeiros, L., Spurgers, K., Logothetis, C., and McDonnell, T. J. (2005) *Mod Pathol* **18**(4), 577-584.
[44] McClain, K. L., Cai, Y. H., Hicks, J., Peterson, L. E., Yan, X. T., Che, S., and Ginsberg, S. D. (2005) *Amino Acids*.
[45] Nambiar, P. R., Nakanishi, M., Gupta, R., Cheung, E., Firouzi, A., Ma, X. J., Flynn, C., Dong, M., Guda, K., Levine, J., Raja, R., Achenie, L., and Rosenberg, D. W. (2004) *Cancer Res* **64**(18), 6394-6401.
[46] Nagai, H., Terada, Y., Tajiri, T., Yabe, A., Onda, M., Nagahata, T., Ezura, Y., Minegishi, M., Horiguchi, M., Baba, M., Konishi, N., and Emi, M. (2004) *J Hum Genet* **49**(5), 246-255.
[47] Matsui, H., Suzuki, K., Hasumi, M., Koike, H., Okugi, H., Nakazato, H., and Yamanaka, H. (2003) *Anticancer Res* **23**(1A), 195-200.

[48] Alevizos, I., Mahadevappa, M., Zhang, X., Ohyama, H., Kohno, Y., Posner, M., Gallagher, G. T., Varvares, M., Cohen, D., Kim, D., Kent, R., Donoff, R. B., Todd, R., Yung, C. M., Warrington, J. A., and Wong, D. T. (2001) *Oncogene* **20**(43), 6196-6204.

[49] Stagliano, N. E., Carpino, A. J., Ross, J. S., and Donovan, M. (2001) *Ann N Y Acad Sci* **947**, 344-349.

[50] Ginsberg, S. D., Elarova, I., Ruben, M., Tan, F., Counts, S. E., Eberwine, J. H., Trojanowski, J. Q., Hemby, S. E., Mufson, E. J., and Che, S. (2004) *Neurochem Res* **29**(6), 1053-1064.

[51] Ramaswamy, S., Tamayo, P., Rifkin, R., Mukherjee, S., Yeang, C. H., Angelo, M., Ladd, C., Reich, M., Latulippe, E., Mesirov, J. P., Poggio, T., Gerald, W., Loda, M., Lander, E. S., and Golub, T. R. (2001) *Proc Natl Acad Sci U S A* **98**(26), 15149-15154.

[52] Dybkaer, K., Iqbal, J., Zhou, G., and Chan, W. C. (2004) *Clin Lymphoma* 5(1), 19-28.

[53] Nambiar, S., Mirmohammadsadegh, A., Bar, A., Bardenheuer, W., Roeder, G., and Hengge, U. R. (2004) *Expert Rev Mol Diagn* **4**(4), 549-557.

[54] Petty, R. D., Nicolson, M. C., Kerr, K. M., Collie-Duguid, E., and Murray, G. I. (2004) *Clin Cancer Res* **10**(10), 3237-3248.

[55] Yamada, S., Ohira, M., Horie, H., Ando, K., Takayasu, H., Suzuki, Y., Sugano, S., Hirata, T., Goto, T., Matsunaga, T., Hiyama, E., Hayashi, Y., Ando, H., Suita, S., Kaneko, M., Sasaki, F., Hashizume, K., Ohnuma, N., and Nakagawara, A. (2004) *Oncogene* **23**(35), 5901-5911.

[56] Mintz, M. B., Sowers, R., Brown, K. M., Hilmer, S. C., Mazza, B., Huvos, A. G., Meyers, P. A., Lafleur, B., McDonough, W. S., Henry, M. M., Ramsey, K. E., Antonescu, C. R., Chen, W., Healey, J. H., Daluski, A., Berens, M. E., Macdonald, T. J., Gorlick, R., and Stephan, D. A. (2005) *Cancer Res* **65**(5), 1748-1754.

[57] MacDonald, T. J., Brown, K. M., LaFleur, B., Peterson, K., Lawlor, C., Chen, Y., Packer, R. J., Cogen, P., and Stephan, D. A. (2001) *Nat Genet* **29**(2), 143-152.

[58] Khatua, S., Peterson, K. M., Brown, K. M., Lawlor, C., Santi, M. R., LaFleur, B., Dressman, D., Stephan, D. A., and MacDonald, T. J. (2003) *Cancer Res* **63**(8), 1865-1870.

[59] Hoek, K., Rimm, D. L., Williams, K. R., Zhao, H., Ariyan, S., Lin, A., Kluger, H. M., Berger, A. J., Cheng, E., Trombetta, E. S., Wu, T., Niinobe, M., Yoshikawa, K., Hannigan, G. E., and Halaban, R. (2004) *Cancer Res* **64**(15), 5270-5282.

[60] Dr*aghici, S. (2003) *Data analysis tools for DNA microarrays*. In., Chapman & Hall/CRC, Boca Raton, Fla..

[61] Caplen, N. J., Parrish, S., Imani, F., Fire, A., and Morgan, R. A. (2001) *Proc Natl Acad Sci U S A* **98**(17), 9742-9747.

[62] Elbashir, S. M., Harborth, J., Lendeckel, W., Yalcin, A., Weber, K., and Tuschl, T. (2001) *Nature* **411**(6836), 494-498.

[63] Elbashir, S. M., Lendeckel, W., and Tuschl, T. (2001) *Genes Dev* **15**(2), 188-200.

[64] Hammond, S. M., Boettcher, S., Caudy, A. A., Kobayashi, R., and Hannon, G. J. (2001) *Science* **293**(5532), 1146-1150.

[65] Yu, J. Y., DeRuiter, S. L., and Turner, D. L. (2002) *Proc Natl Acad Sci U S A* **99**(9), 6047-6052.

[66] Brummelkamp, T. R., Bernards, R., and Agami, R. (2002) *Science* **296**(5567), 550-553.

[67] Brummelkamp, T. R., Bernards, R., and Agami, R. (2002) *Cancer Cell* **2**(3), 243-247.

[68] Ng, S. S. W., Tsao, M. S., Chow, S., and Hedley, D. W. (2000) *Cancer Res* **60**(19), 5451-5455.

[69] Arlt, A., Gehrz, A., Muerkoster, S., Vorndamm, J., Kruse, M. L., Folsch, U. R., and Schafer, H. (2003) *Oncogene* **22**(21), 3243-3251.

[70] Duxbury, M. S., Ito, H., Benoit, E., Waseem, T., Ashley, S. W., and Whang, E. E. (2004) *Cancer Res* **64**(11), 3987-3993.

[71] Harris, J. C., Gilliam, A. D., McKenzie, A. J., Evans, S. A., Grabowska, A. M., Clarke, P. A., McWilliams, D. F., and Watson, S. A. (2004) *Cancer Res* **64**(16), 5624-5631.

[72] Duxbury, M. S., Ito, H., Benoit, E., Zinner, M. J., Ashley, S. W., and Whang, E. E. (2003) *Biochem Biophys Res Commun* **311**(3), 786-792.

[73] Duxbury, M. S., Ito, H., Zinner, M. J., Ashley, S. W., and Whang, E. E. (2004) *Oncogene* **23**(8), 1539-1548.

[74] Duxbury, M. S., Ito, H., Benoit, E., Zinner, M. J., Ashley, S. W., and Whang, E. E. (2004) *Surgery* **136**(2), 261-269.

[75] Paddison, P. J., Silva, J. M., Conklin, D. S., Schlabach, M., Li, M., Aruleba, S., Balija, V., O'Shaughnessy, A., Gnoj, L., Scobie, K., Chang, K., Westbrook, T., Cleary, M., Sachidanandam, R., McCombie, W. R., Elledge, S. J., and Hannon, G. J. (2004) *Nature* **428**(6981), 427-431.

[76] Paddison, P. J., Cleary, M., Silva, J. M., Chang, K., Sheth, N., Sachidanandam, R., and Hannon, G. J. (2004) *Nat Methods* **1**(2), 163-167.

[77] Berns, K., Hijmans, E. M., Mullenders, J., Brummelkamp, T. R., Velds, A., Heimerikx, M., Kerkhoven, R. M., Madiredjo, M., Nijkamp, W., Weigelt, B., Agami, R., Ge, W., Cavet, G., Linsley, P. S., Beijersbergen, R. L., and Bernards, R. (2004) *Nature* **428**(6981), 431-437.

[78] Sidransky, D. (2002) *Nat Rev Cancer* **2**(3), 210-219.

[79] van 't Veer, L. J., Dai, H., van de Vijver, M. J., He, Y. D., Hart, A. A., Bernards, R., and Friend, S. H. (2003) *Breast Cancer Res* **5**(1), 57-58.

In: Trends in Genome Research
Editor: Clyde R. Williams, pp. 25-85
ISBN 1-60021-027-9

Chapter 2

Genomic Diversity of Extremophilic Gram-Positive Endospore-Forming *Bacillus*-Related Species

Hideto Takami
Microbial Genome Research Group
Japan Agency for Marine-Earth Science and Technology (JAMSTEC), Yokosuka, Japan

Abstract

A great number of aerobic endospore-forming Gram-positive *Bacillus* species have been isolated on a number of occasions from a variety of terrestrial and deep-sea environments, including the Mariana Trench which has a depth of 10,897 m. Some of these *Bacullus* species are known to have various capabilities for adapting to extreme environments. In fact, *Bacillus*-related species can grow in a wide range of environments— at pH 2-12, at temperatures between 5 and 78°C, in salinity from 0 to 30% NaCl, and under pressures from 0.1 Mpa to at least 30 Mpa. We are now exploring how these adaptive capabilities, as reflected in their genomes, were acquired and what intrinsic genomic structures are present in *Bacillus*-related species that have allowed them to adapt to such a wide range of environments. To answer these questions, we initiated a genome sequencing project in early 1998 and have to present determined the entire genomic sequences of three extremophilic bacilli: alkaliphilic *Bacillus halodurans*, extremely halotolerant and alkaliphilic *Oceanobacillus iheyensis*, and thermophilic *Geobacillus kaustophilus*. We provide the first comparative analysis of the extremophilic bacillar genomes with those of three other phylogenetically related mesophilic and neutrophilic bacilli, *B. subtilis*, *B. anthracis* and *B. cereus*, in order to highlight the commonality and diversity of the bacillar genome.

Introduction

Aerobic endospore-forming Gram-positive *Bacillus* species have a nearly ubiquitous distribution in nature, having been isolated from various terrestrial soils and deep-sea sediments. In 1996, mesophilic and neutrophilic *Bacillus* species such as *B. cereus* and *B.*

subtilis and thermophilic *Geobacillus kaustophilus, G. stearothermophilus,* and *G. thermocatenulatus* (formally *B. kaustophilus, B. stearothermophilus,* and *B. thermocatenulatus*), showing more than 98% similarity in 16S rDNA sequences, were isolated from deep-sea sediment collected from a depth of 10,897 m at the bottom of the Challenger Deep[104]. In addition, it was reported in 1999 that several halophilic or extremely halotolerant alkaliphilic strains, which are similar to *B. halodenitrificans* or *Salibacillus marismortui* (formally *B. marismortui*), had been isolated from a depth of 1050 m on the Iheya Ridge [105]. Among these extremely halotolerant alkaliphilic deep-sea isolates, strain HTE831 was identified as a member of a newly designated genus and species, *Oceanobacillus iheyensis*. It turns out that many extremophilic *Bacillus*-related species including alkaliphiles, halophiles and thermophiles, thrive in extreme environments very different from the high hydrostatic pressures and low temperatures found in the *in situ* conditions of deep-sea sampling sites [105, 106]. *Bacillus*-related species are known to thrive in a wide range of environments: pH 2-12, temperatures around 5-78°C, salinity from 0 to 30%-NaCl [98], and pressures from 0.1 Mpa (atmospheric pressure) to at least 30 MPa (pressure at a depth of 3000 m) [62, 105]. Thus, these extremophilic *Bacillus*-related species possess adaptive capabilities to extreme environments, those with high or low temperature, high or low pH, and high salinity [84, 105, 106], and we have been interested in their adaptation mechanisms to various extreme environments along with their evolutionary processes.

We initiated a whole-genome sequencing project of alkaliphilic *Bacillus halodurans* C-125 in 1998 as a first step to understanding the adaptation mechanisms to various extreme environments [108-113] and have published the first report for genome sequencing of extremophilic *Bacillus* species in 2000 with special emphasis on the genomic comparison with *B. subtilis* [115] after whole genome analysis of 168 non-extremophilic (mesophilic and neutrophilic) *B. subtilis* species in a collaboration project between Japan and the European Community in 1997 [57]. Subsequent to the *B. halodurans* genome sequencing project, we attempted to determine the entire genomic sequences of two other extremophilic *Bacillus*-related species, extremely halotolerant and alkaliphilic *O. iheyensis* HTE831 [117] and thermophilic *G. kaustophilus* HTA426 [120], which have been isolated from deep-sea environments.

This chapter will provide comparative analysis of the genomes of these extremophilic bacilli with those of 3 other phylogenetically related non-extremophilic bacilli, *B. subtilis* [57], *B. anthracis* [85], and *B. cereus* [41], in order to highlight the extremophilic features of the genomes.

1. Phylogenetic Classification of Bacilli

Since genus *Bacillus* defined as Gram-positive, aerobic, spore-forming, and motile rod-shaped bacteria is a very broad genus [98], some of *Bacillus* species have been designated in new gerera such as *Alicyclobacillus* [128], *Amphibacillus* [76], *Brevibacillus* [93], *Geobacillus* [75], *Halobacillus* [100], *Oceanobacillus* [62], and *Salibacillus* [126]. Phylogenetic analysis of 16S RNA for species in genus *Bacillus* and species in the new genera reclassified from *Bacillus* (*Bacillus*-related species) shows clustering of species possessing similar phenotypic properties such as alkaliphily, halophily, and thermophily

(Figure 1). However, each of the clusters is phylogenetically close to each other, even for those exhibiting different extremophilic phenotypes. Thus, we are very intrigued by questions of how the adaptive capabilities, which are reflected in their genomes, to extreme environments were acquired and what intrinsic genomic structure of *Bacillus*-related species allows them to adapt to such a wide range of environments.

2. Estimation of the Genome Size of Extremophilic *Bacillus*-Related Species

2.1. Alkaliphilic Bacillus Halodurans

Alkaliphilic *Bacillus halodurans* strain C-125 (JCM9153) [107] was isolated from soil in 1970 [38] and is characterized as a β-galactosidase [39] and xylanase producer [34]. Among our collection of alkaliphilic *Bacillus* isolates, this strain has been the most thoroughly characterized, physiologically, biochemically, and genetically [35], and it was used as a representative strain for genetic analysis. Generally, alkaliphilic *Bacillus* strains cannot grow at pH below 6.5, but grow well at pH above 9.5. Facultative alkaliphilic *B. halodurans* can grow at pH 7-10.5 if sodium ions are supplied at a sufficiently high concentration (1–2 %) in the medium. Over the past three decades, our studies have focused on the enzymology, physiology, and molecular genetics of alkaliphilic microorganisms. Industrial applications of these microbes have been investigated and some enzymes such as proteases, amylases, cellulases and xylanases have been commercialized [36, 114].

The chromosomal DNA from *B. halodurans* C-125 was isolated by the following procedure. *B. halodurans* C-125 was grown in 100 ml of NII medium [103] for 4-5 h until reaching mid-logarithmic phase. Cells from 500 μl of culture were harvested by centrifugation, washed once in TE buffer, resuspended in the same volume of TE buffer (50°C), and mixed with 500 μl of 2% PFC agarose pre-warmed at 50°C. The resulting suspension was poured into a mould chamber (BioRad, Hercules, CA, USA). Solidified blocks were immersed in 10 ml of TE buffer containing 40 mg of lysozyme and incubated at 37°C for 2 h. After washing the blocks in TE buffer twice, they were incubated at 50°C in 10 ml of TE buffer containing 8 mg of Proteinase K (Gibco BRL, MD, USA) overnight. The blocks were washed once in TE buffer and then incubated in TE buffer containing 1 mM PMSF for 1 h at room temperature. They were then washed thrice more in TE buffer. The blocks containing chromosomal DNA were stored in TE buffer at 4°C until use.

Restriction endonucleases recognizing 8-bp sequences, *Asc*I (5'-GG/CGCGCC-3') and *Sse*8387I (5'-CCTGCA/GG-3'), were tested for their ability to digest the chromosome of strain C-125, and were found to generate 18 and 19 resolvable fragments, respectively [108]. The intensity of each resolvable band was analyzed using the *pdi* Desk Top Scanner System (*pdi* Inc., NY, USA). In addition, genome size was estimated by first digesting chromosomal DNA with I-*Ceu*I, which recognizes a specific sequence of 26 bases (5'-TAACTATAACGGTCCTAA/GGTAGCGA-3') within the *rrn* operons and yields eight fragments ranging in size 6.5 to 3250kb [74]. The sizes of these fragments were determined

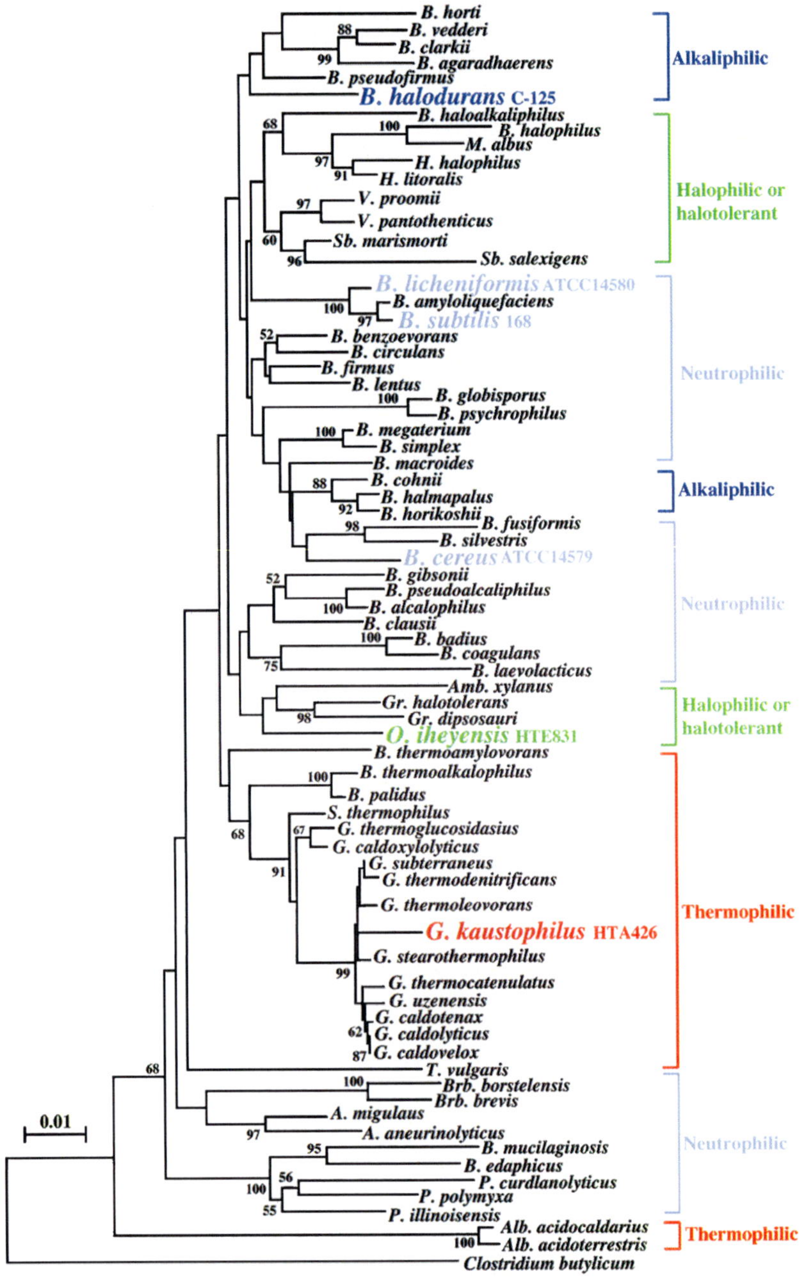

Figure 1. Phylogenetetic tree of Bacillaceae based on 16S rDNA sequences. Phylogenetic positions was generated using the neighbor-joining method with available sequences of Bacillaceae. The numbers indicate bootstrap probability values supporting the internal branches after 1000 replications. Bootstrap probability values less than 50 were omitted. Bar=0.01 Knuc unit. The sequenced and published species are colored by blue (alkaliphilic), green (halophilic or halotolerant), gray (neutrophilic) and red (thermophilic). Abbreviations: *A., Aneurinibacillus; Alb., Alicyclobacillus; Amb., Amphibacillus; B., Bacillus; Brb., Brevibacillus; G., Geobacillus; Gb., Gracilibacillus; H., Halobacillus; M., Marinococcus; O., Oceanobacillus; P., Paenibacillus; S., Saccharococcus; Sb., Salibacillus; T., Thermoactinomyces; V., Virgibacillus.*

by comparison with size standards on a series of pulsed field gel electrophoresis (PFGE) gels [74, 108], and the mean total size of the *B. halodurans* C-125 genome was estimated to be 4.25 Mb by totaling the lengths of the *Asc*I, *Sse*8387I, and I-*Ceu*I fragments, respectively.

2.2. Extremely Halotolerant and Alkaliphilic *Oceanobacillus Iheyensis*

Extremely halotolerant and alkaliphilic *Oceanobacillus iheyensis* strain HTE831 (JCM 11309, DSM 14371) was isolated from deep-sea sediment collected at a depth of 1,050 m on the Iheya Ridge [106] and characterized as Gram positive, strictly aerobic, rod-shaped, motile by peritrichous flagella, and spore-forming. Strain HTE831 grows at salinities of 0–21% (3.6 M) NaCl at pH 7.5 and 0–18% (3.1 M) at pH 9.5 [62]. The optimum concentration of NaCl for growth is 3% at both pH 7.5 and 9.5. Based on phylogenetic analysis using 16S rDNA sequencing, chemotaxonomy, and physiological characters of strain HTE831, this organism was validated in 2002 as being a member of a new species in a new genus, for which the name *Oceanobacillus iheyensis* was proposed [62, 124].

Chromosomal DNA of *Oceanobacillus iheyensis* HTE831 was prepared for PFGE using agarose plugs by the method as for *B. halodurans* C-125 [108]. PFGE with 1% PFC agarose was performed as previously described [74, 108]. Restriction endonucleases recognizing 8-bp or 6-bp sequences were tested for their ability to digest the chromosome of strain HTE831. *Apa*I (5'-GGGCC/C-3') and *Sse*8387I generated 37 and 25 resolvable fragments, respectively. The sizes of these fragments were determined by comparison with size standards on a series of PFGE gels. The mean total size of the genome of *O. iheyensis* HTE831 was estimated to be 3.6 Mb by totaling the lengths of *Apa*I and *Sse*8387I fragments, respectively [62].

2.3. Thermophilic Geobacillus Kaustophilus

Geobacillus kaustophilus HTA426 (JCM12893) is a thermophilic isolate recovered from deep-sea sediment of the Mariana Trench [104]. This strain is Gram-positive, strictly aerobic, and motile by means of peritrichous flagella. Cell growth of the strain is observed at temperatures of 42-74°C, and the optimum growth temperature is 60°C in LB medium. The pH range for growth of the strain is 4.5-8.0. The growth pattern of *G. kaustophilus* HTA426 is very similar to that of *G. stearothermophilus* (ATCC12980^T), the type species of genus *Geobacillus,* in terms of temperature and pH [119].

Digestion with four restriction endonucleases recognizing an 8-bp sequences was performed on *G. kaustophilus* HTA426 (Figure 2). *Sgr*AI (5'-CPu/CCGGPyG-3') generated at least 20 resolvable fragments and produced a digestion pattern similar to that of the type strain of *G. kaustophilus* (DSM7263^T), while the digestion patterns produced with the three other enzymes, *Pme*I (5'-GTTT/AAAC-3'), *Sse*8387I, and *Pac*I (5'-TTAAT/TAA-3'), differed between these two strains. It was particularly notable that the DSM7263^T genome was not digested with *Sse*8387I, whereas this enzyme generated at least 11 resolvable fragments from the *G. kaustophilus* HTA426 genome (Figure 2). On the other hand, digestion of the HTA426 genome with I-*Ceu*I yielded nine fragments ranging in size from 19.4 to 1621 kb and the total size of the *G. kaustophilus* HTA426 genome was estimated to be 3.5 Mb [119].

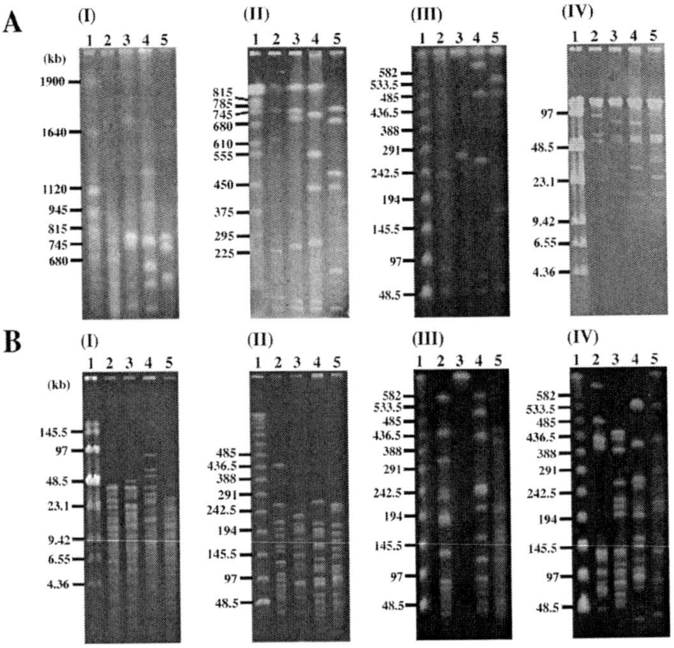

Figure 2. Pulsed-field gel electrophoretic patterns of endonuclease digestions of chromosomal DNAs of *G. kaustophilus* HTA426 and *G. stearothermophilus* HTA462 and comparison with those of the type strains. A: Digestion patterns for I-*Ceu*I: (I) Fragments ranging in size from 700 to 1900 kb; (II) fragments ranging in size from 200 to 800 kb; (III) fragments ranging in size from 50 to 500 kb; (IV) fragments ranging in size from 5 to75 kb. B: Digestion patterns for (I) *Sgr*AI ; (II) *Pme*I; (III) *Sse*8387I; (IV) *Pac*I. Lane 1, Molecular size marker; lane 2, HTA426; lane 3, *G. kaustophilus* DSM7263^T; lane 4, HTA462; 5, *G. stearothermophilus* ATCC12980^T.

3. Determination of Genome Sequences of Extremophilic Bacilli

3.1. Whole Genome Shotgun Sequencing of Three Extremophilic Bacilli

The genomes of *B. halodurans* C-125, *O. iheyensis* HTE831, and *G. kaustophilus* HTA426 were basically sequenced by the whole genome sequencing method [26]. Briefly, aliquots (10 to 20 μg) of chromosomal DNA were fragmented into 1-2 kb pieces by a Bioruptor UCD-200TM (Tosho Denki, Tokyo, Japan) or a HydroShear (GeneMachines, CA, USA) and then prepared and sequenced to produce a whole genome shotgun library as previously described [115, 117, 120]. DNA sequences determined by a MegaBace1000 (Amersham Biosciences, NJ, USA) and ABI PRISM377 DNA sequencer (Perkin Elmer, CT, USA) were assembled into contigs using Phrap (http://bozeman.mbt.washington. edu/phrap.docs/phrap.html) with default parameters. The assembly of shotgun clones from the whole genome of *O. iheyensis* is summarized in Figure 3. The assembly using Phrap yielded 330 contigs at a statistical coverage of 5.9-fold. The 2000 sequences obtained from reverse-end shotgun cloning and from both ends of genomic libraries ranging from 4-6 kb. In addition, 1000 to 2000 sequences from both ends of 20-kb insert in λ-phage clones were also assembled to bridge the remaining contigs. These sequences were assembled with consensus sequences derived from the contigs of random-phase sequences using Phrap and then the contigs were reduced to 105 by this step (Figure 3). Gaps between contigs were closed by shotgun sequencing of large fragments, which bridged the contigs of random-phase sequences. The final gaps were closed by direct sequencing of the products amplified by long accurate PCR [115, 117, 120].

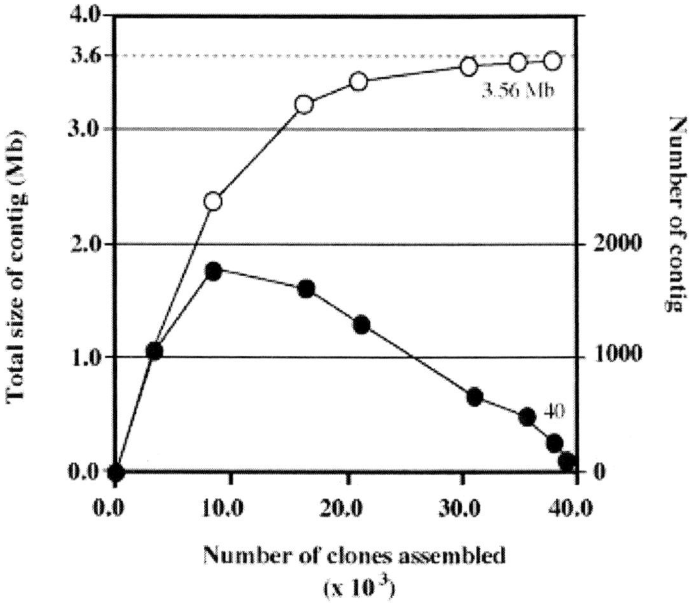

Figure 3. Assembly of shotgun clones from whole genome analyis of alkaliphilic and extremely halotolerant *Oceanobacillus iheyensis* HTE831. Closed circle: Total size of constructed contig. Closed square: Number of constructed contig.

3.2. Gene Finding and Annotation

The predicted protein-coding regions were initially determined by searching for open reading frames (ORFs) longer than 100 codons using the GenomeGambler program, a semi-automated genome analysis systemdeveloped to support this whole-genome sequencing project [90]. GenomeGambler reduces the time and effort required to annotate thousands of protein coding sequences (CDSs) identified in the microbial genome by automating three major routines: analyzing assembly results provided by genome assembler software, annotating CDSs, and searching for homology. All processes and options are manipulated through a WWW browser that enables scientists to share their genome analysis results without choosing computer operating system. A new GenomeGambler system called MetaGenomeGambler^{LITE}, which has just been developed in a collaborative project with in silico Biology Inc. (http://www.insilicobiology.co.jp; Yokohama, Japan) and will be released through this company soon, is a stand-alone system that will make it unnecessary to communicate with a server in the annotation process.

Coding potential analysis of the entire genome was performed with the GeneHackerPlus program using hidden Markov models [130] trained with a set of ORFs longer than 300 nucleotides from either *B. halodurans*, *O. iheyensis*, or *G. kaustophilus* before analyzing sequences from the respective species. This program evaluates codon usage for a series of two amino acids. The Shine-Dalgarno (SD) sequence (UCUUUCCUCCACUAG), which is complementary to the one found at the 3' end of the 16S rRNA, for the three extremophilic bacilli used in this study was identical to that of *B. subtilis*. Searches of protein databases for amino acid similarities were performed using BLAST2 sequence analysis tools [2] with subsequent comparison of CDSs showing significant homology ($>10^{-5}$ significance) using Lipman-Pearson algorithm [82]. Significant similarity was defined as at least 30% identity observed over 60% of the CDS, although those CDSs showing <30% identity over > 60% of the protein were also included in analysis.

Table General features 1. *G. kaustophilus* genome and its comparison of the *Bacillus* -relatedwith

General features	***G. kausto-philus* HTA426**	***O. iheyensis* HTE831**	***B. halodurans* C-125**	***B. cereus* ATCC14579**		***B. Anthracis* Ames**	***B. subtilis* 168**
Chromosome							
Size (base pairs)	3,544,776	3,630,528	4,202,352	5,411,809		5,227,293	4,214,630
G+C content (mol%)							
Total genome	52.1	35.7	43.7	35.3		35.4	43.5
Coding region	52.9	36.1	44.4	35.9		36.0	43.4
Non-coding region	47.0	31.8	39.8	32.7		32.6	43.6
Predicted CDS number	3,498	3,496	4,066	5,234		5,311	4,106
Average length (bp)	862	883	879	835		794	896
Coding region (%)	86	85	85	81		81	87
Initiation codon (%)							
AUG	75.2	79.5	78	75.3		83.1	78
GUG	13.5	7.8	12	11.9		9.1	9
UUG	11.3	12.7	10	12.8		7.8	13
Stable RNA (%)	1.70	1.04	1.02	1.2		1.09	1.27
Number rrn operon of	9	7	8	13		11	10
Mean G+C content	58.5	52.7	54.2	52.6		52.6	54.4
Number of tRNA	87	69	78	108		86	86
Mean G+C content	59.1	58.8	59.5	59.2		59.1	58.2
Plasmid	pHTA426	-----	-----	pBClin	15pX01	pX02	-----
Size (base pairs)	47,890	----	----	15,100	181,677	94,829	----
G+C content (mol%)	44.2	----	----	38.1	32.5	33.0	----
Non-coding region	44.5	----	----	38.4	33.7	34.2	----
Coding region	43.8	----	----	35.4	29.7	30.6	----
Predicted CDS number	42	----	----	21	217	113	----
Average length (bp)	906	----	----	645	645	639	----
Coding region (%)	79.5	----	----	89.8	77.1	76.2	----
Initiation codon (%)		----	----				----
AUG	64.3	----	----	75.3	75.3	75.3	----
GUG	21.4	----	----	11.9	11.9	11.9	----
UUG	14.3	----	----	12.8	12.8	12.8	----

4. Genomic Features of Extremophilic Bacilli

4.1. Alkaliphilic *B. Halodurans*

4.1.1. General Features

The genome of *B. halodurans* is a single circular chromosome [108] consisting of 4,202,352 bp with an average G+C content of 43.7% (coding region, 44.4%; non-coding region, 39.8%) (Figure 4 and Table 1). Based on analysis of skew in the ratio of G-C to G+C (G-C/G+C), we estimated that the site of termination of replication (*terC*) is located nearly 2.2-2.3 Mb (193°) from the replication origin, but we could not identify the gene encoding the replication termination protein (*rtp*) [115]. Several A+T- and G+ C-rich islands are likely to reveal the signature of transposons or other inserted elements (Figure 5). We identified 4,066 protein-coding sequences (CDSs) (Table 1) with an average size of 879 bp. Coding sequences covered 85% of the chromosome, and we found that 78% of the genes in *B. halodurans* started with ATG, 10% with TTG and 12% with GTG, as compared with 87%, 13% and 9%, respectively, in the case of *B. subtilis*. Proteins of *B. halodurans* predicted from 4066 CDSs were estimated to range in size from 1,188 to 199,106 Da for a total of 32,841 Da: non-redundant proteins with assigned biological role, 2,141 (52.7%); conserved proteins of unknown function, 1,182 (29.1%); and no database match for 743 (18.3%) in comparisons with protein sequences from other organisms, including *B. subtilis* (Figure 6). Among the CDSs found in the *B. halodurans* genome, 2,310 (56.8%) were widely conserved in organisms including *B. subtilis* and 355 (8.7%) matched protein sequences found only in *B. subtilis* (Figure 6). The ratios CDSs conserved among the various organisms including *B. subtilis* were 80.5% and 49.7% for functionally assigned CDSs and CDSs matched with hypothetical proteins from other organisms, respectively. Of the non-redundant CDSs with a biological role, 23.8% matched hypothetical proteins found only in the *B. subtilis* database, showing relatively high similarity values (Figure 6).

The 112 CDSs in the *B. halodurans* genome showing significant similarity to transposase or recombinase from various species such as *Anabena* sp. *Rhodobacter capsulatus*, *Lactococcus lactis*, *Enterococcus faecium*, *Clostridium beijerinckii*, *Staphylococcus aureus* and *Yersinia pseudotuberculosis*, indicate that these species have played an important evolutionary role in horizontal gene transfer and also in internal rearrangement generally occurred in the prokaryotic genomes (Figure 7). These CDSs were categorized into 27 groups by similarity patterns and the genes are spread widely throughout the genome. As shown in Figure 5, at least 11 A+T rich and G+C rich islands containing tranposases (T1-T11) were found in the *B. halodurans* genome. One of the notable features of this genome is that *B. subtilis* has only seven transposons and transposon-related proteins. The G+C content of transposases varies from 37.4 to 49.2% and codon usage in transposases, especially for termination, is obviously different from those of other indigenous genes in *B. halodurans*. Among other bacterial genomes, *Synecosystis* sp. PC6803 [45], *Escherichia coli* MG1655 [9], *Mycobacterium tuberculosis* [19], *Deinicoccus radiodurans* [127], and *Lactococcus lactis* [10] have been to contain many transposase genes, as are found in *B. halodurans* C-125.

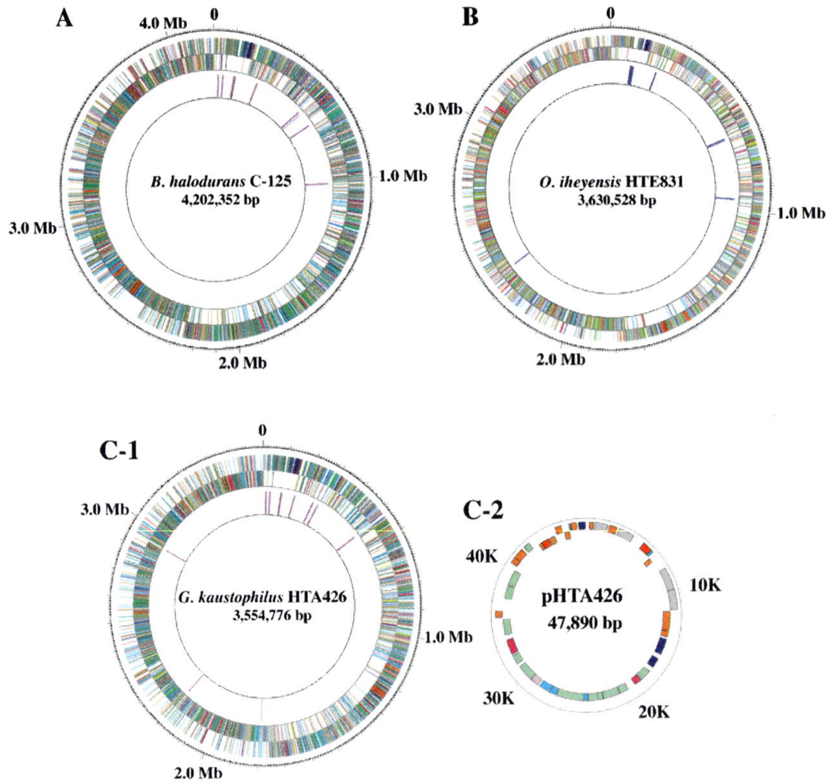

Figure 4. Circular representation of the extremophilic bacillar genomes. A: *Bacillus halodurans* C-125, B: *Oceanobacillus iheyensis* HTE831, C: *Geobacillus kaustophilus* HTA426; (1), chromosome; (2), plasmid pHTA426. The distribution of CDSs is depicted by colored boxes according to the functional category and the direction of transcription (the outer circle is the plus strand; the inner circle is the minus strand; red represents the cell wall, sensors, motility and chemotaxis, protein secretion, cell division, and transformation/competence; magenta represents transport/binding proteins and lipoproteins and membrane bioenergetics; gold represents sporulation and germination; yellow-green represents intermediary metabolism; gray represents DNA replication, DNA restriction/modification and repair, DNA recombination, and DNA packaging and segregation; pink represents RNA synthesis; blue represents protein synthesis; forest green represents miscellaneous functions; sky blue represents conserved CDSs with unknown function; coral represents non-conserved proteins). The third and fourth circles indicate the distribution of rRNA and tRNA in the genome, respectively.

4.1.2. Other Genomic Features

4.1.2.1. Origin of Replication

There are 14 CDSs in the *oriC* region of the *B. halodurans* chromosome. The organization of these CDSs in this region is basically similar to that of other bacteria. In particular, the region from *gidB* to *gyrA* (BH 4060-4066 and BH1-BH7) was found to be identical to that of *B. subtilis*. On the other hand, the 10 CDSs (BH8-BH18), including three CDSs previously identified in the 13.3 kb of *oriC* region [111], between *gyrB* and the *rrnA* operon correspond to the *rrnO* operon in the *B. subtilis* genome, although there is no CDS between *gyrA* and *rrnO* in *B. subtilis*. Out of these 10 CDSs, only one CDS (BH8) was found to have a homologue in another organism, which, interestingly, was not in the genus *Bacillus*, while the others were unique to the *B. halodurans* genome [115].

4.1.2.2. Transcription and Translation

Genes encoding the three subunits (α, β, β') of the core RNA polymerase have been identified in *B. halodurans* along with genes for 20 sigma factors [30]. Sigma factors belonging to the σ^{70} family (σ^A, σ^B, σ^D, σ^E, σ^F, σ^G, σ^H, and σ^K) are required for sporulation and σ^L is well-conserved between *B. halodurans* and *B. subtilis*. Of the 11 sigma factors of the extracytoplasmic function (ECF) family identified in *B. halodurans* and shown in Figure 8, only σ^W is also found in *B. subtilis* while the other 10 (BH640, BH672, BH1615, BH2026, BH3117, BH3216, BH3223, BH3380, BH3632, and BH3882) are unique to *B. halodurans* [115]. These unique sigma factors may play a role in the special physiological mechanisms by which *B. halodurans* is able to adapt to alkaline environments, as it is well known that ECF sigma factors are present in a wide variety of bacteria and that they serve to control the uptake or secretion of specific molecules or ions and to control responses to a variety of extracellular stress signals [61].

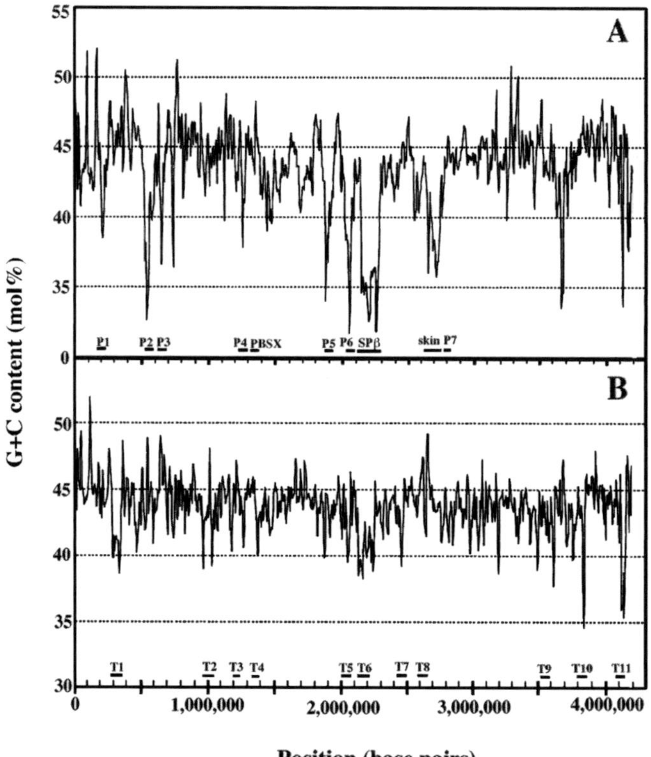

Figure 5. Comparison of G+C profile between the genomes of *B. halodurans* and *B. subtilis*. Distribution of A+T rich islands along the chromosome, in sliding windows of 10,000 nucleotides, with a step of 5,000 nucleotides. Known phages (PBSX, SPβ and skin) are indicated by their names and prophage-like elements in the *B. subtilis* genome are numbered from P1 to P7. A+T-rich or G+C-rich regions containing transposases in the *B. halodurans* genome are also indicated by T1 to T11. A: *B. subtilis*, B: *B. halodurans*.

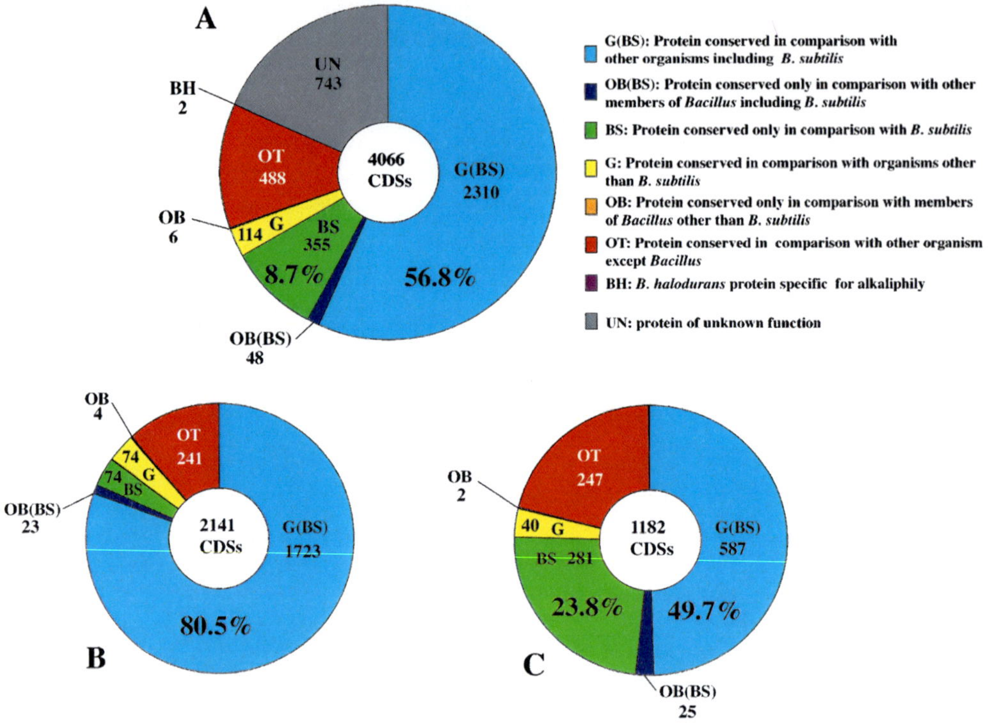

Figure 6. Summary of conserved protein coding sequences (CDSs) identified in the genome of *B. halodurans* C-125. A: all CDSs, B: CDSs with a known functional role, C: CDSs of unknown function.

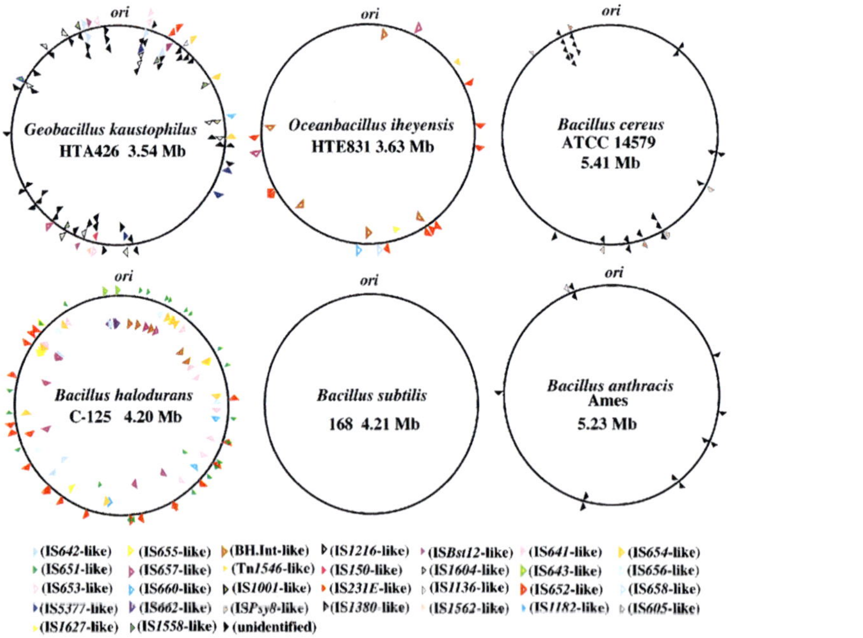

Figure 7. Distribution of major Tpase genes in the 6 bacillar genomes. The Tpase genes categorized into 31 kinds are represented by triangles. The direction of each triangle matches the transcriptional direction. *ori*, region of the chromosomal replication origin.

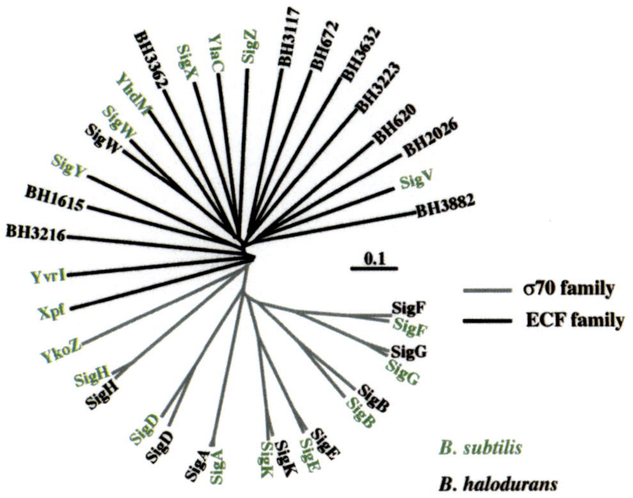

Figure 8. Dendrograms of sigma factors. These unrooted distance dendrograms were generated from the multiple sequence alignment of each paralogue and orthologue between the *B. halodurans* and *B. subtilis* genomes. Bar = 0.1 Knuc unit.

The 79 tRNA species were organized into 11 clusters involving 71 tRNA genes plus 8 single genes without composing the cluster (Table 1), of which six clusters were associated with ribosomal RNA (rRNA) operons. Eight rRNA operons are present in the *B. halodurans* C-125 genome and they are organized identically to those of *B. subtilis* (tRNA-16S-23S-5S, 16S-tRNA-23S-5S, and 16S-23S-5S-tRNA). With respect to tRNA synthetases, the *B. halodurans* C-125 genome lacks the glutaminyl-tRNA synthetase gene (*glnS*), one of two threonyl-tRNA synthetase gene (*thrZ*), and one of two tyrosyl-tRNA synthetase genes (*tyrS*). The *B. subtilis* genome only lacks the glutaminyl-tRNA gene. It is likely that glutaminyl-tRNA synthetase aminoacylates $tRNA^{Gln}$ with glutamate followed by transamidation by Glu-tRNA amidotransferase in both of these *Bacillus* species.

4.1.2.3. Competence and Sporulation

Out of 20 genes related to competence in *B. subtilis*, 13 genes (*cinA, comC, comEA, comEB, comEC, comER, comFA, comFC, comGA, comGB, comGC, comGD*, and *mecA*) that are mainly expressed in the late stage of competence were identified in the *B. halodurans* genome; we could not identify any genes expressed in the early stage of competence. Among six genes whose products are known to serve as components of DNA transport machinery, only three genes (*comGB, comGC,* and *comGD*), but not the other 3 genes known to be well-conserved in *B. subtilis,* were identified in *B. halodurans* C-125. Actually, competence has not been experimentally demonstrated in C-125, despite our attempts to use standard and modified methods along with adjusting culture conditions such as pH, temperature and medium for transformation. It has been clarified that this is due to the absence of some genes required for expression of competence, especially those expressed in the early stage such as *comS*, *srfA*, and *rapC.*

Only 68 genes related to sporulation were identified in the *B. halodurans* C-125_genome, in contrast with 138 genes found in the *B. subtilis* genome. Although the minimum set of genes required for sporulation was well-conserved, as in the case of *B. subtilis,* the *B.*

halodurans C-125 genome lacks some genes encoding key regulatory proteins (the response regulator for aspartate phosphatase and the phosphatase regulator) and the spore coat protein for sporulation conserved in the *B. subtilis* genome. In particular, the *rap* (*rapA-K*) and *phr* (*phrA, phrC, phrE-G, phrI,* and *phrK*) genes were not found in the *B. halodurans* C-125 genome, suggesting that another type(s) of regulatory genes may act to control of sporulation in *B. halodurans* C-125, and that these may act in a manner identical to or different from that in *B. subtilis,* as we have observed sporulation in *B. halodurans.*

4.1.2.4. Cell Walls

The peptidoglycan of alkaliphilic *B. halodurans* C-125 appears to be similar to that of neutrophilic *B. subtilis*. However, the cell wall components in C-125 are characterized by an excess of hexosamines and amino acids, compared to those of *B. subtilis*. Glucosamine, muramic acid, D- and L-alanine, D-glutamic acid, meso-diaminopimelic acid, and acetic acid were found in cell wall hydrolysates [35]. Although some variation was found in the amide content of peptidoglycan isolated from alkaliphilic *Bacillus halodurans* C-125, the pattern of variation was similar to that known to occur in *B. subtilis*. All genes related to peptidoglycan biosynthesis such as *mraY, murC-G, cwlA, ddlA*, and *glnA* and confirmed to be present in the *B. subtilis* genome were also conserved in the C-125 genome [35]. A bacitracin-resistance gene found in the *B. subtilis* genome is duplicated in the C-125 genome (BH474 and BH1538). On the other hand, although *tagH* and *tagG* genes were identified in *B. halodurans* C-125, 13 other genes for teichoic acid biosynthesis found in *B. subtilis* (*dltA-E, ggaA, ggaB, tagA-C, tagE, tagF*, and *tagO*) are missing in the *B. halodurans* genome. *B. halodurans* also lacks six genes (*tuaB-tuaF* and *tuaH*) for teichuronic acid biosynthesis, but retains *tuaA* and *tuaG* which are absent in *B. subtilis* [115]. In addition to peptidoglycan, the cell wall of alkaliphilic *B. halodurans* is known to contain certain acidic polymers, such as galacturonic acid, glutamic acid, aspartic acid, and phosphoric acid. A teichuronopeptide (TUP) is present as a major structural component of the cell wall of *B. halodurans* C-125 and is a copolymer of polyglutamic acid and polyglucuronic acid. Thus, the negative charges on acidic non-peptidoglycan components may permit the cell surface to absorb sodium and hydronium ions and to repel hydroxide ions, and, as a consequence, may contribute to permitting the cells to grow in alkaline environments. A mutant defective in TUP synthesis grows slowly at alkaline pH. The upper limit of pH for growth of the mutant is 10.4, whereas that for the parental strain C-125 is 10.8. The *tupA* gene encoding TUP has been cloned from *B. halodurans* C-125 chromosomal DNA [4], and in this study, it has been clarified that *B. halodurans* C-125 has no paralogue of *tupA* in its genome and that the orthologue of *tupA* can not be found in the *B. subtilis* genome.

4.1.2.5. Membrane Transport and Energy Generation

For growth under alkaline conditions, *B. halodurans* C-125 requires Na^+in the surrounding environment for effective solute transport across the cytoplasmic membrane. According to the chemiosmotic theory, a proton-motive force is generated across the cytoplasmic membrane by electron transport chain or by extrusion of H^+ derived from ATP metabolism through the action of ATPase. We identified four types of ATPases (preprotein translocase subunit, class III heat-shock ATP-dependent protease, heavy metal-transporting ATPase, and cation-transporting ATPase). These ATPases are well-conserved between *B. halodurans* and *B. subtilis*.

Through a series of analyses such as a BLAST2 search, clustering analysis by the single linkage method examining all 8,166 CDSs identified in the *B. halodurans* C-125 and *B. subtilis* genomes, and multiple alignment, 18 CDSs were grouped into the category of antiporter- and transporter-related protein genes in the *B. halodurans* C-125 genome. In this analysis, five CDSs were identified as candidate Na^+/H^+ antiporter genes: BH1316, BH1319, BH2844, BH2964, and BH3946 [115]. However, we could not identify any gene encoding antibiotic-resistance proteins in the *B. halodurans* C-125 genome, whereas the *B. subtilis* genome has nine different such genes. Eleven genes encoding multidrug resistance proteins were identified in the *B. halodurans* C-125 genome, 6 fewer than in the *B. subtilis* genome. A non-alkaliphilic mutant strain (mutant 38154) derived from *B. halodurans* C-125, which is useful as a host for cloning genes related to alkaliphily, has been isolated and characterized [56]. A 3.7-kb DNA fragment (pALK fragment) from the parent strain restored the growth of mutant 38154 under alkaline pH conditions. This fragment was found to contain CDS BH1319, which is one of the Na^+/H^+ antiporter genes in *B. halodurans*. The transformant was able to maintain an intracellular pH lower than the external pH and the cells expressed an electrogenic Na^+/H^+ antiporter driven only by $\Delta\psi$ (membrane potential, interior negative) [35, 56]. *B. subtilis* has an orthologue (*mprA*) of BH1319 and a *mprA*-deficient mutant of *B. subtilis* has been shown to be a sodium-sensitive phenotype [52]. On the other hand, a mutant of strain C-125 with a mutation in BH1317 adjacent to BH1319 has been isolated and shown to have an alkali-sensitive phenotype, although whether the Na^+/H^+ antiporter encoded by BH1317 is active in this mutant has not yet been confirmed experimentally. In addition, it has been reported that BH2819, the function of which is unknown and which is unique to the *B. halodurans* C-125 genome, is also related to the alkaliphilic phenotype [3].

B. halodurans C-125 has a respiratory electron transport chain and its basic gene set is conserved compared with that of *B. subtilis*, but the gene for cytochrome *bd* oxidase (BH3974 and BH3975) is duplicated in the *B. halodurans* C-125 genome. It is also clear that the two genes for *bo3*-type cytochrome *c* oxidase (BH739 and BH740) absent from *B. subtilis* are present in the *B. halodurans* C-125 genome. The *B. halodurans* C-125 genome has an F_1F_0-ATP synthase operon with an identical gene order (ε subunit-β subunit-γ subunit-α subunit-δ subunit-subunit b-subunit c-subunit a) to that seen in *B. subtilis*. In addition to the F_1F_0-ATP synthase operon, the operon for a Na^+-transporting ATP synthase and the operon for flagellar-specific ATP synthase are also conserved between *B. halodurans and B. subtilis* [115].

4.1.2.6. ABC Transporters

Members of the superfamily of adenosine triphosphate (ATP)-binding-cassette (ABC) transport systems couple the hydrolysis of ATP to the translocation of solutes across biological membranes [92]. ABC transporter genes are the most frequent class of protein-coding genes found in the *B. halodurans* genome, as in the case of *B. subtilis*. They must be extremely important in Gram-positive bacteria such as *Bacillus*, as these bacteria have an envelope consisting of a single membrane. ABC transporters protect such bacteria from the toxic action of many compounds. Through a series of analyses described above, 75 genes coding for ABC transporter/ATP-binding proteins were identified in the *B. halodurans* genome (Figure 9). In this analysis of the *B. halodurans* genome, 67 CDSs were categorized as ATP-binding protein genes, although 71 ATP-binding protein genes have been identified in the *B. subtilis* genome [57]. We found that *B. halodurans* has eight more oligopeptide ATP-binding proteins, but four fewer amino acid ATP-binding proteins, than *B. subtilis*

(Figure 9). We could not find any other substantial difference between *B. halodurans* and *B. subtilis* in terms of the other ATP-binding proteins although it should be noted that the specificity of some of these proteins is not known. The genes for oligopeptide ATP-binding proteins (BH27, BH28, BH570, BH571, BH1799, BH1800, BH2077, BH2078, BH3639, BH3640, BH3645, BH3646, AppD, and AppF) are distributed throughout the *B. halodurans* C-125 genome [115]. We speculate that these may enhance survival under highly alkaline conditions although there is no direct evidence to support this. On the other hand, 43 CDSs were identified as ABC transporters/permeases in the *B. halodurans* genome. Surprisingly, *B. halodurans* has only one amino acid permease in contrast with the 12 present in the *B. subtilis* genome. In addition, it is clear that *B. halodurans* lacks the sodium permease gene present in *B. subtilis,* whereas *B. subtilis* lacks the nickel permease gene present in *B. halodurans* [115].

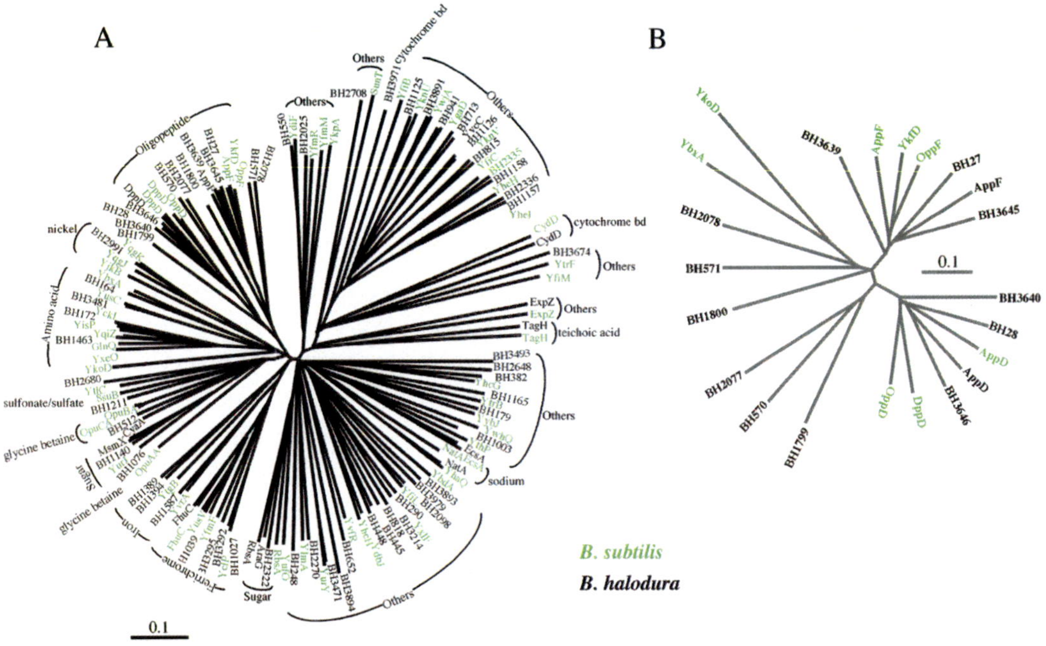

Figure 9. Dendrograms of members of the ABC transporter family of *B. halodurans* and *B. subtilis*. A: ATP-binding protein family, B: oligopeptide ATP-binding protein family. These unrooted dendrograms were generated in the same manner as those in Figure 8. Bar = 0.1 Knuc unit

4.2. Extremely Halotolerant and Alkaliphilic *O. Iheyensis*

4.2.1. General Features

The genome of *O. iheyensis* is single circular chromosome consisting of 3,630,528 bp with an average G+C content of 35.7% (coding region, 36.1%; non-coding region, 31.8%) (Figure 1 and Table 1) [117]. Based on analysis of skew in the ratio of G-C to G+C (G-C/G+C), we estimated that the site of termination of replication (*terC*) is located nearly 1.77-1.78Mb (176°) from the replication origin. We identified 3,496 CDSs, with an average size of 883 bp. Coding sequences covered 85% of the chromosome, and we found that 78% of the genes in *O. iheyensis* started with ATG, 8% with GTG, and 12% with TTG, which are quite similar to values for *B. subtilis* and *B. halodurans*, whose whole genomic sequences have been completely elucidated (Table 1). Proteins of *O. iheyensis* predicted from coding sequences were estimated to range in size from 2,714 to 268,876 Da for a total of 32,804 Da. Following comparison with sequences in a non-redundant protein database, 1972 (56.4%) had an assigned biological role, 1069 (30.6%) were identified as conserved proteins of unknown function, and 456 (13%) had no database match. The 69 tRNA species organized into 10 clusters involving 63 genes plus six single genes (Table 1), of which five clusters were associated with rRNA operons. Seven rRNA operons are present in the *O. iheyensis* HTE831 genome and they are organized identically to those of *B. subtilis* and *B. halodurans* (16S-23S-5S, 16S-23S-5S-tRAN and tRNA-16S-23S-5S).

4.3. Thermophilic *G. Kaustophilus*

4.3.1. General Features

The genome of *G. kaustophilus* comprises a single circular chromosome consisting of 3,554,776 bp and a 47,890-bp plasmid (with mean G+C contents of 52.1% and 44.2%, respectively (Table 1 & Figure 4) [120]. We identified 3,498 CDSs, with a mean size of 862 bp and found that coding sequences cover 86% of the chromosome. Following comparison with sequences in a non-redundant protein database, 1914 CDSs (54.7%) had an assigned biological role and 1096 CDSs (31.3%) were identified as conserved proteins of unknown function. We found that 75.2% of the genes started with ATG, 13.5% with GTG, and 11.3% with TTG; these values are similar to those of other *Bacillus*-related species, except that the ratio of ATG (83.1%) in the initiation codon of *B. anthracis* is a little bit higher than that of the others (Table 1).

In the plasmid designated pTHA426, 42 CDSs with a mean size of 902 bp were identified (Figure 4); the CDSs were much larger than those identified in the plasmids of *B. cereus* (645 bp) and *B. anthracis* (639-645 bp). There is a difference in the pattern of the initiation codon between the circular chromosome and the plasmid of *G. kaustophilus*. The ratio of ATG in the chromosome is more than 11% higher and the ratio of GTG is 8% lower than for the corresponding ratios in the plasmid (Table 1). The number of predicted proteins having biological roles was 24 (57.1%). The *G. kaustophilus* genome was found to contain 9 copies of the rRNA operon and 87 tRNA species organized into 11 clusters involving 81 genes plus 6 single genes.

5. Construction of the "ExtremoBase" Genome Database

A new database, called the "ExtremoBase", was specifically established as a repository for genomic sequences of extremophilic *Bacillus*-related species *B. halodurans* C-125, *O. iheysnsis* HTE831, and *G. kaustophilus* HTA426 and is accessible at http://www.jamstec.go.jp/jamstec-e/bio/en/top.html (Figure 10).

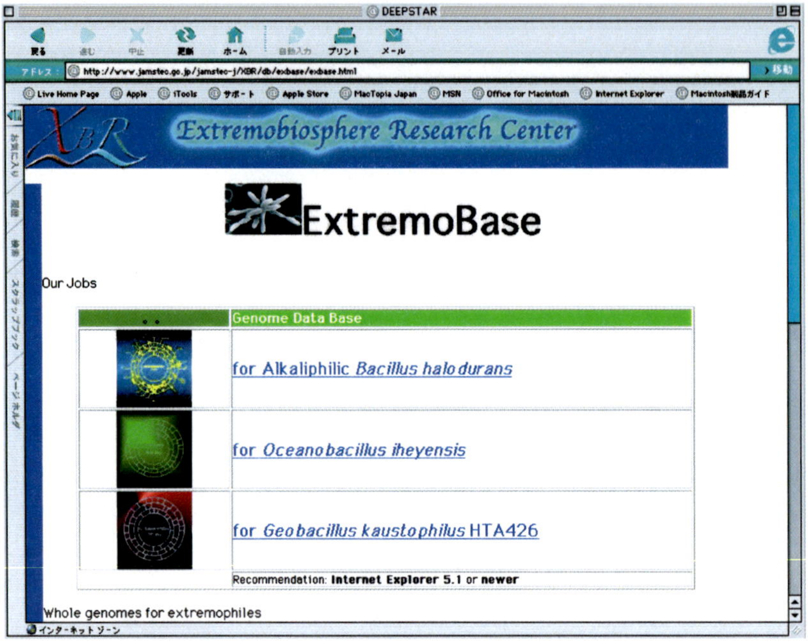

Figure 10. Genome database interface for extremophiles "ExtremoBase".

6. Transposable Elements in Extremophilic Bacillar Genomes

6.1. IS Elements and Group II Intron in the *B. Halodurans* Genome

We identified and characterized sixteen types of new insertion sequence (IS) elements with or without terminal inverted repeats (IRs) and with or without target site duplication (TSD), which is a direct repeat (DR). Many of IS elements belonged to known families, but a few appeared to belong to new IS families and group II introns. Their locations are shown in Figure 11 [116].

6.1.1. IS Elements with IRs that Generate TSD

Ten kinds of IS elements were found to have IRs and flanked by TSD. One at position 746586~747990 bp, in the genome (Figure 11) had imperfect IRs of 18 bp in length, of which the distal 14-bp sequences with 8-bp palindromic structure matched perfectly (Figure 12). The IS element designated as IS*641* was flanked by a 9-bp TSD (Figure 12). IS*641*, which is 1405 bp in length, shows 68% identity with the nucleotide sequence of IS*4Bsu*1 [72] belonging to the IS*4* family [49] and the Tpase of IS*641* shows 70.3% similarity to that of IS*4Bsu*1. The DDE motif, which is conserved in most Tpases and other enzymes capable of catalyzing cleavage of DNA strands [65, 83], was found in the Tpase of IS*641*: D (amino acid (a.a.) 124) D (a.a. 193), E (a.a. 293) and K (a.a. 300). These findings support the view that IS*641* should be categorized as a new member of the IS*4* family (Table 2). The genome of strain C-125 has two other copies of IS*641* (IS*641*-01 and IS*641*-03) with truncation and deletion, respectively, in an IS*641* segment.

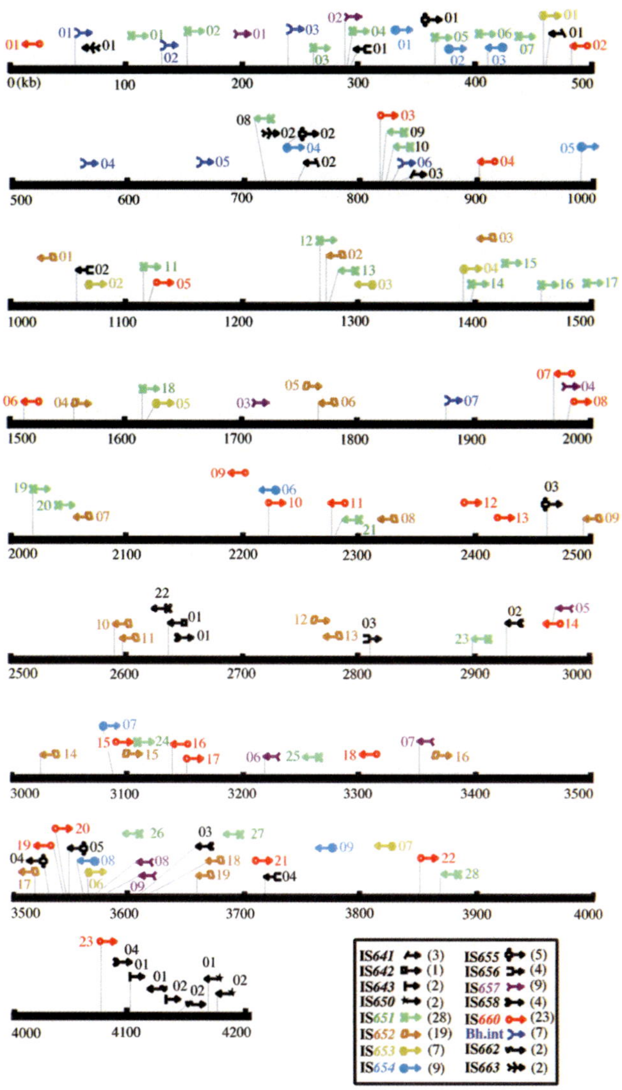

Figure 11. Distribution of IS elements and group II introns in the *B. halodurans* C-125 genome. Arrows indicate the direction of the ISs and the number in parentheses gives the copy number of each element.

The IS element at position 2641523~2642666 bp (Figure 11) has imperfect IRs of 26 bp length (Figure 12). This IS element (1142 bp), designated as IS*642*, was flanked by DRs with a TA sequence (Figure 12). IS*642* showed 43.5 % identity with the nucleotide sequence of IS*630*, which duplicates the TA sequence at the target site [116]. There are two open reading frames (ORFs) overlapping at 545 ~ 597 bp in IS*642*. It is evident that this occurred due to a frameshift mutation because the first and second ORFs are both similar to the Tpase of IS*630,* showing 23.5% and 27.2% similarity, respectively. The DDE motif was found in the Tpase segment encoded by the region straddling the frameshift mutation, as in the case of IS*630*. These results support the view that IS*642* is a new member of the IS*630* family (Table 2).

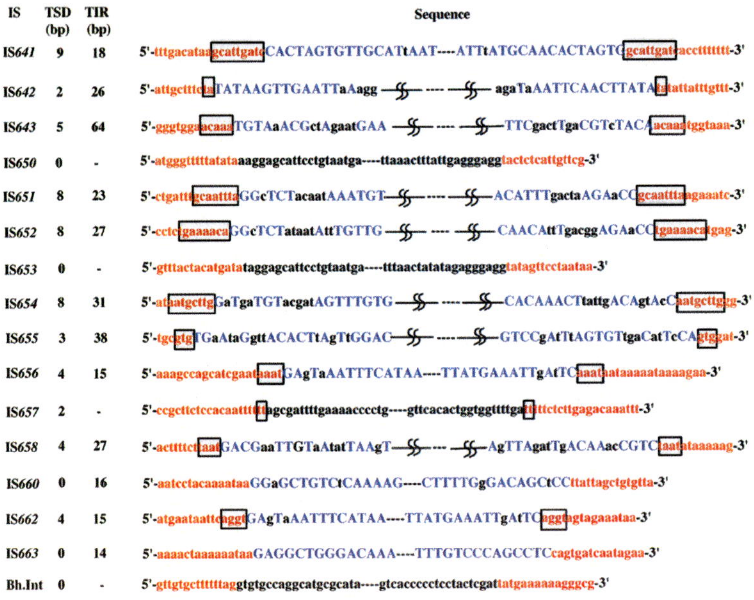

Figure 12. Terminal inverted repeats (IRs) and target site duplication (TSD) of each element identified in the *B. halodurans* genome. IRs are shown in capitals and TSD are boxed.

Table 2. New IS elements and group II intron identifiedin the *B. halodurans* genome

IS	Size (bp)	TSD[a] (bp)	IR (bp)	No. of IS elements			Family[c]
				Total IS	IS with ends[b]	Truncated IS	
IS*641*	1405	9	18	3	2 (0)	1	IS*4*
IS*642*	1142	2 [TA]	26	1	1 (0)	0	IS*630*
IS*643*	2485	5	64	2	1 (0)	1	IS*21*
IS*650*	1929	0	—	2	1	1	IS*650*/IS*653* *
IS*651*	1384	8	23	28	22 (5)	6	IS*L3*
IS*652*	1461	8	27	19	19 (6)	0	IS*L3*
IS*653*	1805	0	—	7	7	0	IS*650*/IS*653* *
IS*654*	1384	8	31	9	9 (1)	0	IS*256*
IS*655*	1221	3	38	5	5 (0)	0	IS*3*
IS*656*	1558	4	15	4	4 (1)	0	IS*656*/IS*662* *
IS*657*	734	2 [TT]	—	9	8 (0)	1	IS*200*/IS*605*
IS*658*	1058	4	27	4	3 (0)	1	IS*30*
IS*660*	1963	0	16	23	6	17	IS*1272**
IS*662*	1566	4	15	2	2 (0)	0	IS*656*/IS*662* *
IS*663*	1980	0	14	2	1	1	IS*1272**
				7	5	2	Group II intron

[a] The target site sequence is shown in [ ]
[b] IS elements with two intact the IS elements without ends. Numbers in patentheses show the IS elements without a target site duplication.
[c] New IS families proposed are shown by asterisks.

In addition, eight other new IS elementswith terminal IRs that generate a TSD were identified: IS*643* (2485 bp, IS*21* family [36]); IS*651* (1384 bp, IS*L3* family); IS*652* (1461 bp, 43.3% identity to IS*651*); IS*654* (1384 bp, IS*256* family); IS*655* (1221 bp, IS*3* family); IS*658* (1058 bp, IS*30* family [20]); and IS*656* (1558 bp, 67.7% identity to IS*662* (1566 bp)). Two ISs (IS*656* and IS*662*) did not show significant similarity to any other IS elements reported to date [116], and were consequently categorized as members of a new IS family designated IS*656*/IS*662* family (Table 2). Note that some intact members of the IS elements described above were found to lack the flanking DRs of target site sequence (Table 2). This indicates that genome rearrangements have occurred through transpositional recombination mediated by IS elements. The existence of truncated members of each of the IS elements described above and below indicates the occurrence of internal rearrangements of the genome, probably through illegitimate recombination.

6.1.2. IS Elements with IRs that Do not Generate TSD

The IS element, designated as IS*663*, with IRs of 14 bp in length is present in the *B. halodurans* C-125 genome (Figure 12). An intact element (1980 bp) shows 42.2% identity to the nucleotide sequence of IS*660* (1963 bp) with IRs of 16 bp in length. The putative Tpase of IS*663* shows 45.5% similarity to that of IS*660*, suggesting that these two IS elements are related to each other. IS*660* and IS*663* show 52.7 and 59.5% identity, respectively, with the nucleotide sequence of an unclassified IS element, IS*1272*, from *Staphylococcus haemolyticus* [5]. In addition, these two ISs (IS*660* and IS*663*) show 42 and 49% identity, respectively, with an unclassified IS element, IS*1182* from *Staphylococcus aureus* (accession no. L43098). These results suggest that IS*660* and IS*663*, as well as IS*1272* and IS*1182*, can be grouped into a new IS family (designated IS*1272* family; Table 2). It is notable that many copies of IS*660*, including various truncated forms, are widely distributed throughout the *B. halodurans* C-125 genome, suggesting that IS*660* may be the oldest IS element present in the genome and that its wide distribution may have occurred through complicated internal rearrangements of the *B. halodurans* C-125 genome.

6.1.3. IS Elements Lacking IRs

Three IS elements lacking IRs, designated IS*657*, IS*650*, and IS*653*, were found to be present in the *B. halodurans* C-125 genome (Figure 12; Table 2). The first IS element, IS*657*, was flanked by a 2-bp TSD that is similar to that found in IS*605* (62.5% similarity) despite IS*605* (1880 bp) being much longer than IS*657* (734 bp) and there only being 42% identity between these nucleotide sequences [15]. These results support the view that IS*657* is a new member of the IS*200*/IS*605* family [8, 15]. There are seven other copies of intact IS*657* (IS*657*-02~05 and IS*653*-07~09) and one truncated copy of IS*657* (IS*657*-06) (Figure 11 and Table 2). The second IS element, IS*650* (1929 bp), showed 43.9% identity to the nucleotide sequence of the third IS element, IS*653* (1805 bp). A putative Tpase in IS*650* showed 78.2% similarity to that of IS*653*, indicating these two ISs are closely related to each other. However, these two did not show significant similarity to any other IS elements reported to date, suggesting that they should be categorized as members of a new IS family (designated IS*650*/IS*653* family; Table 4). There are six other copies of IS*653* (IS*653*-02~07).

6.1.4. Group II Intron

Group II introns are catalytic RNAs that function as mobile genetic elements by inserting themselves directly into target sites in double-stranded DNA [1, 6, 67]. The IS element designated Bh.Int lacks both IRs and TSD (Figure 12). This element (1883 bp) shows 47.6% identity to the nucleotide sequence of the group II intron of *Clostridium difficile* [70]. The protein coding sequence (CDS) of Bh.Int is similar to the putative reverse transcriptase-maturase-transposase of group II introns of *C. difficile*, showing 47.5% similarity. The CDS of Bh.Int also showed significant similarity to group II introns from *Sphingomonas aromaticivorans* (38.4%) [88] and *Pseudomonas putida* (25.7%) (accession no. Y18999).

Among these putative reverse transcriptase-maturase-transposases (RT), the amino acid sequence GTPQGG is well-conserved as a consensus sequence. Thus, IS*653* should be categorized as a new member of the group II introns. The *B. halodurans* C-125 genome contains four other copies of the element (Bh.Int-02~05) and two truncated copies of Bh.Int (Bh.Int-06~07) (Figure 11 and Table 2).

6.1.5. Species-Wide Distribution of IS Elements and Group II Introns Derived from B. Halodurans *C-125*

Five kinds of IS elements, IS*651*, IS*653*, IS*654*, IS*657*, and IS*663*, were amplified by PCR with the primer sets [116] in 10 strains of *B. halodurans* listed in Table 3. Similarly, four other ISs (IS*650*, IS*652*, IS*655*, and IS*656*) and a group II intron were also amplified by PCR in all strains except for AH-101. On the other hand, all ISs and group II introns not amplified by PCR were detected by Southern blot hybridization, except for IS*641* and IS*662* (Table 3). IS*662*, which is a member of a new IS family proposed in the previous study [116], was not detected in the five strains C3, DSM6939, DSM6940, DSM8718, and DSM9774 (Table 3). PCR amplification and Southern blot hybridization patterns of DSM strains for all ISs and group II intron (Bh.Int) were almost identical, except for those of the type strain of *B. halodurans* (DSM497). Although all ISs and Bh.Int identified in the *B. halodurans* C-125 genome were detected in the type strain, it was suggested that two ISs, IS*643* and IS*658*, were truncated or partial because these IS elements were not amplified by PCR. Thus, since it was confirmed that all insertions except for IS*641* and IS*662* are also present in intact, truncated, or partial forms in the genomes of the other *B. halodurans* strainsi, we concluded that the presence of these IS elements is one characteristic of the species *B. halodurans*.

Table 3. Distribution of IS element and group II intron derived from the C-125 in other strains of *B. halodurnas*

Strain	Size of the fragments amplified by PCR (kb)															
	IS*641*	IS*642*	IS*643*	IS*650*	IS*651*	IS*652*	IS*653*	IS*654*	IS*655*	IS*656*	IS*657*	IS*658*	IS*660*	IS*662*	IS*663*	Bh.Int
C-125	1.3 1.0	1.1	2.4	1.7	1.4	1.4	1.6	1.4	1.2	1.5	0.6	1.0	1.9 1.3	1.3 0.8	2.0	1.8
DSM497T	1.3	1.1	—	1.7	1.4 0.9	1.4	1.7	1.4	1.2	1.5	0.6	s.b.	1.9 1.3	1.3	2.0	1.8 1.2
A59	1.3	4.8	2.4	1.7	1.4 0.9	1.4	1.7 3.2	1.4	1.2	1.5	0.6	2.6	2.7	1.3	2.0	1.8
202-1	1.3 1.0	1.1	2.4	1.7	1.4	1.4	1.6	1.4 2.7	1.2	1.5	0.6	1.0	2.7	1.3 0.8	2.0	1.8
C3	—	1.1	2.4	1.7	1.4	1.4	1.6	1.4	1.2	1.5	0.6	s.b.	s.b.	—	2.0	1.8
AH-101	3.6	s.b.	s.b.	s.b.	1.4	s.b.	1.5	1.2	s.b.	s.b.	0.6	1.0	s.b.	0.4	2.0	s.b.
DSM6939	1.3 1.0	s.b.	2.4	1.7	1.4 0.9	1.4	1.7	1.4	1.2	1.5	0.6	s.b.	s.b.	—	2.0	1.8 0.6
DSM6940	1.3 1.0	s.b.	2.4	1.7	1.4 0.9	1.4	1.7	1.4	1.2	1.5	0.6	s.b.	s.b.	—	2.0	1.8 0.6
DSM8718	1.3 1.0	s.b.	2.4	1.7	1.4 0.9	1.4	1.7	1.4	1.2	1.5	0.6	s.b.	s.b.	—	2.0	1.8 0.6
DSM9774	1.3 1.0	s.b.	2.4	1.7	1.4 0.9	1.4	1.7	1.4	1.2	1.5	0.6	s.b.	s.b.	—	2.0	1.8 0.6

T, type strain of *B. halodurans*; —, not detected by PCR; s.b., not detected by PCR but detected by Southern blot analysis

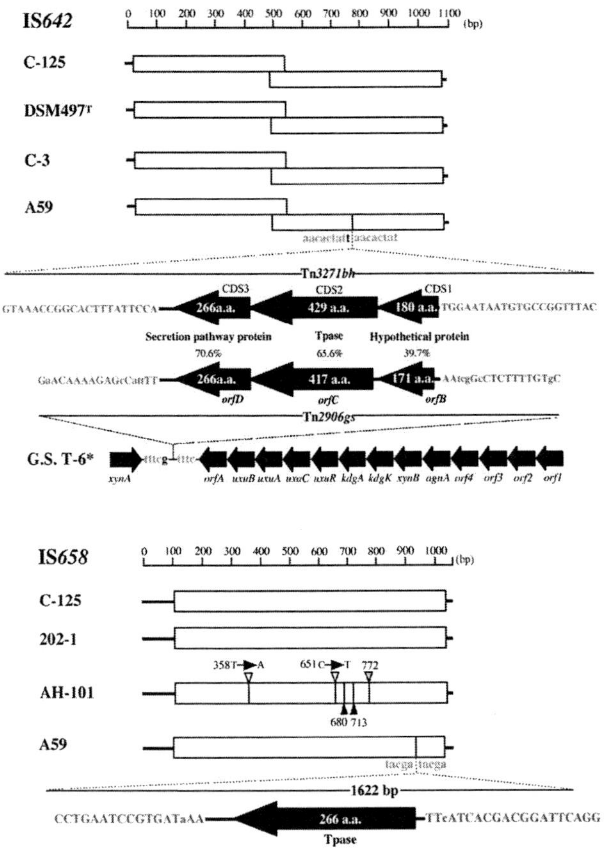

Figure 13. Structure of a new transposon (Tn*3271bh*) within IS*642* and a new IS element (IS*661*) within IS*658* identified in *B. halodurans* A59. IS*642* was detected in the genomes of *B. halodurans* DSM497^{T}, C-3, and A59 by PCR and sequencing. **Geobacillus stearothermophilus* strain T6. IS*658* was detected in the genomes of *B. halodurans* 202-1, AH-101, and A59 by PCR and each amplified fragment was sequenced. Open and closed triangles indicate the frameshift mutation by the substitution and deletion of the nucleotide, respectively. Striped triangle shows a frameshift mutation due to insertion of a nucleotide. Arrows indicate direction of the open reading frame. Terminal IRs and TSD are shown in blue capitals and red letters, respectively.

6.1.6. Characterization of Newly Identified Transposon and IS Element in B. Halodurans *A59*

As mentioned above, IS*642* was amplified by PCR in four strains of *B. halodurans* DSM497, C3, 202-1, and A59, but the PCR fragment of A59 (4.4 kb) was larger than those of the other three strains (1.1 kb). An insertion of a 3271-bp fragment within IS*642* in the A59 genome was confirmed by sequencing of PCR products. The nucleotide sequence of the fragment showed homology with Tpase genes carried by various transposable elements. Three CDSs, which appear to compose tranposon units were identified in the element, and the putative protein deduced from CDS2 comprised 429 amino acids showing 65.6% identity with the amino acid sequence of putative Tpase (*orfC* gene product) identified in the genome of thermophilic *G. stearothermophilus* T-6 [95]. Two other proteins deduced from CDS1 and CDS3 also showed significant identity with the amino acid sequences of *orfB* (39%) and *orfD*

(70.6%) gene products identified in *G. stearothermophilus* T-6 (Figure 13). In addition, the amino acid sequence of the protein deduced from CDS2 showed 44% similarity to that of the *exeA* gene product involved in the general secretion pathway of *Aeromonas hydrophila* [42]. A new transposable element designated Tn*3271bh* was found include IRs and was flanked by TSD, as shown in Figure 13. The transposon Tn*3271bh* has perfect IRs of 21 bp in length with a palindromic structure that is flanked by an 8-bp TSD. Tn*3271bh* was characteristic in that an extra base was added (thymine in this case) to the 3'-end of the TSD located on its left. On the other hand, it appeared that a 2906-bp fragment containing three putative genes (*orfB, orfC*, and *orfD*) in the genome of thermophilic *G. stearothermophilus* T-6 also comprises transposon units, as in alkaliphilic *B. halodurans* A59. This transposon unit, designated Tn*2906gs,* was newly identified in the *G. stearothermophilus* T-6 genome in this study. It shown to have imperfect IRs of 18 bp in length flanked by a 4-bp TSD. Like Tn*3271bh,* Tn*2906gs* appears to be able to add an extra base (guanine in this case) to the 3'-end of the TSD located to its left. Although the IRs and TSD sequences are different from each other, it is clear that these two transposon units are very similar. In addition, it was confirmed that the DSM497 genome also contains a Tn*3271bh*-like element in Southern blot analysis using the whole region of Tn*3271bh* as a DNA probe. Thus, these findings indicate that this kind of transposon can be disseminated in the genome of *Bacillus*-related species inhabiting a wide range of growth environments, such as alkaliphiles and thermophiles.

IS*658* was amplified by PCR in the three strains 202-1, AH-101, and A59, as well as in C-125, but the A59 PCR fragment (2.6 kb) was larger than those of the three other strains (1.1 kb). The insertion of a 1622-bp fragment within IS*658* in the A59 genome was confirmed by sequencing the PCR fragment. The nucleotide sequence of the fragment showed homology with Tpase genes carried by an IS*1380*-like element. The amino acid sequence of the putative protein deduced from CDS identified in the fragment showed 40% similarity to Tpase of the IS*1380*-like element identified in the genome of *Streptococcus pneumoniae* [37]. A new IS element, designated IS*661*, belonging to the IS*1380* family [121] showed perfect IRs with a palindromic structure and was flanked by a 5-bp TSD (Figure 13). On the other hand, Southern blot analysis showed that of all the strains examined in this study, only the *B. halodurans* DSM497 genome incorporates IS*661*.

6.1.7. Bacilli-Wide Distribution of IS Elements and Group II Introns Derived from B. Halodurans *C-125*

Thirteen kinds of IS elements and Bh.Int were amplified by PCR from the genome of *B. alkalophilus* with the same primer set as for *B. halodurans* C-125, although two other ISs, IS*643* and IS*658*, were not detected, even by Southern blot analysis. IS*651,* which had the greatest number of copies (28) distributed throughout the *B. halodurans* C-125 genome, was only detected in the *B. alkalophilus* genome. In addition, two ISs (IS*656* and *IS662*) belonging to the IS*656*/IS*662* family, which was proposed as a unique new IS family in the previous study, were detected from *B. halodurans* C-125 [116] by PCR only in *B. alcalophilus*, whereas IS*650* and IS*653* belonging to another new IS family (IS*650*/IS*653*) were also detected by Southern blot analysis in other bacilli, such as *B. clausii*, *B. vedderi*, *B. firmus*, and *B. thermoalkalophilus*. Thus, these findings suggest that *B. alkalophilus* is very closely related to *B. halodurans*, based on the distribution of ISs and group II introns, although the phylogenetic relationship between the two species based on 16S rDNA sequence analysis is not very close (Figure 14). A total of 19 *Bacillus*-related species, excluding *B. alkalophilus*, were found to lack the five IS elements IS*642*, IS*651*, IS*654*, IS*656*, and IS*662*. No ISs and Bh.Int identified in the *B. halodurans* genome were not detected in five other *Bacillus*-related species: alkaliphilic *Bacillus gibsonii*; thermophilic *G. stearothermophilus*; and neutrophilic *Paeniobacillus illinoisensis*, *Paeniobacillus polymyxa*, and *Paeniobacillus lautus* (Figure 14).

Table 4. IS family identified in the genome of *Bacillus*-related species

IS family	No. of members identified in genomes of:			Reference
	O. iheyensis	Other *Bacillus*-related strains		
IS*3*	1 (IS*672*)	*B. thuringiensis* sub. *aizawai* *B. thuringiensis*, *B. halodurans*	4	[24, 33, 97, 116]
IS*4*	0	*B. thuringiensis* sub. *thuringiensis*, *B. halodurans*, *B. subtilis natto*, *G. stearothermophilus**	15	[54, 60, 64, 72, 116, 129]
IS*5*	1 (IS*671*)		0	
IS*6*	0	*B. thuringiensis* sub. *israelensis* *B. thuringiensis* sub. *fukuokaensis* *B. cereus*	4	[12, 21, 97]
IS*21*	0	*B. thuringiensis* sub. *thuringiensis* *B. halodurans*, *G. stearothermophilus**	5	[60, 116, 129]
IS*30*	1 (IS*670*)	*B. halodurans*	1	[116]
IS*110*	0	*B. halodurans*	2	[116]
IS*200*/IS*605*	1 (IS*669*)	*B. halodurans*	1	[116]
IS*256*	0	*B. halodurans*	1	[116]
IS*481*	0	*G. stearothermophilus**	1	[95]
IS*630*	0	*B. halodurans*, *G. stearothermophilus**	2	[48, 116]
IS*650*/IS*653*	0	*B. halodurans*	1	[116]
IS*656*/IS*662*	0	*B. halodurans*	1	[116]
IS*660*/IS*1272*	0	*B. halodurans*	1	[116]
IS*982*	0	*B. thuringiensis*, *B. stearothermophilus*	2	[48, 132]
IS*L3*	2 (IS*667*) (IS*668*)	*B. halodurans*	2	[116]

*Geobacillus stearothermophilus

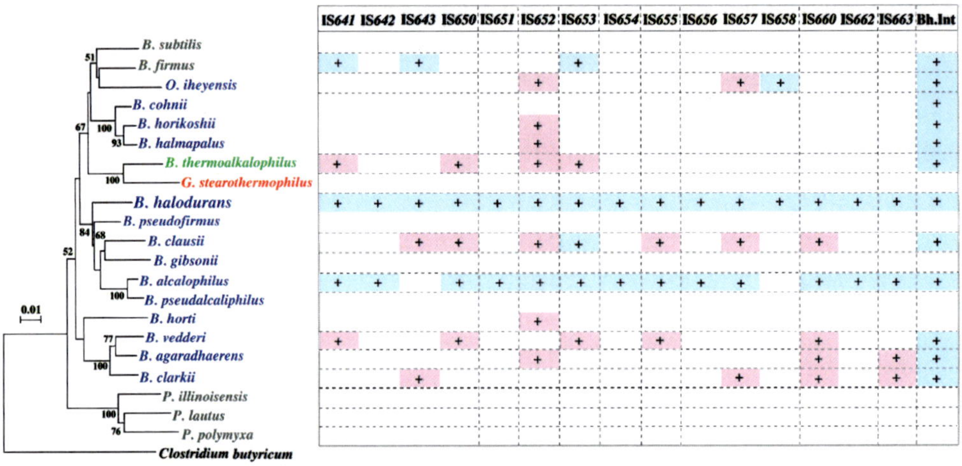

Figure 14. Phylogenetic relationship based on 16S rDNA sequences of *Bacillus*-related species possessing IS elements and a group II intron identified in *B. halodurans* C-125. Blue, alkaliphile; Gray, neutrophile; Red, thermophile; Green, thermophilic alkaliphile. The detected ISs and a group II intron are indicated by plus. Each element confirmed by PCR and Southern blot analysis is marked with light blue and pink, respectively. Bootstrap probability values of less than 50% were omitted. *Clostridium butyricum* MW8 served as an outgroup. Bar = 0.02 Knuc unit. Accession numbers for 16S rDNA sequences are *C. butyricum*, AJ002592; *B. subtilis*, AJ276351; *B. firmus*, D16268; *B. pseudofirmus*, X76439; *B. chonii*, AB023412; *B. horikoshii*, AB043865; *B. halmapalus*, X76447; *B. thermoalkalophilus*, Z26931; *G. stearothermophilus*, AJ284817; *B. clausii*, X76440; *B. gibsonii*, X76446; *B. alcalophilus*, X76436; *B. pseudoalkalophilus*, X76449; *B. horti*, D87035; *B. vedderi*, Z48306; *B. agaradhaerens*, X76445; *Paenibacillus illinoisensis*, D85397; *P. lautus*, D78473; *P. polymyxa*, AJ320493.

On the other hand, three ISs (IS*641*, IS*643*, and IS*653*) and Bh.Int were amplified by PCR with the same size as those from *B. halodurans* C-125 from the genome of neutrophilic *B. firmus* which is phylogenetically distant from *B. halodurans* (Figure 14). Although IS*652* was not amplified from the genomes of 19 *Bacillus*-related species, excluding *B. alkalophilus*, by PCR it was detected by Southern blot analysis in eight species: *B. clausii*, *B. clarkii*, *B. halmapalus*, *B. horikoshii*, *Bacillus chonii*, *B. thermoalkalophilus*, *Bacillus horti*, and *O. iheyensis*. Bh.Int with the exactly same size as that from *B. halodurans* C-125 was amplified by PCR in 11 out of 20 *Bacillus*-related species, in contrast to the IS elements, of which most were not detected by PCR (Figure 14). From these findings, it is clear that five kinds of IS elements, IS*650* (IS*650*/IS*653* family [116]), IS*652* (IS*L3* family [28]), IS*653* (IS*650*/IS*653* family), IS*657* (IS*200*/IS*605* family [8□15]), and IS*660* (IS*1272*/IS*660* family [5, 116]), and Bh.Int are widely disseminated among at least four *Bacillus*-related species, without correlation to the phylogenetic relationships based on 16S rDNA sequences or to their growth environments.

6.2. IS Elements, Transposon, and Group II Introns in the *O. Iheyensis* Genome

Six kinds of new ISs, IS*667* to IS*672*, a group II intron (Oi.Int), and an incomplete transposon (Tn*8521oi*) were identified in the 3,630,528-bp genome of the extremely halotolerant and alkaliphilic *O. iheyensis* HTE831 [102]. Of 19 ISs identified in the *O. iheyensis* HTE831 genome, seven were truncated, indicating the internal rearrangement of the genome (Figure 15). All ISs, except IS*669*, generated a 4- to 8-bp duplication of the target-site sequence, and these ISs carried 23- to 28-bp IRs. Sequence analysis newly placed four ISs (IS*669*, IS*670*, IS*671*, and IS*672*) in separate IS families (IS*200*/IS*605*, IS*30*, IS*5*, and IS*3*, respectively). IS*667* and IS*668* were also characterized as new members of the IS*L3* family. Most ISs found in the *O. iheyensis* HTE831 genome belonged to known IS families reported in other *Bacillus* strains, but aside from the IS5 family, IS*671* was the first to be identified in a bacillus genome (Table 4). On the other hand, IS belonging to the IS*4* family, the most common type of ISs found in bacilli, were not found in the *O. iheyensis* HTE831 genome. IS elements belonging to the IS*L3* family have been reported only in *B. halodurans* C-125 to date, but two other new members (IS*667* and IS*668*) showing significant similarities to those identified in strain *B. halodurans* C-125 were found in the *O. iheyensis* HTE831 genome in this study.

This element (1889 bp in length) is 66% identical to the nucleotide sequence of the group II intron of *B. halodurans* designated Bh.Int [116]. The amino acid sequence deduced from the CDS of Oi.Int was 62% identical to the putative RT of the Bh.Int. It is known that all group II introns are classified into two major subgroups, IIA and IIB [59], and Oi.Int placed in subgroup IIB, as shown in Figure 16. Domain I is the largest among all intron domains, if the optional ORF looping out in domain IV is excluded from consideration. Domain I is involved in the alignment of the 5' splice site (GUGUG) and the recognition of intron-specific target DNA, EBS1 and EBS3. Domain V is the most highly conserved primary sequence within the RNA core of the group II intron and plays a key role in splicing. Domain V binds domain I extensively to form a catalytic core with long-range tertiary interaction. In domain V of Oi.Int, potential tertiary parings (ζ–ζ', λ–λ', and κ–κ') were identified in a consensus model [59]. Domain VI forms a relatively variable structure. Most of the group II introns have a bulging A on the 3' side of the basal helix of domain VI, at either seven or eight nucleotides from the 3' splice site (Figure 16). A branch point of Oi.Int was found seven nucleotides from the 3' splice site (AU). These findings support the view that Oi.Int should be categorized as a new member of the group II intron class, although the splicing of Oi.Int has not been confirmed experimentally.

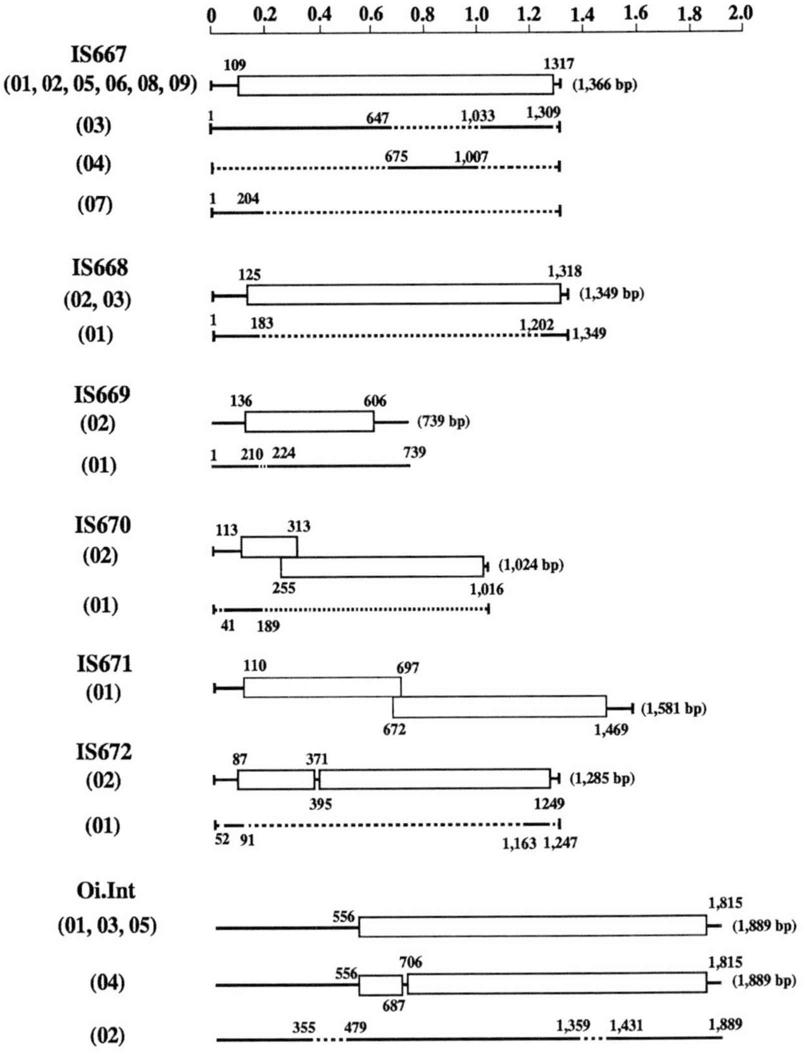

Figure 15. Structure of each IS element and the group II intron identified in the *O. iheyensis* genome. The box shows the Tpase or RT of each element and the numbers beside each box indicate the position of the Tpase in the element. The black lateral bar indicates the elements identified in the genome. The black dashed lines indicate deleted parts of the element. The small vertical bar at the end of the element denotes IRs. The partial IS elements lacking terminal sequence and shorter than 100 bp are not shown.

A trace of the 8521-bp transposon unit, designated Tn*8521oi*, is present in the *O. iheyensis* HTE831 genome. A *ger* gene cluster comprising three CDSs (OB481, OB482, and OB483) was found in the Tn*8521oi* element (Figure 17A). The *O. iheyensis* HTE831 genome has two other paralogous gene clusters located at 73° and 114° (*oriC* region at 12 o'clock assigned to 0°), respectively, on the circular chromosome. The genome of *B. subtilis* 168 has five gene clusters (*gerA*, *gerB*, *gerK*, *yndDEF*, and *yfkQRT*) orthologous to the *ger* gene cluster introduced into the *O. iheyensis* HTE831 genome by Tn*8521oi*, although the *gerBC* gene product did not show significant homology to the amino acid sequence of the putative corresponding protein (OB481) in the fifth gene cluster located at 315° (Figure 17B). The spores are thought to recognize germinants such as L-alanine, L-valine, L-asparagine, glucose, fructose, and KCl through receptor proteins encoded by the *gerA* family of operons, which includes *gerA*, *gerB*, and *gerK* [69]. The *O. iheyensis* HTE831 genome has only three paralogous *ger* gene clusters, even when one acquired by the insertion of Tn*8521oi* is included, in contrast to five in *B. subtilis* and four in *B. halodurans* (Figure 17B). Although it is unclear what role these three *gerA*-like operons identified in the *O. iheyensis* HTE831 genome play in spore germination, and no experimental data for the frequency of germination from *O. iheyensis* spores has been obtained, these genomic characteristics of the *ger* gene cluster presumably imply a low frequency of spore germination in *O. iheyensis*. On the other hand, a low frequency of spore formation in generally rich media has been observed in strain HTE831 [62]. Thus, *O. iheyensis*, a low-frequency spore producer, may have no serious problems in spore germination under enriched conditions, even if the number of paralogous *gerA*-like operons is smaller than that of high-frequency spore formers.

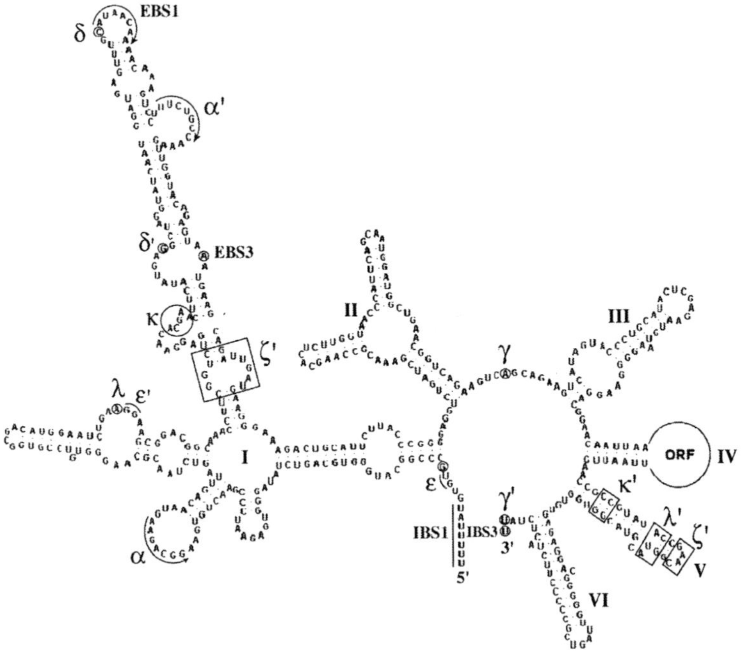

Figure 16. Secondary-structure model of Oi.Int. The model was constructed by comparative analysis with a consensus group II intron structure model combined with RNA folding analysis using the MFOLD program (http://bioweb.pasteur.fr/seqanal/interfaces/mfold-simple.html). Roman numberals correspond to the six major structural domains of the group II introns. Potential tertiary pairings are designated α-α', δ-δ', ε-ε', γ-γ', ζ-ζ', κ-κ', λ-λ' and EBS1-IBS1. EBS3 represents a potential tertiary pairing with IBS3. ORF is encoded completely within domain IV. An asterisk indicates the lariat branch point A. Group II intron splicing occurs through the following two-step transesterification: the 2'-OH group of a conserved intron adenosine residue in domain VI attacks the phosphodiester bond at the 5' splice site, forming a lariat form of the intron that contains the 2'-5' linkage and releasing the 5' exon; then, the 3'-OH librated at the end of the upstream exon attacks the 3' splice site, resulting in exon ligation and intron release.

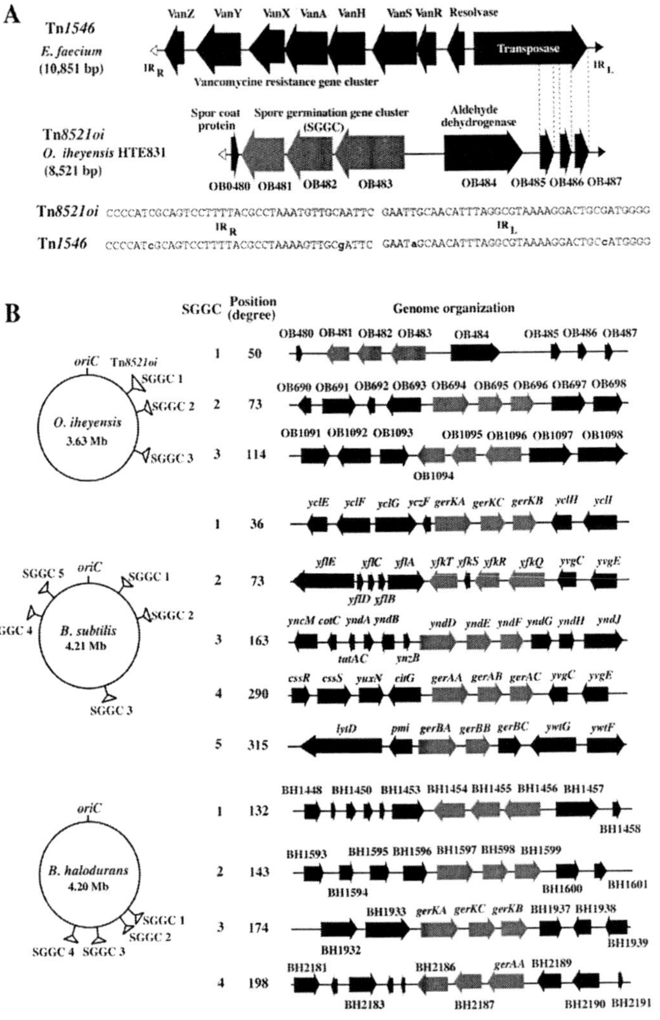

Figure 17. Structure of the transposon-like element containing the spore germination gene cluster (SGGC), and the distribution of SGGCs in bacilli genomes. A: Structure of the transposon-like element identified in the HTE831 genome and comparison with that of Tn*1546*. Gray arrows show spore germination (*ger*)-related genes. B: Distribution of SGGCs in the HTE831 genome and comparison with those of *B. subtilis* 168 and *B. halodurans* C-125. The 12 o'clock position of the *oriC* region is assigned 0°. Gray arrows indicate the *ger*-related gene.

6.3. IS Elements and Group II Intron in the *G. Kaustophilus* Genome

The *G. kaustophilus* genome possessing 91 genes encodes putative transposases (Tpases) categorized into 31 groups, which appear to be carried by various ISs. Although the number of groups was slightly greater than that in *B. halodurans* (27 groups), the number of genes was fewer than the 112 found in the *B. halodurans* genome. However, the total number of Tpase genes in the *G. kaustophilis* genome is much greater than that of four other sequenced bacilli, *B. subtilis* (none), *O. iheyensis* (21 genes), *B. cereus* (28 genes), and *B. anthracis* (12 genes) (Figure 7). A total of 43 of the Tpase genes in the *G. kaustophilus* genome were similar to the sequences present in the genomes of thermophilic bacteria such as *G.*

stearothermophilus [129], *Thermoanaerobacter tengcongensis* [6], and *T. maritima* [77]. The remaining 47 genes were similar to those of mesophilic bacteria such as *B. halodurans*, *O. iheyensis* [102] and *B. cereus*, and also to those of mesophilic archaea such as *Methanosarcina mazeri* [22] and *Methanosarcina acetivorans* [27]. Of the 47 genes, 9 showed significant homology to Tpases carried by IS*642*, IS*653*, and IS*654* identified in the *B. halodurans* genome, which are categorized into the IS*630* family, the IS*650*/IS*653* family, and the IS*256* family, respectively [116]. Further, 26 kinds of ISs, IS*Gka1* to IS*Gka26*, two kinds of group II intron (Gk.Int1 and Gk.Int2), and a transposon (Tn*3095gk*) were identified in the 3,544,776-bp genome of thermophilic *G. kaustophilus* HTA426, and 22 IS elements were categorized into major IS families such as IS*3*, IS*4*, IS*5*, IS*21*, IS*110*, and IS*L3*, and others were filed into 3 new families. Several regions in the *G. kaustophilus* HTA426 genome were highlighted by characteristic G+C content, dinucleotide bias, and codon bias, suggesting direct evidence for horizontal gene transfer. In fact, one of these areas is located in a region of prophage categorized into the *Siphovirus* family.

Two kinds of group II introns, designated Gk.Int1 and Gk.Int2 were identified in the *G. kaustophilus* HTA426 genome. Gk.Int1 (2,782 bp) contains an ORF encoding RT, and its amino acid sequence showed 42% identity to that of a group II intron from *B. cereus*. The amino acid sequence of RT in Gk.Int2 (1,889 bp in length) showed 76% identity to that of Oi.Int identified in the *O. iheyensis* genome [102]. Gk.int1 was found to be inserted into the *recA* gene and to have the ability to splice in at temperatures above 70°C *in vivo* (Figure 18). This is the first prokaryotic group II intron to be found in a housekeeping gene [17].

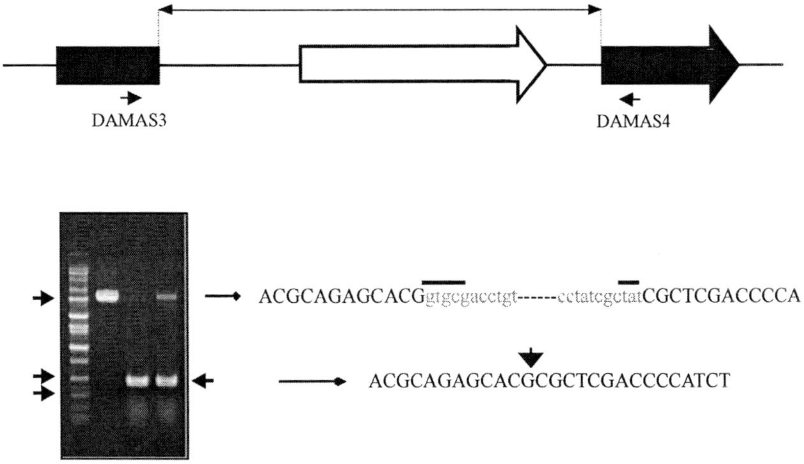

Figure 18. Organization of group II intron-encoded ORFs and splicing of the Gk.Int1 intron. A: Schematic diagram of the *Geobacillus kaustophilus recA* gene. The *recA* gene contains a Gk.Int1 intron of 2,782 bp in length. Thick arrows indicate the locations of the primers used. B: *in vivo* and *in vitro* splicing of the Gk.Int1 intron. (1) Electrophoretic analysis of the *recA* product after the splicing of Gk.Int1. Lane 1: PCR product obtained from the *G. kaustophilus* chromosomal DNA with the DAMAS3 and DAMAS4 primers; Lane 2: *in vivo*; Lane 3: *in vitro*. (2) The DNA sequence of the 5' and 3' junction sites of the Gk.Int1 intron. The bold lines above the sequence correspond to the G2I splice-site consensus sequences. The bottom nucleotide is the sequence of the spliced *recA* RT-PCR product. The thick arrow indicates the splice junction of *recA*.

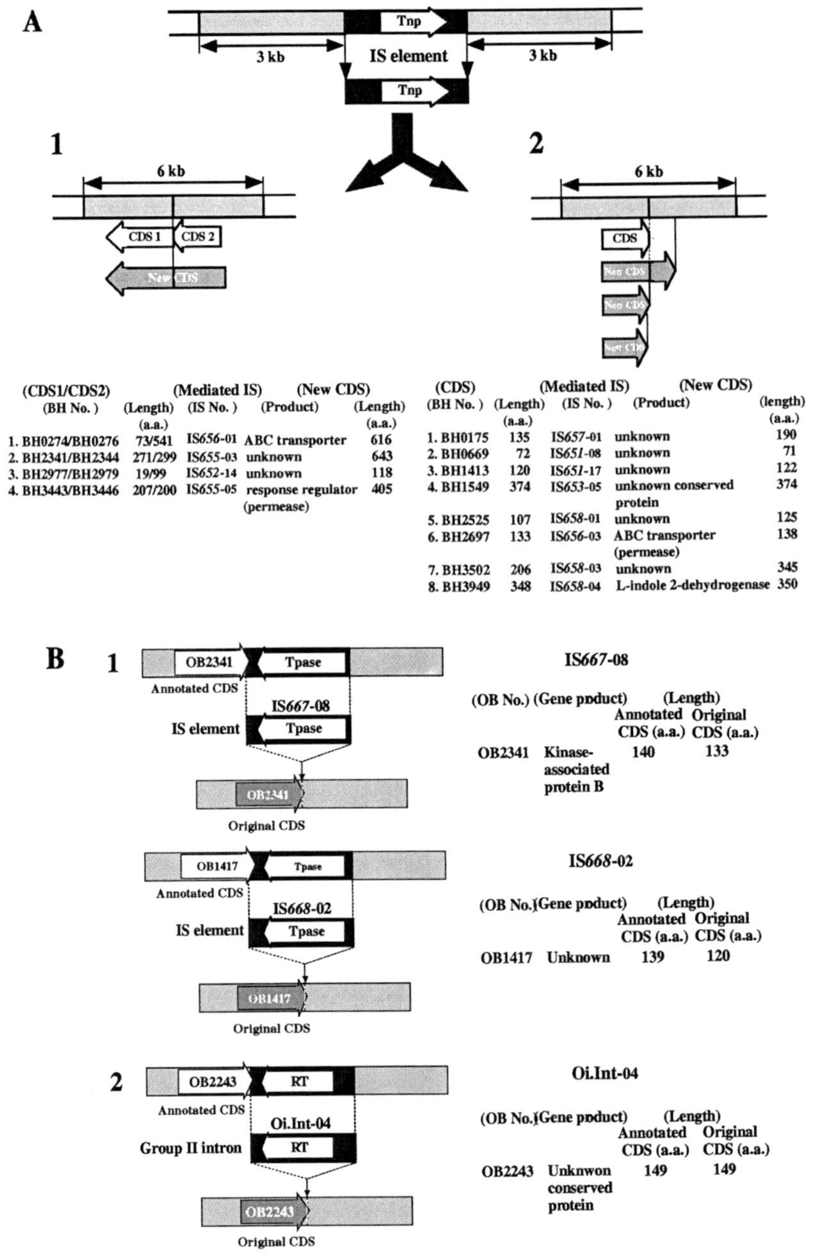

Figure 19. Alteration of protein-coding regions mediated by ISs and the group II intron. A: *B. halodurans* C-125, (1) The case in which CDS 1 and CDS 2 identified on either side of the Tpase coding region in the IS element merge as one CDS upon elimination of the IS element. (2) The case in which an alternation occurred in the C-terminal region of the CDS upon insertion of the IS element. B: *O. iheyensis* HTE83, (1) IS elements. (2) Group II intron. An alteration occurs in the *C*-terminal region of the protein-coding sequence (CDS) upon insertion of the IS element and a group II intron. Black and gray boxes indicate the insertion sequences (IS or group II intron) and the HTE831 chromosome, respectively. Dark-gray arrows represent original CDSs before insertion of the IS elements and group II intron.

6.4. Behavior of IS Elements in the Extremophilic Bacillar Genomes

To investigate how protein coding regions are affected by ISs in the genome, the CDS in the regions adjacent to each IS were analyzed. The nucleotide sequence of the 3-kb region upstream and that of the 3-kb region downstream of each of all intact IS elements identified in this study were extracted from the entire genome sequence through the ExtremoBase web. A 6-kb sequence, from which an IS region was excised, was searched for CDS using the BLAST2X program.

In the case of the *B. halodurans* genome, at least 12 CDSs were likely affected by insertion of 7 kinds of IS elements (IS*651*, IS*652*, IS*653*, IS*655*, IS*656*, IS*657*, and IS*658*), although most of the IS elements widely distributed throughout the genome were inserted in non-coding regions. Examples shown in Figure 19A-1 include two CDSs (CDS 1 and CDS 2) on either side of the Tpase gene which were identified as originating from one CDS, suggesting that it had been divided into two parts by an IS insertion. The gene encoding an ABC transporter (permease) comprising 616 a.a. appeared to have been divided into two genes encoding BH0274 (73 a.a.) and BH0276 (541 a.a.) by IS an insertion. Similarly, the gene for a response regulator (a member of the Arac/xylS family) appeared to have been divided into two genes encoding BH3443 (207 a.a.) and BH3446 (200 a.a.). In addition, two other genes of unknown function were also each presumably divided into two genes, BH2341 (271 a.a.) and BH2344 (299 a.a.) in the first case, and BH2977 (19 a.a.) and BH2979 (99 a.a.) in the second case (Fig 19A-1). On the other hand, eight CDSs located upstream of Tpase also seemed to be affected by ISs, as shown in Figure 19A-2. Six CDSs (BH0175, BH1413, BH2525, BH2697, BH3502, and BH3949) were likely produced by the truncation of the original CDS by an IS insertion. Thus, among 89 intact ISs of 16 kinds identified in this study, 12 intact IS elements of 7 kinds consequently seem to have affected a CDS by their insertion.

On the other hand, two CDSs, OB2341 and OB1417, identified in the *O. iheyensis* genome appear to have been produced by the truncation of the original CDS by an IS insertion (Figure 19B-1). OB2341 has been annotated as a kinase-associated protein B, but the function of OB1417 is still unknown. The gene encoding OB1417 appears to have been elongated by 59 bases through the insertion of IS*668*-02, and in the case of OB2341, the size of the original gene product (133 a.a.) appears to have increased to 140 a.a. with the insertion of IS*667*-08. Thus, among the 12 intact ISs of six kinds identified in this study, two intact IS elements of two kinds consequently appear to have each affected CDS by their insertion.

In addition, the CDS OB2243 located downstream from the RT of Oi.Int-04 was found to be affected by insertion through retrohoming or retrotransposition (Figure 19B-2), although three other intact Oi.Ints were inserted in noncoding regions, as in the case of Bh.Int identified in the *B. halodurans* genome [116]. The example of a group II intron inserted in the coding sequence region is very unusual, even in other bacterial genomes [11, 25]. In fact, Oi.Int-04 was inserted at the position between the 2nd and 3rd letter in the 149th codon of OB2243, consequently producing a stop codon (TAG). Despite no example having been identified to date of a group II intron insertion in the coding region with opposite transcriptional direction to the coding sequence, another stop codon (TAA) will occur at the same position in place of TAG due to the intrinsic nucleotide sequence of the genome, and, eventually, no change will occur in the amino acid sequence of OB2243._However, it has not yet been confirmed that self-splicing of Oi.Int-04 occurs in the *O. iheyensis* HTE831 genome.

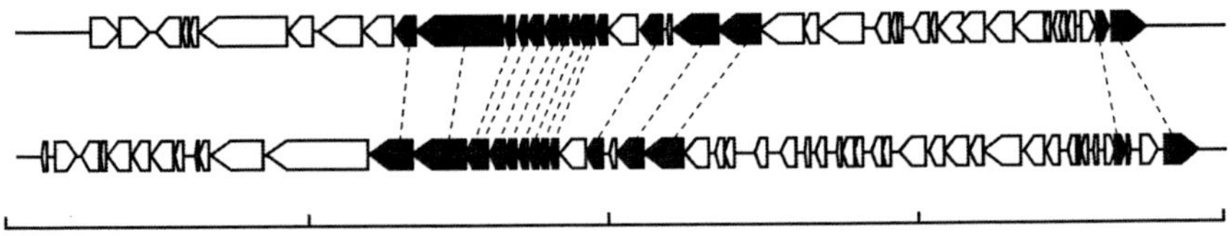

BH3517	hypothetical protein	1	SpyM3_1312	putative minor structural protein
BH3518	phage-related protein	2	SpyM3_1313	putative platlet-binding protein, minor tail fiber protein
BH3519	hypothetical protein	3	SpyM3_1314	hypothetical protein
BH3520	conserved hypothetical protein	4	SpyM3_1315	hypothetical protein
BH3521	conserved hypothetical protein	5	SpyM3_1316	hypothetical protein
BH3522	hypothetical protein	6	SpyM3_1317	hypothetical protein
BH3523	hypothetical protein	7	SpyM3_1318	hypothetical protein
BH3524	hypothetical protein	8	SpyM3_1319	hypothetical protein
BH3525	hypothetical protein	9	SpyM3_1320	hypothetical protein
BH3526	hypothetical protein	10	SpyM3_1321	conserved hypothetical protein
BH3529	hypothetical protein	11	SpyM3_1323	hypothetical protein
BH3531	conserved hypothetical protein	12	SpyM3_1325	hypothetical protein
BH3532	conserved hypothetical protein	13	SpyM3_1326	conserved hypothetical protein
BH3550	conserved hypothetical protein	14	SpyM3_1351	putative cI-like repressor, metallo-prtoeinase motif
BH3551	phage integrase	15	SpyM3_1354	putative phage integrase

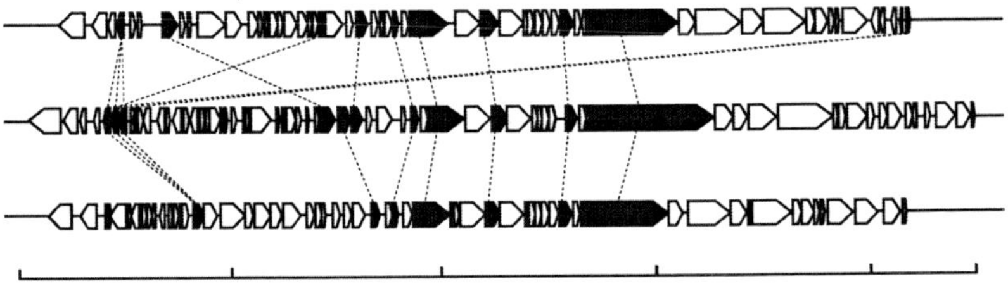

SpyM3_0684	putative repressor	1	GK0492	transcriptional repressor of PBSX genes	14	SpyM3_0964	conserved hypothetical protein
SpyM3_0736	conserved hypothetical protein	2	GK0492	transcriptional repressor of PBSX genes			
SpyM3_0684	putative repressor	3	GK0493	transcriptional regulator	15	SpyM3_0964	conserved hypothetical protein
SpyM3_0701	putaive immunity repressor protein	4	GK0493	transcriptional regulator			
SpyM3_0736	conserved hypothetical protein	5	GK0493	transcriptional regulator			
SpyM3_0684	putative repressor	6	GK0494	transcriptional repressor of PBSX genes	16	SpyM3_0964	conserved hypothetical protein
SpyM3_0687	putative repressor	7	GK0519	phage associated-antirepressor			
			GK0521	phage-related protein	17	SpyM3_0950	conserved hypothetical protein
SpyM3_0704	putative recombinase	8	GK0522	DNA integration/recombination/invertion protein			
SpyM3_0708	conserved hypothetical protein	9	GK0526	Phage-related, Zn finger domain containing protein	18	SpyM3_0948	conserved hypothetical protein
SpyM3_0710	conserved hypothetical protein	10	GK0528	phage-terminase large subunit of lambdaBa02	19	SpyM3_0946	conserved hypothetical protein
SpyM3_0712	conserved hypothetical protein	11	GK0530	serine protease (phage related-protein, ClpP family)	20	SpyM3_0942	putative ClpP protease
SpyM3_0719	putative major tail protein	12	GK0536	phage-related protein of bacteriophage phi-105 ORF34	21	SpyM3_0935	conserved hypothetical protein
SpyM3_0722	conserved hypothetical protein	13	GK0539	phage-related protein of bacteriophage phi-105 ORF36	22	SpyM3_0932	conserved hypothetical protein

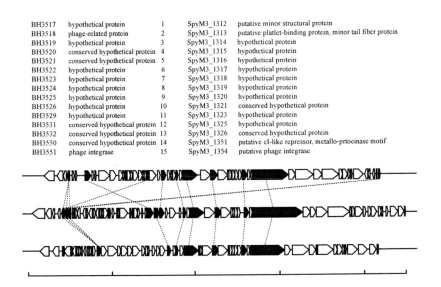

Figure 20. Comparison of bacteriophage region identified in the extremophilic bacillar genomes with those of *Streptococcus pyogenes* M3. A: *B. halodurans* (Bha35X). B: *G. kaustophilus* (Gka462P). DR, direct repeat. SpyM3, *S. pyogenes* prophage. ( ), NCBI ID number for each prophage.

6.5. Bacteriophage

Sequence analysis of the *B. halodurans* genome revealed a complete prophage, showing the typical genome organization of the Sfi11-like siphovirus with sequence matches over the head and tail genes to *Streptococcus pyogenes* M3 prophage 315.5 (Figure 20A) [13, 14]. As in a number of other prophages, an isolated adenine methyltransferase gene was detected between the DNA replication module and the DNA-packaging module. More interestingly, however, the presence of a type II restriction endonuclease and associated cytosine-specific methyltransferase located between the phage lysinand the *attR* site was confirmed. Possession of the prophage thus confers a potentially new restriction modification system on the lysogenic cell.

The *G. kaustophilus* genome contains at least 21 putative phage-associated genes, which are similar to *S. pyogenes*, *Lactococcus lactis*, *B. subtilis*, and *Clostridium perfringens*. These genes are distributed within an approximately 40-kb region corresponding to the 535-575 kb region from the *oriC* of the *G. kaustophilus* genome. The sequence similarity and the organization of the phage-associated genes in the genome are comparatively similar to those of prophage 315.1 identified in *S. pyogenes* M3 as well as *B. halodurans* (Figure 20B). On the other hand, the genomes of *B. halodurnas* and *G. kaustophilus* do not contain intact prophages, such as SPβ, PBSX, and skin, as have been found in the *B. subtilis* genome [57]. It was confirmed that *B. halodurans* and *G. kaustophilus* contain the gene for sigma K in a complete form, which in *B. subtilis* is divided into two parts, *spoIVCB* (N-terminal) and *SpoIIIC* (C-terminal) by the prophage (skin element). Similarly, no active prophages identified in the *B. subtilis* genome were found in the *O. iheyensis* genome, although the genome also contains at least 27 putative phage-associated genes.

6.6. Comparative Analysis of Transposable Elements Disseminated among Bacilli

6.6.1. IS Elements

IS*643* belonging to the IS*21* family [86] was amplified by PCR with a primer set designed for *B. halodurans* C-125 from eight strains of *B. firmus* and *B. halodurans* including C-125 (Tables 3 and Figure 14). Although the nucleotide sequences of the putative Tpase of IS*643* showed extremely high identity to each other (ranging from 99.4% to 100%) among seven strains of *B. halodrunas* (C-125, 202-1, C3, DSM6939, DSM6940, DSM8718, and DSM9774), the Tpases from these seven strains showed relatively low identity with those of 2 other strains, *B. halodurans* A59 (81.2–81.5%) and *B. firmus* (80.2–80.6%). A similar tendency was noted at the amino acid sequence level of Tpase of the IS element.

IS*651* and IS*652* belonging to the IS*L3* family [28] were amplified by PCR from all strains of *B. halodurans,* except for AH-101 and *B. alkalophilus*, respectively (Tables 3 and Figure 14). The putative Tpases of IS*651* showed 97.9–99.8% identity in nucleotide sequence and 97.8–99.5% identity in amino acid sequence to each other of the nine (C-125, DSM497^T, A59, 202-1, C3, DSM6939, DSM6940, DSM8718, and DSM 9774) strains, and these nine strains also showed a similar range of identity with that of *B. alcalophilus* at both levels although strain AH-101 did not show significant homology to those of 9 strains. On the other hand, the nucleotide sequences of putative Tpases of IS*652* from the 10 strains showed remarkable identity to each other, ranging from 99.4% to 100%. On the other hand, the nucleotide sequence of the putative Tpase of the IS*652*-like element from *O. iheyensis* obtained in the previous study [117] showed lower identity of 62.7–63.2% with each of the 10 strains.

IS*653* belonging to the IS*650*/IS*653* family was amplified by PCR from all strains of *B. halodurans*, *B. alcalophilus*, *B. clausii*, and *B. firmus*. The putative Tpase of IS*653* from the strains of *B. halodurans* obtained from DSMZ, *B. alcalophilus*, and *B. firmus* showed 99.3–100% identity in nucleotide sequence and 98.1–100% identity in amino acid sequence. The nucleotide sequence of the Tpase of IS*653* from *B. halodurans* C-125 was identical with those from strain C3 and strain 202-1 but showed comparatively low identities with those from A59 (74%) and AH-101 (73%). Thus, Tpases of IS*653* identified in the genomes of 10 *B. halodurans* strains and in three other species were found to have become the most diversified among all ISs detected in bacilli genomes in this study.

6.6.2. Group II Introns

Group II introns occur in mitochondrial and chloroplast genomes of fungi and plants and in cyanobacteria, proteobacteria, and Gram-positive bacteria [7, 25]. Although the best-characterized bacterial group II intron is the L1.LtrB intron of *Lactococcus lactis* ML3, there are fewer known examples of group II introns in Gram-positive bacteria, especially in bacilli, than in Gram-negative bacteria [11, 25]. In a previous study, we identified a group II intron designated Bh.Int in the genome of *B. halodurans* C-125 and showed that the genome contains five copies of the element and two truncated copies of Bh.Int [116]. Surprisingly, Bh.Int with exactly the same size was amplified by PCR with a primer set for *B. halodurans* C-125 from 11 species out of 21 *Bacillus*-related species, a result contrasting with that of other IS elements (Table 3 and Figure 14). The nucleotide sequence of the putative RT of Bh.Int showed very high identity, ranging from 98.4% to 99.9%, with each other among 11 species (*B. halodurans*, *B. alcalophilus*, *B. agaradhaerens*, *B. clarkii*, *B. clausii*, *B. cohnii*, *B. halmapalus*, *B. horikoshii*, *B. thermoalcalophilus*, *B. vedderi*, and *B. firmus*), whereas there was no particular trend for the same species with regard to phylogenetic relationship based on 16S rDNA sequence and each species is randomly dispersed in the phylogenetic tree. On the other hand, the nucleotide sequence of the RT of the Bh.Int-like element identified in the *O. iheyensis* genome showed only 62.5–63.2% identity with those of others listed in Figure 14 and was clearly phylogenetically distant from the 11 other species. It is thought that the mobile group II introns may have evolved from a preexisting autocatalytic intron that acquired an open reading frame, perhaps from another retroelement, or from a preexisting retroposon that acquired ribozyme activity, enabling it to function as a self-splicing intron [7]. Therefore, it is suggested that the RT of the Bh.Int-like element was acquired in the *O. iheyensis* genome via a different route from the case of other bacilli.

Alkaliphilic *Bacillus pseudofirmus* is one of the most phylogenetically closely related species to *B. halodurans* based on 16S rDNA sequence analysis. However, the *B. pseudofirmus* genome does not possess any Bh.Int-like elements. What is the difference between group II intron-containing and intronless genomes? This is a most fundamental and interesting question regarding the distribution of the group II introns in bacteria. It is presumably correct to state that there is no single adequate explanation for the current distribution of group II introns in bacteria. However, it can be expected that some answers will be found in bacterial genomic sequences, which continue to be elucidated.

7. Orthologous Analysis of the Genome of *Bacillus*-Related Species

The genomes of extremophilic *Bacillus*-related species represent a unique opportunity to investigate the genes that underlie the capabilities to adapt to extreme environments. The first issue is addressed by comparing the orthologous relationships among the proteins deduced from all CDSs identified in the genomes of six bacilli and two other Gram-positive bacteria, *Staphylococcus aureus* [58] and *Clostridium acetobutylicum* [79]. Orthologous groups in the Gram-positive bacterial species were established based on the all-against-all similarity results of applying the clustering program on the MBGD database [123]. The common orthologs conserved in all *Bacillus*-related genomes were then identified for use in the construction of multiple alignments. Since these orthologs generally display complicated mutual relationships, such as many-to-many correspondences and fusion or fission of domains, we selected only those orthologs with one-to-one correspondences without domain splitting, in order to simplify the analysis.

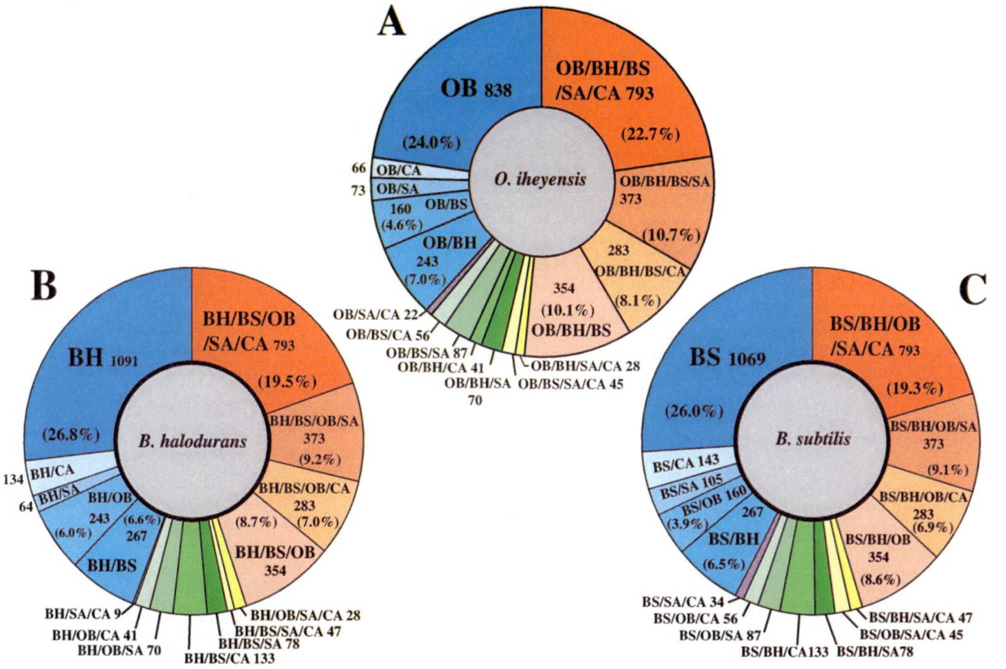

Figure 21. Summary of orthologous relationships among the proteins deduced from all CDSs identified in the bacilli genomes and in other major Gram-positive species. A: *O. iheyensis* genome. B: *B. halodurans* genome. C: *B. subtilis* genome. Abbreviations: OB: *Oceanobacillus iheyensis* [118], BH: *Bacillus halodurans* [116], BS: *Bacillus subtilis* [58], SA: *Staphylococcus aureus* [59], CA: *Clostridium acetobutylicum* [80].

Out of 3,496 proteins identified in the *O. iheyensis* genome, 838 putative proteins (24.0%) had no orthologous relationship to proteins encoded in the four other genomes (Figure 21), 793 proteins (22.7%) were orthologous to five Gram-positive bacterial species, 354 (10.1%) were identified as common proteins only among *Bacillus*-related species, and 243 putative proteins (7.0%) were common only to the two alkaliphiles, *O. iheyensis* and *B. halodurans*. As shown in Figure 21, the trend of orthologous relationships was almost the same in the case of analyses based on each *Bacillus*-related species, although the genome size of *O. iheyensis* is 600 kb smaller than that of the other two *Bacillus* genomes. In addition, orthologous relationships emerged in comparisons with all combinations among the five genomes used in this study (Figure 21). The putative proteins characterized on the basis of orthologous relationships were assigned to the functional categories used for *B. subtilis*.

Out of 838 putative proteins lacking orthologous relationship to the four other Gram-positive species, 390 were orphans showing no significant similarity of amino acid sequence to any other protein and 448 were conserved in other organisms, of which 174 had no known function. A total of 60 proteins were classified as transport/binding proteins and lipoproteins (category 1.2), the most abundant category. Nearly half of these proteins are ABC transporter-related proteins (Figure 22). Many of the orthologs, which were shared between two to four species in the comparison were also grouped into this category, indicating that some of these transport-related proteins contribute to the distinguishing characteristics of subsets of Gram-positive bacteria. Further, 1803 putative proteins identified as orthologs by comparative analyses with the three genomes of *Bacillus*-related species represent about 44.0-51.2% of each genome, and of these, about 980 orthologs are located at similar positions in each genome.

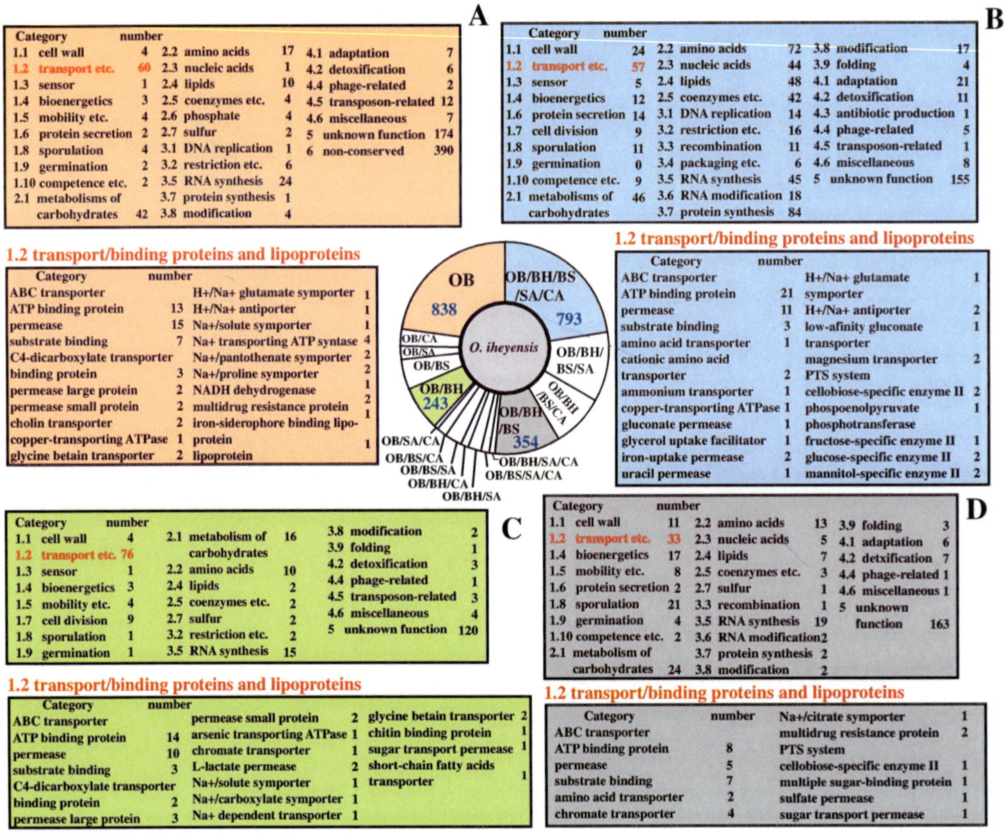

Figure 22. Functional assignment of CDSs based on the orthologous relationships. A: Orphans which have no orthologous relationship to four other Gram-positive species. B: Orthologs identified among the genomes among the genomes of five Gram-positive bacterial species. C: Orthologs identified between *O. iheyensis* and *B. halodurans,* both alkaliphiles. D: Orthologs identified among the genomes of three *Bacillus* related species. The functional categories used at the *B. subtilis* genome database (SubtiList: http://www.pasteur.fr/Bio/SubtiList.html) were used in this study.

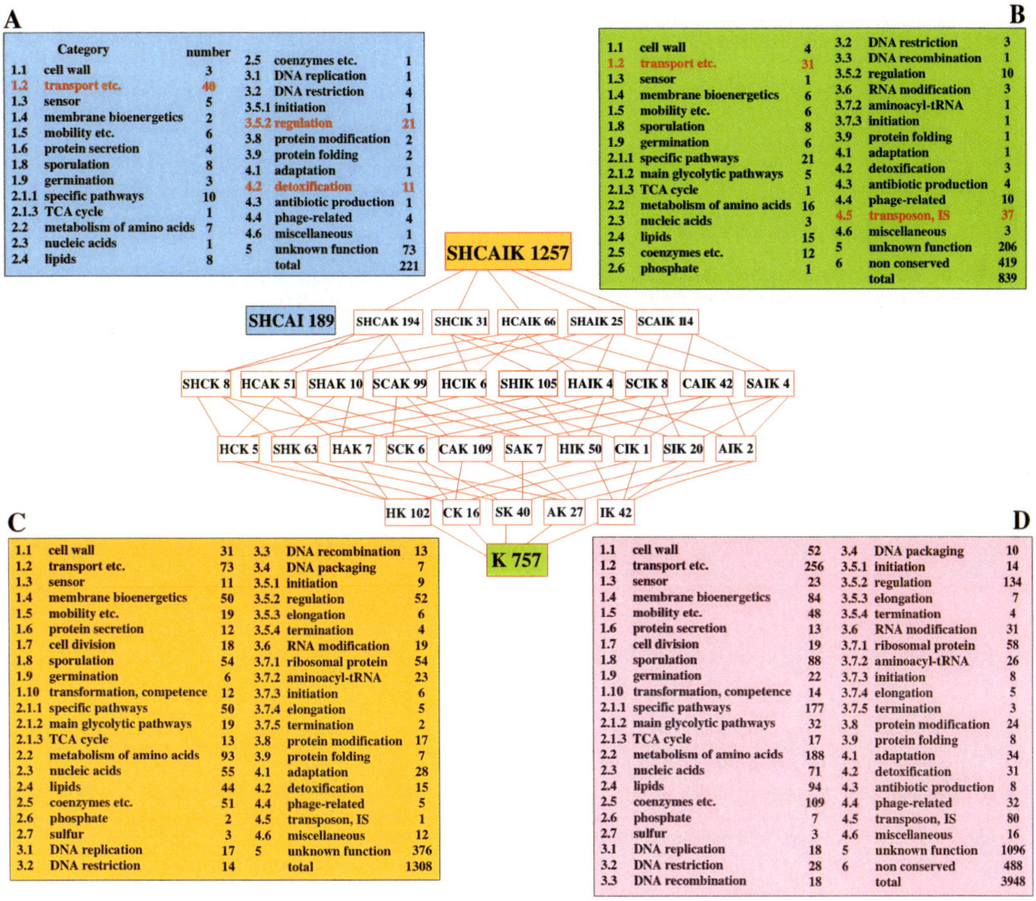

Figure 23. Summary of the orthologous relationships between the six bacillar genomes and the functional assignment of the genes belonging to each group. A: *B. anthracis*, C: *B. cereus*, I: *O. iheyensis*, S: *B. subtilis*, H: *B. halodurans*, K: *G. kaustophilus*. The figure in the box shows the number of orthologous groups for each combination of species. A: Breakdown of the genes (221 genes) categorized into 189 common orthologous groups in all bacilli except for *G. kaustophilus*. B: Breakdown of genes unique to *G. kaustophilus* (839 genes) categorized into 757 groups, which have no orthologous relationships to the other five bacilli. C: Breakdown of the genes (1,308 genes) categorized in to 1257 common orthologous groups in all six bacilli. D: Breakdown of all genes identified in the *G. kaustophilus* genome. Note that the number of orthologous groups dose not coincide with the number of genes, because the paralogous genes of *G. kaustophilus* are included in each orthologous group.

Of 3,498 predicted genes on the *G. kaustophilus* chromosome, unique genes possessing no orthologous relationships to the other five sequenced bacillar genomes accounted for 839 (24%) genes in 757 groups, orphans showing no significant similarity to any other gene products accounted for 488 (14%) genes in 419 groups (Figure 23B and 23D), and genes common to all six sequenced bacillar genomes accounted for 1308 genes in 1257 common orthologous groups. Recently, it was shown that 271 genes are indispensable for the growth of *B. subtilis* in nutritious conditions [51]. Out of the 1308 common genes, 233 show correspondences to the *B. subtilis* essential genes. Through a series of orthologous analyses of the 6 bacilli used in this study, 4 essential genes, *ymaA*, *ydiO*, *tagB*, and *tagF*, associated with purine/pyrimidine biosynthesis, DNA methylation and teichoic acid biosynthesis, were found to be unique to the *B. subtilis* genome. Teichoic acids are composed of cell-wall teichoic acid and lipoteichoic acid [80]. Six genes (*tagA*, tag*B*, *tagD, tagE*, *tagF*, and *tagO*) are known to be associated with teichoic acid biosynthesis in *B. subtilis,* with all genes except t*agE* being essential for growth. The five other *Bacillus*-related species, however, lack some of these genes; remarkably, *G. kaustophilus* lacks all genes except *tagE*, suggesting that these bacilli may have a different pathway for teichoic acid biosynthesis. The *G. kaustophilus* genome lacks eight more *B. subtilis* essential genes (16 genes in all) associated with H^+/Na^+ antiporter for pH homeostasis, glycyl-tRNA synthetase, inorganic pyrophosphatase, and DNA methyltransferase: *mrpB*, *mrpC*, *mrpF*, glyQ, *glyS*, *menA*, *ppaC*, and *ydiP*.

As shown in Figure 23A, 189 orthologous groups comprising 221 genes are commonly shared among the five mesophilic bacilli, but not by *G. kaustophilus*. In these mesophile specific orthologs, there 20 genes encode ABC transporter (10 ATP-binding proteins, 6 permeases, and 4 substrate-binding proteins) in function category 1.2 (transport/binding proteins and lipoproteins), 20 genes encoding transcriptional regulator (3.5.2, regulation), and 11 genes encoding proteins for immunity to bacteriotoxin-related proteins, toxic anion resistance-related proteins, and catalase (4.2, detoxification) (numbers in Figure 23). This is one of the significant differences between thermophilic *G. kaustophilus* and mesophilic bacillar genomes. The set of 839 unique genes of *G. kaustophilus* comprises 22 individual ABC transporter genes (10 ATP-binding proteins, 7 permeases, and 5 substrate-binding proteins), whereas only six and three genes are categorized into categories 3.5.2 and 4.2, respectively (Figure 23B).

G. kaustophilus shares 1773-2014 orthologous genes with the other five bacilli, corresponding to 53.4%-62.0% of all genes in the *G. kaustophilus* HTA426 genome. If the relative physical distribution of orthologous genes in the genomes between *G. kaustophilus* and other *Bacillus*-related species is the same, a diagonal line should appear from lower left to upper right in Figure 24. However, many orthologous genes deviate from the line although the physical distributions of the orthologous genes between *G. kaustophilus* and *B. subtilis* and those between *G. kaustophilus* and *O. iheyensis* are largely collinear (Figure 24B, D). The differences in the physical distributions of orthologous genes within the genomes presumably are a result of minor inversion and horizontal gene transfer. On the other hand, 1056 common orthologous genes possessing one-to-one correspondences among the six bacilli and t represent 23.7-36% of each genome. Most of the common genes were found to be distributed in collinear regions, but the direction of collinearity of the orthologs between *G. kaustophilus* and *B. cereus* changes at ~28-33° from the *ter* region in both directions (Figure 24C). The physical distribution of orthologous genes between *G. kaustophilus* and *B. halodurans* is very similar to the case of *B. cereus* (Figure 24A), and a similar result has previously been documented in a comparison between *B. subtilis* and *B. halodurans*. It has been reported that the *B. halodurans* genome has an inversion between the regions around 112-153° and 212-240°, due to the behavior of IS elements [115, 116].

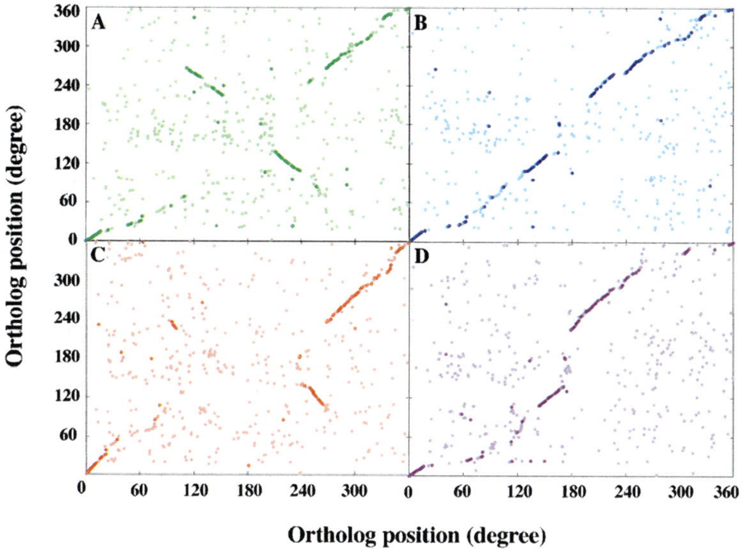

Figure 24. Pairwise comparison of ortholog organization between *G. kaustophilus* (Y axis) and four other bacillar genomes (X axis). A: *G. kaustophilus* and *B. halodurans*. B: *G. kaustophilus* and *B. subtilis*. C: *G. kaustophilus* and *B. cereus*. D: *G. kaustophilus* and *O. iheyensis*. Light-colored dots represent the orthologs showing one-to-one correspondences between the two genomes. Dark-colored dots, which represent the common orthologs across the six bacillar genomes, are overlaid on the light-colored dots.

8. Genomic Features Related to Extremophilic Phenotypes

8.1. Alkaliphic Phenotype

8.1.1. Candidate Genes Involved in Alkaliphily

Generally, alkaliphilic *Bacillus* strains cannot grow or grow poorly under conditions of neutral pH, but grow well at pH above 9.5 [35]. *O. iheyensis* grows in pH up to 10 with a broad optimum pH range for growth from 7.0 to 9.5 [62]. Over the past three decades, alkaliphilic microorganisms have been studied to elucidate their adaptation mechanisms to alkaline environments. As shown in Figure 22C, 243 orthologs were identified between the only two alkaliphiles (*O. iheyensis* and *B. halodurans*) and of these, 76 genes were grouped into category 1.2 [117] (Figure 22). These included various ABC transporters, and transporters associated with C_4-dicarboxylate, organic osmotic solute transport and Na^+ uptake (Figure 25). The ABC transporters could be categorized into three groups based on substrate specificity. All five genes encoding ABC transporters for branched-chain amino acids identified in the *O. iheyensis* genome showed orthologuous relationships to only *B. halodurans* among the five Gram-positive species compared. These particular transporters could be important for alkaliphily. Branched-chain amino acids such as leucine, isoleucine, and valine are believed to be converted to L-glutamate in the presence of 2-oxoglutarate and pyridoxal 5-phosphate by a branched-chain amino acid aminotransferase [44, 91]. This protein is widely distributed in various organisms including *O. iheyensis*. Since L-glutamic acid should be negatively charged at pH higher than its pKa (3.9 or 4.3), the converted L-glutamic acid and its accompanying proton could contribute to the acidification of the alkaliphilic *Bacillus* cytoplasm, the pH of which is maintained at around 8 to 8.5, even though pH outside of the cell is around 10.5 [35, 55]. Twenty-one genes encoding oligopeptide ABC transporters were identified in the *O. iheyensis* genome compared to 28 for *B. halodurans*, 29 for *C. acetobutylicum* and in contrast to only 11 genes in *B. subtilis* [79]. However, only six of the genes identified in *O. iheyensis* showed orthologous relationships between only the two alkaliphiles. Similar to the case of ABC transporters for branched-chain amino acids, these transport systems are presumably active in the uptake of oligopeptides during growth under alkaline pH conditions. Thus, they can contribute to the acidification of the cytoplasm if acidic amino acids, such as glutamic acid and aspartic acid, are released by digestion of the incorporated oligopeptide by a peptidase, or if they are converted to free amino acids by digestion by aminotransferase. These acidic amino acids are an important resource of protons and for acidic polymers in the cell wall.

The cell wall is crucial in alkaliphilic *Bacillus* species because their protoplasts lose stability in alkaline environments [35]. Alkaliphilic *Bacillus* species contain certain acidic polymers containing galacturonic acid, gluconic acid, glutamic acid, asparatic acid, and phosphoric acid. The amount of acidic polymers is known to increase during growth under alkaline pH conditions. The Donnan equilibrium theory of electrolytes between an anionic polymer layer and the bulk aqueous phase was applied to cell wall systems, with a reduction in pH at the cell wall-membrane boundary [122]. According to this calculation, the pH values estimated inside the polymer layer (cell wall) are more acidic than those of the surrounding environment by 1-1.5 units. Teichuronopeptide (TUP) is a co-polymer of polyglutamic acid, which is one of important components in the cell wall of the alkaliphilic *B. halodurans* [35] and actually contributes to the regulation of pH homeostasis in the cytoplasm. The putative protein (OB2920) showing significant similarity to *tupA* gene product involved in TUP biosynthesis of *B. halodurans* [115] is shared only between the two alkaliphiles (Figure 25). To date, no homolog of *tupA* has been identified in any other organism, except for two alkaliphiles.

Likewise, alkylphosphonate ABC transporters common to only the two alkaliphiles are not found in the three other Gram-positive species. In all, four genes encode alkylphosphonate ABC transporters (two permeases and one ATP-binding and one phosphonate binding protein), and these are shared between *O. iheyensis* and *B. halodurans*. *E. coli* has been known for some time to cleave carbon-phosphorus (C-P) bonds in unactivated alkylphosphonates [18]. When an alkylphosphonate, such as methylphosphonate, is degraded by bacterial C-P lyase ($CH_3PO_3^{2-} \rightarrow CH_4 + HPO_4^{2-}$), the resultant monohydrogen phosphate ion is utilized as a source of phosphorus for growth [71]. On the other hand, in the case of mitochondria, monohydrogen phosphate ion is an important substrate and exchanges itself for dicarboxylates, such as malate and succinate, by means of the dicarboxylate carrier [53]. It is unclear whether these alkylphosphonate ABC transporters contribute to the regulation of pH homeostasis of the bacterial cytoplasm because the C-P lyase gene has not been identified in the genomes of either alkaliphile.

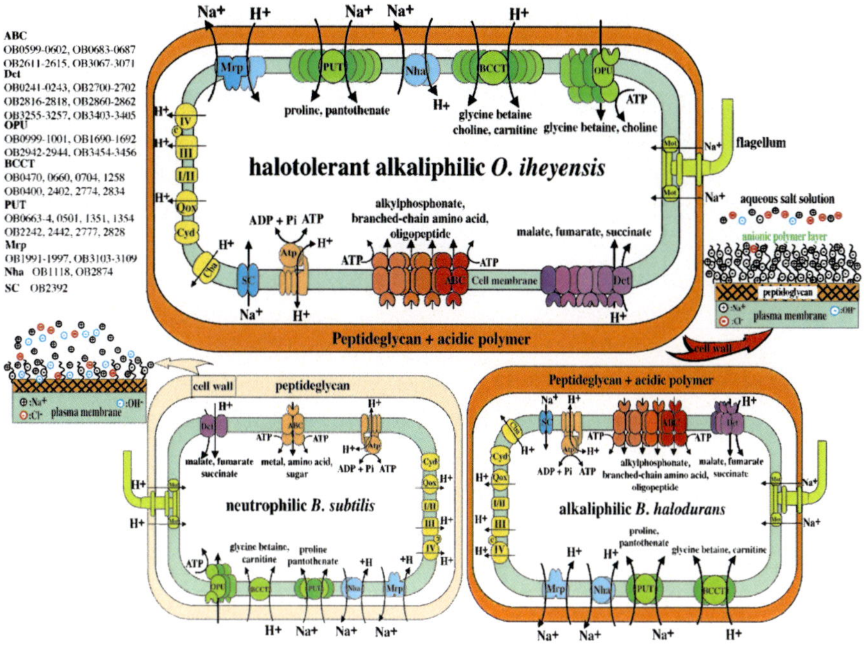

Figure 25. Overview of putative major transport systems that govern alkaliphily and extreme halotolerance in *O. iheyensis*. Overview of the cell wall system and the enzymes involved in the respiratory chain (yellow) are also shown. Transporters are grouped by category of trasport/binding proteins and lipoprotein: sodium cycle (blue), organic osmotic solutes such as glycine betaine, choline, carnitine, proline, and pantothenate (green), carboxylic acids such as malate, fumarate, and succinate (purple), and peptides and amino acids (red). ABC transport systems are shown as composite figures of oval, circular and sickle shape. The gene number of *O. iheyensis* corresponding to each component of the transporter is described below or above each figure. Abbreviations: Atp, F_1F_0 ATP synthase; Abc, ABC transporter; Bcct, glycine betaine, carnitine/H^+ symporter; Cba, cytochrome *c* oxidase (*bo3*-type); Cyd, cytochrome *bd* oxidase; I, NADH dehydrogenase, II, succinate dehydrogenase; III, menaquinol cytochrome *c* oxidoreductase; IV, cytochrome *caa3* oxidase; Dct, C_4-dicarboxylate transport system; Mrp, Na^+/H^+ antiporter; Mot, channel for energization of motility; Nha, Na^+/H^+ antiporter; Opu, glycine betaine ABC transporter; Pan, Pantothenate/Na^+ symporter; Put, proline/Na^+ symporter; Qox, cytochrome *aa3* quinol oxidase; Sc, voltage-gated sodium channel.

O. iheyensis possesses a total of 18 genes encoding six sets of C_4-dicarboxylate carriers, which are all grouped into the DctA family [43]. Of these, seven genes encoding two sets of C_4-dicarboxylate carriers and one permease large protein are shared only between *O. iheyensis* and *B. halodurans* (Figure 25). The other 11 genes encoding three C_4-dicarboxylate binding proteins, two permease large proteins and two permease small proteins are unique among the five Gram-positive species. Although the seven shared proteins showed highest similarity among the alkaliphiles, the other 11 unique proteins showed significant similarity to those of Gram-negative strains such as *Sinorizobium meiloti*, *Salmonella typhimurium*, and *Pseudomonas aeruginosa*. In aerobic bacteria, dicarboxylate transport carriers catalyze uptake of C_4-dicarboxylates in a H^+- or Na^+ symport [43]. This transport system may play a role in the regulation of pH homeostasis and the sodium cycle of the alkaliphilic bacterial cytoplasm.

The Na^+ cycle plays an important role in the remarkable capacity of aerobic alkaliphilic *Bacillus* species [55] for pH homeostasis. The capacity for pH homeostasis directly reflects the upper pH limit of growth. The first major player in the alkaliphile Na^+ cycle is the Na^+/H^+

antiporter, which achieves net H^+ accumulation coupled to Na^+ efflux. Na^+/H^+ antiport activity also represents an important mechanism for maintaining low intracellular sodium concentrations in halophilic or halotolerant aerobic bacteria [125]. The major antiporter for pH homeostasis is thought to be the Mrp-encoded antiporter, first identified in *B. halodurans*. Mrp could function as part of a complex with six other gene products. The *O. iheyensis* genome possesses 14 genes encoding two sets of Mrp-related proteins and all 14 genes showed various orthologous relationships among 4/5 Gram-positive species but not *C. acetobutylicum*. The genome contains two genes for additional antiporters including NhaC, a property, which is shared among all five Gram-positive species. These antiporters presumably play fundamental roles in the pH homeostasis of the bacterial cell.

The second major player of the Na^+ cycle is Na^+ re-entry via the Na^+/solute symporter and presumably the ion channel associated with the Na^+-dependent flagella motor [55]. Two genes encoding a Na^+/solute symporter and a Na^+-dependent transporter are shared only between *O. iheyensis* and *B. halodurans*. These alkaliphile-specific transporters could also be important for Na^+ re-entry, although there is no experimental evidence for such a function under alkaline pH conditions. One of new findings of the genome sequencing project of *B. halodurans* was the discovery of the first prokaryotic voltage-gated sodium channel in the alkaliphilic *B. halodurans* initially based on the sequences of transmembrane domains [87] and later confirmed experimentally to be activated by voltage and selective for sodium, although it is inhibited by calcium channel blockers. A putative protein (OB2392) identified in *O. iheyensis* shows significant similarity to this sodium channel. Because this sequence is hardly detected in other prokaryotic genomes except for the two alkaliphiles, voltage-gated channels could be a common characteristic of alkaliphilic *Bacillus*-related species. This channel likely provides a transient supply of Na^+ for the sodium cycle under both alkaline and neutral pH conditions [16]. Recently, it has been confirmed that the voltage-gated sodium channel deficient mutant lost alkaliphily in another alkaliphilic *Bacillus* species, *B. pseudofirmus* [40].

Totally, 32 putative proteins associated with flagella were identified in the *O. iheyensis* genome and all of these proteins, except for one, were well-conserved among the three *Bacillus*-related species. Alkaliphile motility is Na^+-coupled and is observed only in cells growing at highly alkaline pH ranges [55]. In fact, *O. iheyensis* is extremely motile under alkaline pH conditions. Therefore, these flagella-associated proteins identified in the *O. iheyensis* genome are likely to work as Na^+-channels for Na^+ entry at high pH to ensure an adequate supply of Na^+ for the increased antiport coupled to H^+ accumulation (Figure 25). This is in contrast to H^+-driven flagella motors present in neutrophilic *B. subtilis* [94]. On the other hand, there are no major differences in the proteins associated with the terminal oxidase of respiratory chain between neutrophilic *B. subtilis* and the two other alkaliphilic bacilli, although *B. subtilis* is missing cytochrome *bd* oxidase while this enzyme is conserved in both alkaliphilies as well as the thermophile *G. stearothermophilus* (http://www.genome.ou.edu/bstearo.html).

We highlighted the genes involved in alkaliphilic phenotype based on comparative analysis with three *Bacillus* species and two other Gram-positive species through this paper. However, out of 243 genes shared only between the two alkaliphiles (OB/BH), the functions of 120 genes still remain unknown, as shown in Figure 22C. Therefore, it will be necessary to analyze gene expression patterns under alkaline and neutral pH conditions to clarify the genes responsible for alkaliphilic phenotype.

8.2. Extreme Halotolerant Phenotype

8.2.1. Candidate Genes Involved in the Extreme Halotolerance

Bacteria subjected to sudden increases in osmolarity respond with an adaptive response that is characterized by two distinct phases. The key physiological role of compatible solute accumulation as an adaptive response of *B. subtilis,* which can grow in the medium containing NaCl up to 7% [98], to high osmolarity environments has been firmly established. *B. subtilis* responds to a sudden increase in external osmolarity by an initial rapid uptake of K^+, followed by the accumulation of large amounts of compatible solute proline through *de novo* synthesis. The genome of *O. iheyensis*, which can grow at salinities of 0- 21% (3.6 M) at pH 7.5 and 0-18% (3.1 M) at pH 9.5 [62], contains two putative proteins showing significant similarity to both Na^+ and K^+ transporters from various bacterial species [47]. These two proteins could play a major role in the initial rapid uptake of K^+. *B. subtilis* uses a high-affinity and substrate-specific transport system, OpuE (osmoprotectant uptake), to transport proline efficiently for osmoprotective purposes [47]. The OpuE transporter consists of a single component and is a member of the sodium/solute symporter family (SSF). The *O. iheyensis* genome possesses 5 genes encoding Na^+/proline symporters (there are 4 in *B. subtilis*) as well as 3 more genes for Na^+/pantothenate symporters, which is other member of the SSF (there is only one in *B. subtilis*). *B. subtilis* employs transporters to scavenge glycine betaine from the environment up to cellular levels that surpass 1 M in osmotically stressed cultures [47]. Also, glycine betaine can be synthesized when the precursor choline is provided to the cell. The glycine betaine and choline ABC transport systems comprise an ATP-binding protein, permease and substrate-binding protein, and a secondary glycine betaine transporter comprising a single component. There are no large differences in the glycine betaine and choline ABC transport systems between the moderately halotolerant *B. subtilis* and extremely halotolerant *O. iheyensis*, although *O. iheyensis* has one more set of glycine betaine ABC transport systems (Figure 25). The principal difference is found in the glycine betaine transporter, as well as in the choline/H^+ and carnitine/H^+ symporters, between the moderate and extremely halotolerant bacilli. In contrast to only one glycine transporter in *B. subtilis*, the *O. iheyensis* possesses 6 genes encoding glycine betaine transporter and one each of choline/H^+ and carnitine/H^+ symporters. *O. iheyensis* must fully employ a large number of osmoprotectant transporters (Figure 25) in order to survive in neutral or alkaline hypersaline environments that surpass 3 M NaCl.

8.3. Thermophilic Phenotype

8.3.1. Candidate Genes Involved in Thermophily

Although neither the upper temperature limit for bacterial life, nor what specific factors determine this limit, are not clear, it is generally assumed that the limit will be dictated by molecular instability. In fact, DNA duplex stability is apparently achieved at high temperatures through elevated salt concentrations, polyamines, cationic proteins, and supercoiling, rather than the manipulation of G+C ratios [78]. RNA stability is enhanced by covalent modification, and the secondary structure is probably also critical. We identified some genes which seem to be involved in the stabilization of DNA and RNA among a set of unique *G. kaustophilus* genes: protamine, spermidine/spermine synthase, tRNA methyltransferase (MTase), and rRNA MTase [120].

DNA topology is affected by the interaction with cationic proteins, numerous examples of which have been identified in hyperthermophiles. The small basic proteins bind DNA *in vitro* with substantial increases in T_m and have been variously shown to bend DNA or to form nucleosome structures [78]. Protamine is a protein replacing histones that binds DNA in sperm in a way that allows higher condensation of DNA than is possible with histones. Surprisingly, a gene (GK 1739) was found to show significant similarity (51%) to sperm protamine P1 from *Phascolarctos cinereus* (Koala bear). This marks the first discovery of a prokaryotic protamine-like gene in prokaryotes [120]. Archaeal histones belonging to the HMf family are homologs of eukaryal nucleosome core histones, and have been shown to bind to and compact archaeal DNA both *in vitro* and *in vivo* [99]. Histone-like proteins from *Sulfolobus* [29] have no eukaryal homologs, but, like the HMf proteins, they also compact DNA and increase the T_m of DNA *in vitro*. Therefore, the protamine P1-like protein identified in *G. kaustophilus* presumably behaves similarly to archaeal histone-like proteins in supporting life at high temperatures.

Polycationic polyamines, which increase the T_m of DNA and protect ribosomes from thermal inactivation *in vitro*, have been observed in hyperthermophiles. The polyamines participate in many cellular processes through their binding to DNA, RNA, and phospholipids, not only in thermophiles but also in mesophiles. There is an interesting report showing that most spermines and spermidines exist as a polyamine-RNA complexes in mesophilic *E. coli* cells [68]. Comprehensive analysis of the polyamines in hundreds of bacterial and archaeal species, from mesophiles to hyperthermophiles, has been carried out [31, 32, 50]. The results show that some kinds of polyamine, such as norspermine and norspermidine, occurred mainly in hyperthermophilic Archaea [78]. A hyperthermophilic bacterium, *Thermus thermophilus*, produced unusual polyamines (homocaldohexamine) in addition to norspermine and norspermidine, and inactivation of the basic genes related to polyamine synthesis, such as *speA*, *speB*, and *speE*, resulted in a loss of the hyperthermophilic phenotype (growth defect at 78°C) [81]. Thus, it is thought that these polyamines may play unique roles in supporting hyperthermophilic life. On the other hand, thermophilic *Geobacillus* species do not produce polyamines specific to hyperthermophiles, but produce spermine as a major polyamine; spermine is not produced by mesophilic *Bacillus*-related species, such as *B. halodurans*, *B. subtilis* and *B. cereus*, which we used for comparative analysis in this study [32]. The genomes of the five species (*B. halodurans, B. subtilis, B. anthracis, B. cereus*, and *G. kaustophilus*), i.e., all except for *O. iheyensis*, contain a common gene for spermidine synthase, and in addition to the common gene, other unique genes were identified in the *B. anthracis*, *B. cereus* and *O. iheyensis* genomes. Since it became clear that *G. kaustophilus* possesses unique genes for spermine/spermidine synthase and polyamine ABC transporter (permease) among the 6 sequenced bacilli, these genes seem to be strong candidates responsible for thermophily in these bacilli.

All types of cellular RNA contain modified nucleosides, but the largest number and greatest variety are found among tRNAs, and more than 80 different modifications have been identified to date in the tRNAs of various organisms [66]. Modifications consist of simple chemical alterations of the nucleoside (e.g. methylation of the base or ribose, base isomerization, reduction, thiolation or deamination) or more complex hypermodifications. The structural stabilization of ribonucletic acids in hyperthermophiles is particularly important in tRNAs, where there is a requirement for the maintenance of a complex three-dimensional structure. Recently, the inactivation of the gene for tRNA MTase in *Thermus thermophilus* resulting in a thermosensitive phenotype (growth defect at 80°C) has been reported; this suggests a role for the N^1-methylation of tRNA adenosine-58 in the adaptation of life to extreme temperatures [23]. The six bacillar genomes were found to share five orthologous tRNA MTases and four orthologous rRNA MTases, and the *G. kaustophilus* genome was found to contain three more unique tRNA or tRNA/rRNA MTase genes lacking orthologous relationships to the other five bacilli. Thus, these genes also seem to be strong candidates responsible for thermophily, although their specificity in the modification of tRNA is still not clear.

8.3.2. Other Thermophilic Properties

8.3.2.1. Principal Component Analysis

The features of the genomic sequences separating thermophiles and mesophiles can be easily identified through principal component analysis (PCA) (or correspondence analysis, a similar technique) of the amino acid composition and the relative synonymous codon usage, as mentioned previously. In both analyses, the first principal component (PC1) is correlated with the G+C content of the chromosome and the second PC (PC2) is clearly correlated with the optimal growth temperature, allowing thermophiles and mesophiles to be distinguished along the second axis. We attempted PCA in order to confirm whether the *G. kaustophilus* genome has a signature similar to that of other thermophiles (Figure 26). In both analyses, all thermophiles whose genomes have already been reported were located above the boundary distinguishing thermophiles from mesophiles, except *Thermosynochococcus elongatus* [131], whose upper growth temperature limit of 60°C is rather low in comparison to that of other thermophiles. *G. kaustophilus* was located above the boundary in the PCA of amino acid composition, but below the boundary in the PCA of synonymous codon usage. Thus, the *G. kaustophilus* genome is the first complete thermophilic genome that clearly shows different tendencies between the PCAs of synonymous codon usage and amino acid composition.

In the case of the PCA of amino acid composition, we were able to determine the boundary distinguishing thermophiles from mesophiles to be at 0.0164 on the second principal axis. *G. kaustophilus* placed on this boundary, along with the thermophilic *Thermoplasma acidophilum* [89] and *Thermoplasma volcanicum*, which can grow at temperatures of up to 62-67°C [46]. On the other hand, the PC2 positions of the five mesophilic *Bacillus*-related species are below the boundary (Figure 26A). Therefore, the genomes of the six *Bacillus*-related species serve as good resources for studying the mechanisms of thermostabilization of proteins and thermophily of microbes, since the limited number of amino acid changes that affect the differences in PC2 positions (shown in Figure 26) seem to reflect differences in thermophily or thermostability among these six bacilli.

In contrast to the results of the PCA of the amino acid composition, the synonymous codon usage in the *G. kaustophilus* genome does not show any distinguishable thermophilic pattern (Figure 26B). The thermophilic pattern in the synonymous codon usage is probably due to natural selection related to thermophily acting on the nucleotide sequence; it may be related to mRNA thermostability or the stability of codon-anticodon interactions [63, 96]. This pattern also seems to reflect the dinucleotide composition of genomic sequences, which may be related to the molecular flexibility of the DNA; purine-purine (RR) or pyrimidine-

pyrimidine (YY) dinucleotides are predominant in thermophiles [101]. The *G. kaustophilus* genome did not appear to have been subjected to such selective pressure (e.g. the RR+YY value of the *G. kaustophilus* genome (50.7%) was less than that of the *B. subtilis* genome (53.2%)). Specific factors involved in the stabilization of DNA or RNA, of which some are discussed below, might compensate for the lack of this genomic signature.

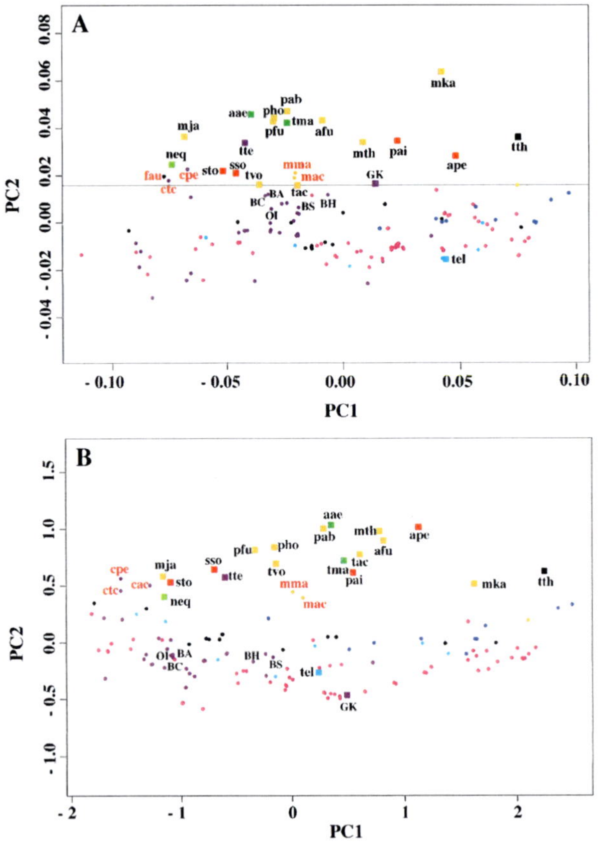

Figure 26. Distribution of *G. kaustophilus* along the first and second axes of PCA. A: Amino acid composition of 150 prokaryotic genomes. B: Synonymous codon usage in 150 prokaryotic genomes. Mesophiles are denoted by circles. Red: crenarchaeota; orange: euryarchaeota; gray: nanoarchaeota; green: hyperthermophilic bacteria; purple: firmicutes; blue: actinobacteria; magenta: proteobacteria; white: cyanobacteria; black: others. Also, aae: *Aquifex aerolicus*; afu: *Archaeoglobus fulgidus*; ape: *Aeropyrum pernix*; mja: *Methanococcus jannaschii*; mka: *Methanopyrus kandleri*; mth: *Methanobacterium thermoautotrophicum*; neq: *Nanoarchaeum equitans*; pab: *Pyrococcus abyssi*; pai: *Pyrobaculum aerophilum*; pfu: *Pyrococcus furiosus*; pho: *Pyrococcus horikoshii*; sso: *Sulfolobus solfataricus*; sto: *Sulfolobus tokodaii*; tac: *Thermoplasma acidophilum*; tel: *Thermosynechococcus elongatus*; tma: *Thermotoga maritima*; tte: *Thermoanaerobacter tengcongensis*; tth: *Thermus thermophilus*; tvo: *Thermoplasma volcanicum*; BA: *B. anthracis*; BC: *B. cereus*; BH: *B. halodurans*; BS: *B. subtilis*; GK: *G. kaustophilus*; OI: *O. iheyensis*. The following mesophilic microorganisms above the boundary are shown in red. ctc: *Clostridium tetani*; cpe: *Clostridium perfringens*; fau: *Fusobacterium nucleatum*; mac: *Methanosarcina acetivorans*; mma: *Methanosarcina mazei.*

Generally, the G+C content in rRNA and tRNA, rather than that of the entire genome, is known to linearly correlate with growth temperature in thermophilic archaea, although discriminating moderate thermophiles from mesophiles through the G+C content in the RNA molecules alone is generally not easy [73]. Indeed, the mean G+C content in the tRNA of the *G. kaustophilus* genome was 59.1%, a value slightly lower than in *B. halodurans* and *B. cereus* (Table 1). On the other hand, the mean G+C content in the rRNA operons in the *G. kaustophilus* genome was found to be 58.5% (Table 1). This value is 4–6 percentage points higher than that of mesophilic *Bacillus*-related species (52.7–54.4%) with maximum temperatures for growth ranging from 42 to 58°C. However, this difference in rRNA was less than the difference in genomic G+C content between *G. kaustophilus* (52.1%) and the mesophilic bacilli (35.3-43.7%), probably due to the stronger constraints imposed on the rRNA operons. We examined the relationship between the G+C content in the 16S rRNA and that in the entire genome and confirmed a clear correlation between these values among various mesophiles (Figure 27). On the other hand, the hyperthermophiles showed apparently higher G+C content in rRNA than did the mesophiles regardless of their genomic G+C contents. The G+C content in 16S rRNA of *G. kaustophilus* was moderately, but still significantly higher, than that of the mesophiles, even when the difference in the genomic G+C content was taken into consideration (Figure 27). Therefore, we concluded that the higher G+C content in rRNA is one of the thermophilc signatures in the *G. kaustophilus* genome.

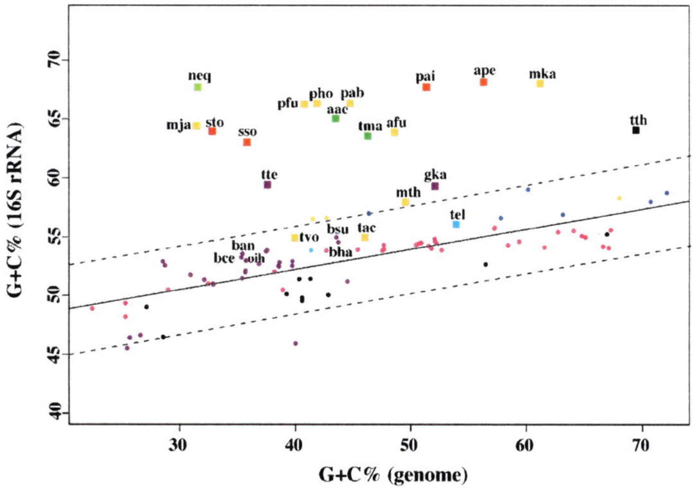

Figure 27. Relationship between G+C content of 16S rRNA and that of the entire genome. The solid line is the regression line calculated using only the mesophilic genomes; the regression equation is $y=0.17x+45.36$, where x and y are the genomic and the rRNA G+C content, respectively. The dashed lines are the upper and lower limits of the 95% prediction interval. The symbols, colors and abbreviated species names are the same as those used in Figure 26.

8.3.2.2. Asymmetric Amino Acid Substitution Pattern

We tried to identify amino acid substitutions showing significant asymmetry between *G. kaustophilus* and other *Bacillus*-related species by using multiple alignments of 1056 common orthologous groups that have one-to-one correspondences across all genomes. The resulting asymmetric substitutions were plotted on the plane generated by the first two principal components (shown in Figure 26) according to the difference in the PC scores yielded by each substitution (Figure 28).

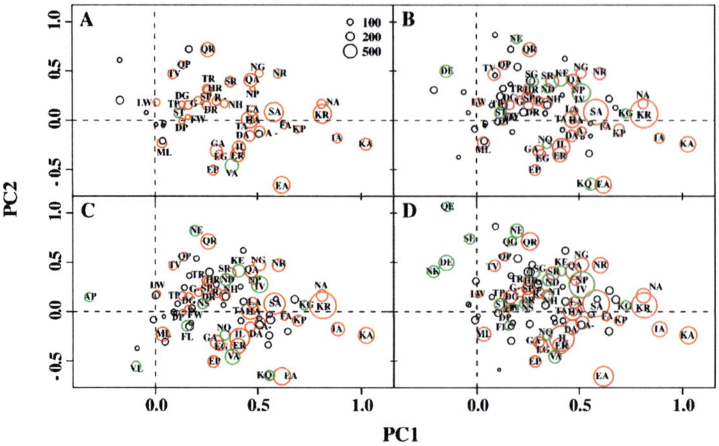

Figure 28. Asymmetric amino acid substitution patterns across *G. kaustophilus* and other mesophilic bacilli, observed in the multiple alignments of 1,056 common orthologous groups with one-to-one correspondences. A: *G. kaustophilus* and *B. halodurans*. B: *G. kaustophilus* and *B. subtilis*. C: *G. kaustophilus* and *B. cereus*. D: *G. kaustophilus* and *O. iheyensis*. Only substitutions are shown (for example, *AB*) whose frequencies are significantly larger than those in the opposite direction (*BA*), where *AB* denotes a substitution pattern in which amino acid *A* in a mesophilic bacillar genome is changed to amino acid *B* in the *G. kaustophilus* genome (see Method). Each substitution is plotted according to the differences in PC1 and PC2 scores yielded by that substitution on the same principal component plane as in Figure 6; note that the same substitution is plotted at the same position in all plots. The area of the circle is proportional to the difference between the number of substitutions from the number in the opposite direction ($n_{AB} - n_{BA}$). Red open circles represent asymmetric substitutions commonly identified in all mesophilic bacillar genomes; green open circles represent species-specific asymmetric substitutions whose difference in number from that in the opposite direction is greater than or equal to 200; black open circles represent other species-specific asymmetric substitutions. The actual substitution pattern (*AB* for the change from the *A* of the mesophilic bacillus to the *B* of *G. kaustophilus*) is shown for each red or green open circle. A dash (-) in the substitution pattern denotes a gap character.

There were 39 asymmetric substitutions commonly identified between *G. kaustophilus* and all other *Bacillus*-related species (red circles in Figure 28). Remarkably, all of these substitutions increased the PC1 scores of the *G. kaustophilus* proteins, corresponding to an increase in the chromosomal G+C content. On the other hand, 24 out of 39 substitutions increased the PC2 scores of the *G. kaustophilus* proteins, presumably corresponding to an increase in the thermostability of the proteins. These substitutions generally increased the content of Arg, Ala, Gly, Val and Pro in the *G. kaustophilus* proteins, while decreasing Gln, Thr, Asn and Ser (Figure 28). However, the overall increase in the PC2 score by these common substitutions was less remarkable than that in the PC1 score.

In contrast, among species-specific asymmetric substitutions (those with larger and smaller differences are represented by green and black circles, respectively, in Figure 28), we were able to find a substantial number of substitutions that increased the PC2 scores of the *G. kaustophilus* proteins, especially when we compared them with those of the *B. subtilis* or *O. iheyensis* proteins (Figure 28). Indeed, eight out of 10 and 15 out of 18 large asymmetric substitutions (green circles) were found in *B. subtilis* and *O. iheyensis* proteins, respectively, were found to increase the PC2 scores of *G. kaustophilus* proteins. In particular, four asymmetric substitutions (QE, SE, DE, and NK) found in the comparison with the *O. iheyensis* genome and located in the upper-left quadrant of the principal component plane cannot be explained by the difference in GC/AT mutation pressure; instead, they are likely to be explained by the difference in selection pressure related to the thermostability of proteins.

Ranking based on the number of asymmetric substitutions (*B. halodurans* (50 substitutions) < *B. subtilis* (82) < *B. cereus* (84) < *O. iheyensis* (92)) was not equivalent to the order based on similarity (*B. subtilis* (64.0%) > *B. cereus* (63.0%) > *B. halodurans* (61.3%) > *O. iheyensis* (57.0%)) for the comparison of the 1,056 orthologous protein sequence alignments for each *Bacillus*-related species and *G. kaustophilus*. Therefore, the difference in Figure 28 cannot be explained by the difference in evolutionary distance alone.

The observation that all common asymmetric substitutions between *G. kaustophilus* and other *Bacillus*-related species increased the PC1 scores indicates that the observed substitution bias is mainly due to the GC/AT directional mutation pressure [101], which itself cannot be considered as a direct cause of the thermostabilization of proteins in general. Indeed, as indicated in Figure 26 as well as in the previous studies [73], increase in G+C content seems to be a process completely independent from that of thermoadaptation. One of the plausible explanations is that accelerated amino acid changes caused by the GC/AT mutation pressure, combined with subsequent natural selection, facilitated the adaptation of *G. kaustophilus* to an environment with higher temperature through the increase in the thermostability of all its proteins. Similarly, Nishio, *et al.* [78] recently reported that an increase in G+C content in the *Corynebacterium efficiens* genome beyond that in the *Corynebacterium glutamicum* genome could account for the major patterns of asymmetric amino acid substitutions possibly associated with the increase in the thermostability of *C. efficiens*. Thus, this type of scenario might hold more generally for mesophilic bacteria in their adaptation to environments with higher temperatures.

However, by this hypothesis alone, it is difficult to explain the substantial differences in the substitution patterns among mesophilic bacilli. An alternative hypothesis is that the common ancestors of these bacilli have some thermophilic features and that the current mesophilic bacilli have lost these features during the course of evolution. In this case, the difference in substitution patterns among the organisms can be explained as a difference in the extent to which the thermostability of proteins have decreased in each organism. Thus, the position of the *Bacillus*-related species on the PC2 axis in the PCA of the amino acid composition is remarkable; it is located near the boundary distinguishing thermophiles from mesophiles (Figure 26).

Conclusion

Since phylogenetically related *Bacillus*-related species share many genes despite each species having a different capability to adapt to various environments, it is expected that comparative analysis with *Bacillus*-related species is useful for identifying candidate genes associated with the mechanisms of adaptation to these environments. Thus, we attempted to identify the genes involved in extremophilic phenotypes such as alkaliphily, halotolerance, and thermophily based on comparative analysis with the genomes of six closely related *Bacillus*-related species and two other Gram-positive bacteria. Consequently, we were able to identify strong candidate genes responsible for extremophily that were unique or common genes among the *Bacillus*-related species. However, nearly half of the genes in each of the sets are of unknown function, and other candidate genes for extremophily may yet be discovered among these genes. Further comparative analyses using other *Bacillus*-related species with various phenotypic properties are required as a second step in uncovering hidden capacity for extremophily.

Through a series of bacillar genome analyses, the presence of transposable elements such as ISs, group II introns, and transposons in the genomes of extremophilic *Bacillus*-related species contrasted to their absence in the *B. subtilis* 168 genome. Some of those elements were common to all bacilli, without correlation to phenotypic properties or phylogenetic placement using 16 rDNA sequences. Thus, it is thought that the transposable elements are certainly one of the important factors responsible for genomic diversity in *Bacillus*, as well as in other bacterial genera.

Acknowledgements

I am grateful to the members of microbial genome research group of JAMSTEC for their cooperation in the extremophilic bacilli genome sequencing projects. Thanks are due to Prof. I. Uchiyama for his great contribution in orthologous analysis. I thank Drs. E. Ohtsubo and C.-G. Han for their help in IS analysis. Finally, I also thank to Profs. K. Horikoshi, S. Kuhara, and N. Ogasawara for their useful suggestions.

Reference

[1] Abarca, F. M. & Toro, N. (2000). Group II introns in the bacterial world. *Mol. Microbiol.* **38**: 917-926.

[2] Altschul, S.F., Madden, T.L., Schaffer, A.A., Zhang, J., Zhang, Z., Miller, W. & Lipman, D.J. (1997). Gapped BLAST and PSI-BLAST: a new generation of protein database search programs. *Nucleic Acids Res.*, **25**: 3389-3402.

[3] Aono, R., Hashimoto, M., Hayakawa, A., Nakamura, S. & Horikoshi, K. (1992). A novel gene required for the alkaliphily of the facultative alkaliphilic *Bacillus* sp. strain C-125. *Biosci. Biotechnol. Biochem.*, **56**: 842-844.

[4] Aono, R., Ito, M. & Machida, T. (1999). Contribution of the cell wall component teichuronopeptide to pH homeostasis and alkaliphily in the alkaliphile *Bacillus lentus* C-125. *J. Bacteriol.* **181**: 6600-6606.

[5] Archer, G.L., Thanassi, J.A., Niemeyer, D.M. & Pucci, M.J. (1996). Characterization of IS*1272*, an insertion sequence-like element from *Staphylococcus haemolyticus*. *Antimicrob. Agents Chemother.* **40**: 924-929.

[6] Bao, Q., Tian, Y., Li, W., Xu, Z., Xuan, Z., Hu, S., Dong, W., Yang, J., Chen, Y., Xue, Y., Xu, Y. *et al.* (2002). A complete sequence of the *Thermoanaerobacter tengcongensis* genome. *Genome Res.* **12**: 689-700.

[7] Belfort, M., Derbyshire, V., Parker, M.M., Cousineau, B. & Lambowitz, A.M. (2002). In Craig, N. L., Crigie, R., Gellert, M., Lambowitz, A.M. (Eds.), *Mobile DNA* II, pp. 761–783. Washington, D.C., USA: American Society for Microbiology Press.

[8] Beuzon, C.R. & Casadesus, J. (1997). Conserved structure of IS*200* elements in *Salmonella*. *Nucleic Acids Res.* **25**: 1355-1361.

[9] Blattner, F. R., Plunkett III, G., Bloch, C.A., Perna, N.T., Burland, V., Riley, M., Collado-Vides, J., Glasner, J.D., Rode, C.K., Mayhew, G.F. *et al.* (1997). The Complete Genome Sequence of *Escherichia coli* K-12. *Science* **277**: 1453-1462.

[10] Bolotin, A., Mauger, S., Malarme, K., Ehrlich, S.D. & Sorokin, A. (1999). Low-redundancy sequencing of the entire *Lactococcus lactis* IL1403 genome. *Antonie Van Leeuwenhoek* **76**: 27-76.

[11] Bonen, L. & Vogel, J. (2001). The ins and outs of group II introns. *Trens Genet.* **17**: 322-331.

[12] Bourgouin, C., Delecluse, A., Ribier, J., Klier, A. & Rapoport, G. (1988). A *Bacillus thuringiensis* subsp. *israelensis* gene encoding a 125-kilodalton larvicidal polypeptide is associated with inverted repeat sequences. *J. Bacteriol.* **170**: 3575-3583.

[13] Canchaya, C., Proux, C., Fournous, G., Bruttin, A. & Brüssow, H. (2003). Prophage genomics. *Microbiol. Mol. Biol. Rev.* **67**: 238-276.

[14] Canchaya, C., Fournos, G., Chibani-Chennoufi, S., Dillmann, M.-L. & Brüssow, H. (2003). Phage as agents of lateral gene transfer. *Cur. Opin. Microbiol.* **6**: 417-424.

[15] Censini, S., Lange, C., Xiang, Z., Crabtree, J.E., Ghiara, P., Borodovsky, M., Rappuoli, R. & Covacci, A. (1996). *cag*, a pathogenicity island of *Helicobacter pylori*, encodes type I-specific and disease-associated virulence factors. *Proc. Natl. Acad. Sci. USA.* **93**: 14648-14653.

[16] Chahine, M., Pilote, S., Pouliot, V., Takami, H. & Sato, C. (2004). Role of arginine residues on the S4 segment of the *Bacillus halodurans* Na^+ channel in voltage-sensing. *J. Membrane Biol.* **201**: 9-24.

[17] Chee, G.J. & Takami, H. (2005). A prokaryotic group II intron is found between the two exons of a housekeeping gene. *Gene* in press

[18] Chen, C. M., Ye, Q. Z., Zhu, Z. Wanner, B. L. & Walsh, C. T. (1990). Molecular biology of carbon-phosphorus bond cleavage. *J. Biol. Chem.* **265**: 4461-4471.

[19] 19.□Cole, S.T., Brosch, R., Parkhill, J., Garnier, T., Churcher, C., Hsrris, Gordon, D.S.V., Eiglmeier, K., Gas, S., Barry III, C. E. *et al.* (1998). Deciphering the biology of Mycobacterium tuberculosis from the complete genome sequence. *Nature* **393**: 537-544.

[20] Dalrymple, B., Caspers, P. & Arber, W. (1984). Nucleotide sequence of the prokaryotic mobile genetic element IS*30*. *EMBO J.* **3**: 2145-2149.

[21] Delecluse, A., Bourgouin, C., Klier, A. & Rapoport, G. (1989). Nucleotide sequence and characterization of a new insertion element, IS*240*, from *Bacillus thuringiensis israelensis*. *Plasmid* **21**: 71-78.

[22] Deppenmeier, U., Johann, A., Hartsch, T., Merkl, R., Schmitz, R.A., Martinez-Arias, R., Henne, A., Wiezer, A., Bäumer, S., Jacobi, C. et al. (2002). The genome of Methanosarcina mazei: Evidence for lateral gene transfer between bacteria and archaea. *J. Mol. Microbiol. Biotechnol.* **4**: 453-461.

[23] Droogmans, L., Roovers, M., Bujnicki, J.M., Tricot, C., Hartsch, T., Stalon. V. & Grosjean, H. (2003). Cloning and characterization of tRNA (m^1A58) methyl-transferase (Trml) from Thermus thermophilus HB27, a protein required for cell growth at extreme temperatures. *Nucleic Acids Res.* **31**: 2148-2156.

[24] Dunn, M.G. & Ellar, D.J. (1997). Identification of two sequence elements associated with the gene encoding the 24-kDa crystalline component in Bacillus thuringiensis ssp. fukuokaensis: An example of transposable element archaeology. *Plasmid* **37**: 205-215.

[25] Edgell, D.R., Belfort, M. & Shub, D.A. (2000). Barriers to intron promiscuity in bacteria. *J. Bacteriol.* **182**: 5281-5289.

[26] Fleischmann, R. D., Adams, M. D., White, O., Clayton, R. A., Kirkness, E.F., Kerlavage, A. R., Bult, C. J., Tomb, J.F., Dougherty, B. A., Merrick, J. M. *et al.* (1995). Whole genome random sequencing and assembly of *Haemophilus influenzae* Rd. *Science* **269**: 496-512.

[27] Galagan, J., Nusbaum, C., Roy, A., Endrizzi, M.G., Macdonald, P., FitzHugh, W., Calvo, S., Engels R., Smirnov, S., Atnoor, D., Brown, A. et al. (2002). The genome of M. acetivorans reveals extensive metabolic and physiological diversity. *Genome Res.* **12**:, 532-542.

[28] Germond, J.E., Lapierre, L., Delley, M. & Mollet, B. (1995). A new mobile genetic element in Lactobacillus delbrueckii subsp. *bulgaricus*. *Mol. Gen. Genet.* **248**: 407–416.

[29] Green, G.R., Searcy, D.G. & DeLange, R.J. (1983). Histone-like protein in the archaebacterium Sulforlobus acidocaldarius. *Biochim. Biophys. Acta* **741**: 251-257.

[30] Haldenwang, W. G. (1995). The sigma factors in B. subtilis. *Microbiol. Rev.* **59**: 1-30.

[31] Hamana, K., Hamana, H., Niitsu, M., Samejima, K., Sakane, T. & Yokota, A. (1994). Occurrence of tertiary and quaternary branched polyamines in thermophilic archaebacteria. *Microbios* **79**, 109-119.

[32] Hamana, K. (1999). Polyamine distribution catalogues of clostridia, acetogenic anarobes, actinobacteria, bacilli, hekiobacteria and haloanaerobes within Gram-positive eubacteria, -Distribution of spermine and agmatine in thermophiles and halophiles-. *Micobiol. Cult. Coll.* **15**: 9-28.

[33] Hodgman, T. C., Ziniu, Y., Shen, J. & Ellar, D.J. (1993). Identification of a criptic gene associated with an insertion sequence not previously identified in Bacillus thuringiensis. *FEMS Microbiol. Lett.*, **114**: 23-30.

[34] Honda, H., Kudo, T., Ikura, Y. & Horikoshi, K. (1985). Two types of xylanases of alkalophilic Bacillus sp. No. C-125. *Can. J. Microbiol.* **31**: 538-542.

[35] Horikoshi, K. (1999). In Alkaliphiles. Haward Academic Publishers, Amsterdam.

[36] Horikoshi, K. (1999). Alkaliphiles: Some applications of their products for biotechnology. *Microbiol. Mol. Biol. Rev.* **63**: 735-750.

[37] Iannelli, F., Oggioni, M. R. & Pozzi, G. (2002). Allelic variation in the highly polymorphic locus *pspC* of Streptococcus pneumoniae. *Gene* **284**: 63-71.

[38] Ikura, Y. & Horikoshi, K. (1978). Cell free protein synthesizing system of alkalophilic *Bacillus* No. A-59. *Agric. Biol. Chem.* **42**: 753-756.

[39] Ikura, Y. & Horikoshi, K. (1979). Isolation and some properties of β-galactosidase producing bacteria. *Agric. Biol. Chem.* **43**: 85-88.

[40] Ito, M, Xu, H., Guffanti、A.A., Wei、Y., Zvi、L., Clapham, D.E. & Krulwich, T.A. (2004). The voltage-gated Na^+ channel Na_VBP has a role in motility, chemotaxis, and pH homeostasis of an alkaliphilic Bacillus. *Proc. Natl.Acd. Sci. USA* **101**: 10566-10571

[41] Ivanova, N., Sorokin, A., Anderson, I., Galleron, N., Candelon, B., Kapatral, V., Bhattacharyya, A., Reznik, G., Mikhailova, N., Lapidus, A., *et al.* (2003). Genome sequence of *Bacillus cereus* and comparative analysis with Bacillus antracis. *Nature*, **423**: 87-91.

[42] Jahagirdar, R. & Howard, S.P. (1994). Isolation and characterization of a second *exe* operon required for extracellular protein secretion in Aeromonas hydrophila. *J. Bacteriol.* **176**: 6819-6826.

[43] Janausch, I., Zientz, G., E., Tran, Q., Kröger, H.A. & Unden, G. (2002). C_4-dicarbolylate carriers and sensors in bacteria. *Biochim. Biophys. Acta* **1553**: 39-56.

[44] Kagamiyama, H. & Hayashi, H. (2000). Branched-chain amino acid aminotransferase of *E. coli*. *Methods Enzymol.* **324**: 103-113.

[45] Kaneko, T., Sato, S., Kotani, H., Tanaka, A., Asamizu, E., Nakamura, Y., Miyajima, N., Hirosawa, M., Sugiura, M., Sasamoto, S. et al. (1996). Sequence analysis of the genome of the unicellular Cyanobacterium Synechocystis sp. strain PCC6803. II. Sequence determination of the entire genome and assignment of potential protein-coding regions. *DNA Res.* **3**: 109-136.

[46] Kawashima, T., Amano, N., Koike, H., Makino, S., Higuchi, S., Kawashima-Ohya, Y., Watanabe, K., Yamazaki, M., Kanehori, K., Kawamoto, T. et al. (2003). Archaeal adaptation to higher temperatures revealed by genomic sequence of Thermoplasma vo*lcanium*. *Proc. Natl. Acad. Sci. USA* **97**: 14257– 14262.

[47] Kempf, B. & Bremer, E. 1(998). Uptake and synthesis of compatible solutes as microbial stress responses to high-osmolality environments. *Arch. Microbiol.* **170**: 319-330.

[48] Kiel, J.A., Bosels, J.M., Berge, A.M., & Venema, G. (1993). Two putative insertion sequences flank a truncated glycogen branching enzyme gene in the thermophile Bacillus stearothermophilus CU21. *DNA Seq.* **4**: 1-9.

[49] Klaer, R., Kuhn, S., Tillmann, E., Fritz, H.J. & Starlinger, P. (1981). The sequence of IS*4*. *Mol. Gen. Gnet.* **181**: 169-175.

[50] Kneifel, H., Stetter, K.O., Andreesen, J.R., Weigel, H., Köning, H. & Schoberth, S.M. (1986). Distribution of polyamines in representative species of archaebacteria. *System. Appl. Microbiol.* **7**: 241-245.

[51] Kobayashi, K. Ehrlich, S.D., Albertini, A., Amati, G., Andersen, K.K., Arnaud, M., Asai, K., Ashikaga, S., Aymerich, S., Bessineres, P. *et al.* (2003). Essential Bacillus subtilis genes. *Proc. Natl Acad. Sci. USA* **100**: 4678–4683.

[52] Kosono, S., Morotomi, S., Kitada, M. & Kudo, T. (1999). Analyses of a Bacillus subtilis homologue of the Na+/H+ antiporter gene which is important for pH homeostasis of alkaliphilic Bacillus sp. C-125. *Biochim. Biophys. Acta*. **1409**: 171-175.

[53] Krämer, R. & Palmieri, F. (1992). Metabolite carriers in mitochondria. In Ernster, L. (ed.), New Comprehensive Biochemistry: Molecular Mechanisms in Bioenergetics. vol. 23, pp. 359-384. Amsterdam, the Nether lands, Elsevier Science Publishers B.V.

[54] Kronstand, J. & Whiteley, H.R. (1984). Inverted repeat sequences flank a Bacillus thuringiensis crystal protein gene. *J. Bacterial.* **160**: 95-102.

[55] Krulwich, T.A., Ito, M. & Guffanti, A.A. (2001). The Na^+-dependence of alkaliphily in Bacillus. *Biochim. Biophys. Acta*, **1505**: 156-168.

[56] Kudo T, Hino, M., Kitada, M. & Horikoshi, K. (1990). DNA sequences required for the alkalophily of Bacillus sp. strain C-125 are located close together on its chromosomal DNA. *J. Bacteriol.* **172**: 7282-7283.

[57] Kunst, F., Ogasawara, N., Mozer, I., Albertini, A. M., Alloni, G., Azevedo, V., Bertero, M. G., Bessieres, P., Bolotin, A., Borchert, S. *et al.* (1997). The complete genome sequence of the Gram-positive bacterium Bacillus subtilis. *Nature* **390**: 249-256.

[58] Kuroda, M., Ohta, T., Uchiyama, I., Baba, T., Yuzawa, H., Kobayashi, I., Cui, L., Oguchi, A., Aoki, K., Nagai, Y. *et al.* (2001). Whole genome sequencing of meticillin-resistant *Staphylococcus aureus*. *LANCET* 357: 1225-1240.

[59] Lehman, K. & Schmidt, U. (2003). Group II introns: Structure and catalytic versatility of large natural ribozymes. *Crt. Rev. Biochem. Mol. Biol.* **38**: 249-303.

[60] Lereclus, D., Ribier, J., Kiler, A., Menou, G, & Lecadet, M.-M. (1984). A transposon-like structure related to the δ-endotoxin gene of Bacillus thuringiensis. *EMBO J.* **3**: 2561-2567.

[61] Lonetto, M.A., Brown, K.L., Rudd, K.E. & Buttner, M.J. (1994). Analysis of the Streptomyces coelicolor sigE gene reveals the existence of a subfamily of eubacterial RNA polymerase sigma factors involved in the regulation of extracytoplasmic functions. *Proc. Natl. Acad. Sci. USA* **91**: 7573-7577.

[62] Lu, J., Nogi, Y. & Takami, H. (2001). Oceanobacillus iheyensis gen. nov., sp. nov., a deep-sea extremely halotolerant and alkaliphilic species isolated from a depth of 1050 m on the Iheya Ridge. *FEMS Microbiol. Lett.* **205**: 291-297.

[63] Lynn, D. J., Singer, G.A.C. & Hickey, D.A. (2002). Synonymous codon usage is subject to selection in thermophilc bacteria. *Nucleic Acids Res.* **30**: 4272-4277.

[64] Mahillon, J., Seurinck, J., Van Rompuy, L., Delcour, J. & Zabeau, M. (1985). Nucleotide sequence and structural organization of an insertion sequence element (IS*231*) *from Bacillus thuringiensis* strain berliner 1715. *EMBO J.* **4**: 3895-3899.

[65] Mahillon, J. & Chandler, M. (1998). Insertion sequence. *Microbiol. Mol. Biol. Rev.* **62**: 725-774.

[66] McCloskey, J.A. and Crain, P.F. (1998). The RNA modification database-1998. *Nucleic Acids Res.* **26**: 196-197.

[67] Michel F. & Ferat, J.L. (1995). Structure and activities of group II introns. *Annu. Rev. Biochem.* **64**: 435-461.

[68] Miyamoto, S., Kashiwagi, K., Ito, K., Watanabe, S. & Igarashi, K. (1993). Estimation of polyamine distribution and polyamine stimulation of protein synthesis in Escherichia *coli. Arch. Biochem. Biophys.* **300**: 63-68.

[69] Moir, A. & Smith, D. A. (1990). The genetics of bacterial spore germination. *Annu. Rev. Microbiol.* 44: 531-553.

[70] Mullant P., Pallen, M., Wilkins, M., Stephen, J.R. & Tabaqchali, S. (1996). A group II intron in a conjugative transposon from the gram positive bacterium Clostridium difficile. *Gene* **174**: 145-150.

[71] Murata, K., Higaki, N. & Kimura, A. (1988). Detection of carbon-phosphorus lyase activity in cell free extracts of Enterobacter aerogenes. *Biochem. Biophys. Res. Commun.* **157**: 190-195.

[72] Nagai, T., Tran, LS. P., Inatsu, Y. & Itoh. Y. (2000). A new IS*4* family insertion sequence, IS*4Bsu*1, responsible for genetic instability of poly-γ-glutamic acid production in Bacillus subtilis. *J. Bacteriol.* **182**: 2387-2392.

[73] Nakashima, H., Fukuchi, S. & Nishikawa, K. (2003). Compositional changes in RNA, DNA and proteins for bacterial adaptation to higher and lower temperatures. *J. Biochem.* **133**: 507–513.

[74] Nakasone, K., Masui, N., Takaki, Y., Sasaki, R., Maeno, G., Sakiyama, T., Hirama, C., Fuji, F. & Takami, H. (2000). Characterization and comparative study of the *rrn* operons of alkaliphilic Bacillus halodurans C-125. *Extremophilies* **4:** 209-214.

[75] Nazina, T. N., Tourova, T. P., Poltaraus, A. B., Novikova, E. V., Grigoryan, A. A., Ivanova, A. E., Lysenko, A. M., Petrunyaka, V. V., Osipov, G. A., Belyaev, S. S. & Ivanov, M.V. (2001). Taxonomic study of aerobic thermophilic bacilli: descriptions of Geobacillus subterraneus gen. nov., sp. nov. and Geobacillus uzenensis sp. nov. from petroleum reservoirs and transfer of Bacillus stearothermophilus, Bacillus thermocatenulatus, Bacillus thermoleovorans, Bacillus kaustophilus, Bacillus thermoglucosidasius and Bacillus thermodenitrificans to Geobacillus as the new combinations G. stearothermophilus, G. thermocatenulatus, G. thermoleovorans, G. kaustophilus, G. thermoglucosidasius and G. thermodenitrific. *Int. J. Syst. Evol. Microbiol.* **51**: 433-446.

[76] Niimura, Y., Koh, E., Yanagida, F., Suzuki, K.-I., Komagata, K., & Kozaki, M. (1990). Amphibacillus xylanus gen. nov., sp. nov., a facultatively anaerobic sporeforming xylan-digesting bacterium which lacks cytochrome, quinone, and catalase. *Int. J. Syst. Bacteriol.* **40**: 297-301.

[77] Nelson, K. E., Clayton, R. A., Gill, S. R., Gwinn, M. L., Dodson, R. J., Haft, D. H., Hickey E. K., Peterson, J. D., Nelson, W. C., Ketchum, K. A. *et al.* (1999). Evidence for lateral gene transfer between archaea and bacteria from gnome sequence of Thermotoga maritima. *Nature* **399**: 323-329.

[78] Nishio, Y., Nakamura, Y., Kawarabayasi, Y., Usuda, Y., Kimura, E., Sugimoto, S., Matsui, K., Yamagishi, A., Kikuchi, H., Ikeo, K. & Gojiobori, T. (2003) Comparative complete genome sequence analysis of the amino acid replacements responsible for the thermostability of Corynebacterium efficiens. *Genome Res.* **13**: 1572-1579.

[79] Nölling, J., Breton, G., Omelchenko, M.V., Makarova, K. S., Zeng, Q., Gibson, R., Lee, H.M., Dubois, J., Qiu, D., Hitti, J. *et al.* (2001). Complete sequence and comparative analysis of the solvent-producing bacterium Clostridium acetobutylicum. *J. Bacteriol.* **183**: 4823-4838.

[80] Neuhaus, F. C. & Baddiley J. (2003). A continuum of anionic charge: Structures and functions of D-alanyl-teichoic acids in gram-positive bacteria. *Microbiol. Mol. Biol. Rev.* **67**: 686-723.

[81] Oshima, T., Hamasaki, N.,Uzawa, T. & Friedman, S.M. (1989). Biochemical functions of unusual polyamines found in the cells of extreme thermophiles. In Goldemberg, S. H. and Algranati, I. D. (Eds.), *The biology and chemistry of polyamines.* pp. 1-10, Oxford, UK, IRL Press,

[82] Pearson, W.R. & Lipman, D.J. (1988). Improved tools for biological sequence comparison. *Proc. Natl. Acad. Sci.USA,* **85**: 2444-2448.

[83] Plasterk, R.H. (1993). Molecular mechanisms of transposition and its control. *Cell* **74**: 781-786.

[84] Priest, F. G. 1993. In *Bacillus subtilis* and other Gram-positive bacteria. Sonenshein, A.L., Hoch, J.A. & Losick, R. (Eds.), pp. 3-16. Washington, DC, USA: ASM Press.

[85] Read, T.D., Peterson, S.N., Tourasse, N., Baillie, L.W., Paulsen, I.T., Nelson, K.E., Tettelin, H., Fouts, D.E., Eisen, J.A., Gill, S.R. et al. (2003). The genome sequence of Bacillus antracis Ames and comparison to closely related bacteria. *Nature* **423**: 81-86.

[86] Reimmann, C., Moore, R., Little, S., Savioz, A., Willetts, N.S. & Haas, D. (1989). Genetic structure, function and regulation of the transposable element IS*21*. *Mol. Gen. Genet.* **215**: 416-424.

[87] Ren, D., Navarro, B., Xu, H., Yue, L., Shi, Q. & Clapham, D. E. (2001). A prokaryotic voltage-gated sodium channel. *Science* **294**: 2372-2375.

[88] Romine, M.F., Stillwell, L.C., Wong, K.-K., S.J., Thurston, Sisk, E.C., Sensen, C., Gaasterland, T., Fredrikson, J.K. & Saffer, J.D. (1999). Complete sequence of a 184-kilobase catabolic plasmid from Sphingomonas aromaticivorans F199. *J. Bacteriol.* **181**: 1585-1602.

[89] Ruepp, A., Graml, W., Santos-Martinez, M.L., Koretke, K.K., Volker, C., Mewes, H. W., Frishman, D., Stocker S., Lupas, A. & Baumeister, W. (2000). The genome sequence of the thermoacidophilic scavenger Thermoplasma acidophilum. *Nature* **407**: 508–513.

[90] Sakiyama, T., Takami, H., Ogasawara, N., Kuhara, S., Kozuki, T., Doga, K., Ohyama, A. & Horikoshi, K. (2000). An automated system for genome analysis to support microbial whole-genome shotgun sequencing. *Biosci. Biotech. Biochem.* **64**: 670-673.

[91] Schadewaldt, P., Hummel, W., Wendel, U., & Adelmeyer, F. (1995). Enzymatic method for determination of branched-chain amino acid aminotransferase activity. *Anal. Biochem.* **230**: 199-204.

[92] Schneuder, E. & Hunke, S. (1998). ATP-binding-cassete (ABC) transport systems: Functional and structural aspects of the ATP-hydrolyzing subunits/domains. *FEMS Microbiol. Rev.* **22**: 1-20.

[93] Shida, O., Takagi, H., Kadowaki, K. & Komagata, K. (1996). Proposal for two new genera, Brevibacillus gen. nov. and Aneurinibacillus gen. nov. *Int. J. Syst. Bacteriol.* **46**: 939-946.

[94] Shioi, J.I., Matsuura, S, & Imae, Y. (1980). Quantitative measurements of proton motive force and motility in Bacillus subtilis. *J. Bacteriol.* **144**: 891-7.

[95] Shulami, S., Gat, O., Sonenshein, A.L., & Shoham, Y. (1999). The glucuronic acid utilization gene cluster from Bacillus stearothermophilus T-6. *J. Bacteriol.*, **181**: 3695-3704.

[96] Singer, G.A.C. & Hickey, D.A. (2003). Thermophilic prokaryotes have characteristic patterns of codon usage, amino acid composition and nucleotide content. *Gene* **317**: 39-47.

[97] Smith, G.P., Ellar, D.J., Keeler, S.J. & Seip, C.E. (1994). Nucleotide sequence and analysis of an insertion sequence from Bacillus thuringiensis related to IS*150*. *Plasmid* **32**: 10-18.

[98] Sneath, P. H. A., Mair, N.S., Sharp, M.E. & Holt, J.G. (1986). In *Bergey's Manual of Systematic Bacteriology*, Vol. 2. Baltimore, USA, Wiliams and Wikins.

[99] Soares, D., Dahlke, I., Li, W.-T., Sandman, K., Hethke, C., Thomm, M. & Reeve, J. (1998). Archaeal histone stability, DNA binding and transcription inhibition above 90°C. *Extremophiles* **2**: 75-81.

[100] Spring, S., Ludwig, W., Marquez, M.C., Ventosa, A. & Schleifer, K.H. (1996). Halobacillus gen. nov., with descriptions of Halobacillus litoralis sp. nov. and Halobacillus trueperi sp. nov., and transfer of Sporosarcina halophila to Halobacillus halophilus comb. nov. *Int. J. Syst. Bacteriol.* **46**: 492-496.

[101] Sueoka, N. (1988). Directional mutation pressure and neutral molecular evolution. *Proc. Natl. Acad. Sci. USA* **85**: 2653-2657.

[102] Takaki, Y., Matsuki, A., Chee, G.J. & Takami, H. (2004). Identification and distribution of new insertion sequences in the genome of the extremely halotolerant and alkaliphilic Oceanobacillus iheyensis HTE831. *DNA Res.* **11**: 233-245.

[103] Takami, H., Kobayashi, T., Aono, R. & Horikoshi, K. (1992). Molecular cloning, nucleotide sequence, and expression of the structural gene for a thermostable alkaline protease from Bacillus sp. No. AH-101. *Appl. Microbiol. Biotechnol.* **38**: 101-108.

[104] Takami, H., Inoue, A., Fuji, F. & Horikoshi, K. (1997). Microbial Flora in the deepest sea mud of Mariana Trench. *FEMS Microbiol. Lett.* **152**: 279-285.

[105] Takami, H., Kobata, K., Nagahama, T., Kobayashi, H., Inoue, A. & Horikoshi, K. (1999). Biodiversity in the deep-sea sites located near the south part of Japan. *Extremophiles* **3**: 97-102.

[106] Takami, H. (1999). Isolation and Characterization of Microorganisms from Deep-sea Mud. In Horikoshi, K. & Tsujii, K. (eds.) Extremophiles in deep-sea environments. pp. 3-26. Tokyo, Japan: Springer-Verlag.

[107] Takami, H. & Horikoshi, K. (1999). Reidentification of facultatively alkaliphilic Bacillus sp. C-125 to *Bacillus halodurans. Biosci. Biotech. Biochem.* **63**: 943-945.

[108] Takami, H, Nakasone, K., Hirama, C., Takaki, Y., Masui, N., Fuji, F., Nakamura, Y. & Inoue, A. (1999). An improved physical and genetic map of the genome of alkaliphilic Bacillus sp. C-125. *Extremophiles* **3**: 21-28.

[109] Takami H, Nakasone, K., Ogasawara, N., Hirama, C., Nakamura, Y., Masui, N., Fuji, F., Takaki, Y., Inoue, A., & Horikoshi, K. (1999). Sequencing of three lambda clones from the genome of alkaliphilic Bacillus sp. strain C-125. *Extremophiles* **3**: 29-34.

[110] Takami, H., Takaki, Y., Nakasone, K., Hirama, C., Inoue, A. & Horikoshi, K. (1999). Sequence analysis of 32kb fragment including the major ribosomal protein gene clusters in alkaliphilic Bacillus sp. strain C-125. *Biosci. Biotechnol. Biochem.* **63**: 452-455.

[111] Takami, H., Masui, N., Nakasone, K. & Horikoshi, K. (1999). Replication origin region of the chromosome of alkaliphilic Bacillus sp. strain C-125. Biosci. Biotechnol. *Biochem.* **63**: 1134-1137.

[112] Takami, H., Takaki, Y., Nakasone, K., Sakiyama, T., Maeno, G., Sasaki, R., Hirama, C., Fuji, F. & Masui, N. (1999). Genetic analysis of the chromosome of alkaliphilic Bacillus halodurans C-125. *Extremophiles* **3**: 227-233.

[113] Takami, H. (1999). Genome analysis of facultatively alkaliphilic Bacillus halodurans C-125. In Horikoshi, K. & Tsujii, K. (eds.) *Extremophiles in deep-sea environments*. pp. 249-284. Tokyo, Japan: Springer-Verlag.

[114] Takami, H. & Horikoshi, K. (2000). Analysis of the genome of an alkaliphilic Bacillus strain from an industrial point of view. *Extremophiles* **4**: 99-108.

[115] Takami, H., Nakasone, K., Takaki, Y., Maeno, G., Sasaki, R., Masui, N., Fuji, F., Hirama, C., Nakamura, Y., Ogasawara, N., Kuhara, S. & Horikoshi, K. (2000).

Complete genome sequence of the alkaliphilic bacterium *Bacillus halodurans* and genomic sequence comparison with *Bacillus subtilis*. *Nucleic Acids Res.* **28**: 4317-4331.

[116] Takami, H., Han, C.G., Takaki, Y. & Ohtsubo, E. (2001). Identification and distribution of new insertion sequences in the genome of alkaliphilic Bacillus halodurans C-125. *J. Bacteriol.* **183**: 4345-4356.

[117] Takami, H., Takaki, Y. & Uchiyama, I. (2002). Genome sequence of Oceanobacillus iheyensis isolated from the Iheya Ridge and its unexpected adaptive capabilities to extremely environments. *Nucleic Acids Res.* **30**: 3927-3935.

[118] Takami, H., Matsuki, A. & Takaki, Y. (2004). Wide-range distribution of insertion sequences identified in *B.* halodurans among bacilli and a new transposon disseminated in alkaliphilic and thermophilic bacilli. *DNA Res.* **11**: 153-162.

[119] Takami, H., Nishi, S., Lu, J., Shimamura, S. & Takaki, Y. (2004). Genomic characterization of thermophilic Geobacillus species isolated from the deepest sea mud of the Mariana Trench. *Extremophiles* **8**: 351-356.

[120] Takami, H., Takaki, Y., Chee, G.J., Nishi, S., Shimamura, S., Suzuki, H., Matsui, S. & Uchiyama, I. (2004). Thermoadaptation trait revealed by the genome sequence of thermophilic Geobacillus kaustophilus. *Nucleic Acids Res.* **32**: 6292-6303.

[121] Takemura, H., Horinouchi, S. & Beppu, T. (1991). Novel insertion sequence IS*1380* from Acetobacter pasteurianus is involved in loss of ethanol-oxidizing ability. *J. Bacteriol.* **173**: 7070-7076.

[122] Tsujii, K. (2002). Donnan equilibria in microbial cell walls: a pH-homeostatic mechanism in alkaliphiles. *Coll. Surf. B. Biopolymer* **24**: 247-251.

[123] Uchiyama I. (2003). MBGD: microbial genome database for comparative analysis. *Nucleic Acids Res.* **31**: 58-62.

[124] Validation List No. 85 (2002). Validation of publication of new names and new combinations previously effectively published outside the IJSEM. *Int. J. Syst. Evol. Microbiol,* **52**: 685-690.

[125] Ventosa, A., Nieto, J. & Oren, A. (1998). A. Biology of moderately halophilic aerobic bacteria. *Microbiol. Mol. Biol. Rev.* 62: 504-544.

[126] Wainø, M., Tindall, B.J., Schumann, P. & Ingvorsen, K. (1999). *Gracilibacillus* gen. nov., description of Gracilibacillus halotolerans gen. nov., sp. nov.; transfer of Bacillus dipsosauri to Gracilibacillus dipsosauri comb. nov., and Bacillus salexigens to the genus Salibacillus gen. nov., as Salibacillus salexigens comb. nov. *Int. J. Syst. Bacteriol.* **49**: 821–831.

[127] White, O., Eisen, J.A., Heidelberg, J.F., Hickey, E.K., Peterson, J.D., Dodson, R.J., Haft, D.H., Gwinn, M.L., Nelson, W.C., Richardson, D.L. et al. (1999). Genome sequence of the radioresistant bacterium Deinococcus radiodurans R1. *Science* **286**: 1571-1577.

[128] Wisotzkey, J. D., Jurtshuk, P., Fox, G. E. Jr., Deinhard, G. & Poralla, K. (1992). Comparative sequences analyses on the 16S rRNA (rDNA) of Bacillus acidocaldarius, Bacillus acidoterrestris, and Bacillus cycloheptanicus and proposal for creation of a new genus, Alicyclobacillus gen. nov. *Int. J. Syst. Bacteriol.* **42**: 263-269.

[129] Xu, K., He, Z.-Q., Mao, Y.-M., Sheng, R.-Q., & Sheng, Z.-J. (1993). On two transposable elements from Bacillus stearothermophilus. *Plasmid*, **29**: 1-9.

[130] Yada, T., Totoki, Y., Takagi, T., & Nakai, K. (2001). A novel bacterial gene-finding system with top-class accuracy in locationg start codons. *DNA Res.* **8**: 97-106.

[131] Yamaoka, T., Satoh, K. & Katoh, S. (1978). Photosynthetic activities of a thermophilic blue-green alga. *Plant Cell Physiol.* **19**: 943-954.

[132] Yu, W., Mierau, I., Mars, A., Johnson, E., Dunny, G. & McKay, L.L. (1995). Novel insertion sequence-like element IS*982* in Lactococci. *Plasmid* **33**: 218-225.

In: Trends in Genome Research
Editor: Clyde R. Williams, pp. 87-117
ISBN 1-60021-027-9

Chapter 3

Targeted Modification of Mammalian Genomes

David A. Sorrell and Andreas F. Kolb
Molecular Recognition Group, Hannah Research Institute, Ayr, KA6 5HL, UK.

Abstract

The stable and site-specific modification of mammalian genomes has a variety of applications in biomedicine and biotechnology. Here we outline two alternative approaches that can be employed to achieve this goal: homologous recombination or site-specific recombination. Homologous recombination relies on sequence similarity (or rather identity) of a piece of DNA that is introduced into a host cell and the host genome. The frequency of homologous recombination is generally markedly lower than the process of random integration. Especially in somatic cells homologous recombination is an extremely rare event. However, strategies involving the introduction of double-strand breaks can increase the frequency of homologous recombination.

Site-specific recombination makes use of enzymes (recombinases, transposases, integrases), which catalyse DNA strand exchange between DNA molecules that have only limited sequence homology. The recognition sites of site-specific recombinases (e.g. Cre or ΦC31) are usually 30 - 40bp. Retroviral integrases only require a specific dinucleotide sequence to insert the viral cDNA into the host genome. Depending on the individual enzyme, there are either innumerable or very few potential target sites for a particular integrase/recombinase in a mammalian genome. A number of strategies have been utilized successfully to alter the site-specificity of recombinases. Therefore site-specific recombinases provide an attractive tool for the targeted modification of mammalian genomes.

1. Introduction

The ability to modify the mammalian genome is crucial to a variety of applications in biomedicine and biotechnology, including human gene therapy and animal transgenesis. The goal of most of these applications is to achieve the long-term stable expression of an introduced transgene or therapeutic gene. The best way to achieve this is by integrating the transgene or therapeutic gene into the genome. In this review we start by discussing the reasons why site-specific integration as opposed to random integration is the best way of achieving the stable long-term expression of an introduced gene. We then outline the major strategies currently available to achieve site-specific genomic modifications, which are based on homologous recombination and site-specific recombination.

2. The Need for Site-Specific Gene Integration

2.1. Commonly Used Methods for Transgene Integration

Numerous approaches have been used to deliver exogenous DNA into mammalian cells for subsequent integration into the chromosomes. These approaches can be broadly categorized into three groups depending on whether the type of delivery system used is physical or chemical, viral or transposon-based.

Physical methods of delivery include electroporation, naked DNA injection, ultrasound, and biolistic particle delivery using a gene gun [1]. Chemical based delivery methods use reagents such as Calcium phosphate, cationic polymers including DEAE-dextran and polyethylenimine (PEI), and liposomes [2, 3]. Although these methods can be very efficient, the introduced genes will generally only be present transiently, and will be integrated into the host genome only in a small minority of cells where they can be abundantly and stably expressed [2].

Several commonly used viral vectors are able to mediate integration of transgenes into the genome. Retroviruses insert their genome (including any embedded transgene) into a distinct dinucleotide sequence at non-specific sites throughout the host genome, but expression of the transgene or therapeutic gene is often rapidly down-regulated due to epigenetic silencing phenomena [4, 5]. One exception to this are lentiviral vectors, which have successfully been used to generate transgenic mice and pigs, and appear to escape epigenetic silencing [6, 7]. Human Adeno-associated virus (AAV) preferentially integrates at a specific site on human chromosome 19, but also exhibits a significant level of random integration [8]. The site-specific integration event, however, is dependent on the viral rep genes (which encode a site-specific recombinase), which are absent in most current AAV-derived vectors in order to allow more space for the transgene(s) of interest [9-11]. In the absence of the rep proteins, integration of the transgene into the host genome is either absent or random.

Finally, transposable elements are potentially useful vehicles for the integration of genes into the genome. One promising example is the *Sleeping Beauty* (SB) transposon, a member of the Tc1/*mariner* family of transposons, which was reconstructed from transposon fossils found in fish genomes [12]. SB has been shown to efficiently deliver transgenes, into TA dinucleotides, at non-specific locations across the chromosomes [12]. However, a physical, chemical or viral system is still needed initially to deliver the transposon vector into the cells.

2.2. Limitations of These Methods - Random Transgene Integration

Irrespective of which of the above gene transfer methodologies are used, the site of integration of a transgene or therapeutic gene cannot normally be predicted. This is problematic for two reasons. Firstly, expression of a transgene or therapeutic gene can be extinguished due to inhibitory influences of the genomic site in which it is integrated [13]. Secondly, the integrated gene can have mutagenic effects by inhibiting or activating host genes at the integration site [14]. This was recently demonstrated in an X-chromosome-linked severe combined immunodeficiency (SCID-X1) gene therapy trial in which two patients developed leukaemia after retroviral vector integration activated a proto-oncogene [14]. Therefore, the ability to insert transgenes or therapeutic genes at a precise location in the mammalian genome would have major benefits for the efficiency of transgenesis and the safety of gene therapy [15, 16].

3. Classical Homologous Recombination-Based Targeting Strategies

Homologous recombination-based targeting (gene targeting) strategies were the first approaches developed to site-specifically modify the mammalian genome [17]. They exploit the ability of a fragment of genomic DNA, when introduced into a mammalian cell, to locate and recombine with a homologous sequence present in the chromosome. These strategies have now become the current method of choice for most targeted modifications of the mouse genome [18]. Mice containing these modifications are generated by targeting the gene of interest in embryonic stem (ES) cells and then incorporating these targeted cells into blastocysts, from which animals containing the targeted gene can be derived [19, 20].

Several different types of targeted modification can be achieved using these approaches. In this section we give an overview of the basic one-step strategies used for the generation of simple knockout or knock-in alleles, including the types of targeting vector that can be used and the selection strategies needed to enrich for homologous recombinants. We then consider more complex two-step strategies that have been used for the creation of more subtle targeted mutations.

3.1. Targeting Vectors for the Generation of Knockout and Knock-in Alleles

A targeting vector is required to deliver the homologous fragment of genomic DNA into the ES cell. These vectors consist of a plasmid backbone, genomic DNA sequences that are homologous to the desired integration site and one or more selection markers. Two types of targeting vector are available.

3.1.1. Replacement Vectors

Replacement vectors are the most common type of vector used (Figure 1) [21, 22]. They consist of a positive selection marker flanked by two regions of chromosomal homology. Additionally, in experiments using a positive-negative enrichment strategy, a negative selection marker is positioned adjacent to one of the homologous arms in the plasmid backbone (see section 4.2.4). The frequency of recombination between the vector and chromosome increases with the total length of homologous DNA sequences used and the ideal length to use in the vector is between 5 – 8 kb [21]. The positive selection marker is usually asymmetrically positioned within the homologous DNA, so that the region of homology in the targeting vector is divided into a short arm and a long arm (Figure 1). This is to facilitate the identification of homologous recombinants by PCR using one primer that anneals to the selection marker and a second primer that anneals to a region of genomic DNA immediately adjacent to the short arm of homology. The short arm is ideally between 0.5 – 2 kb in length, which is sufficient to support recombination without compromising the efficiency of the PCR [21].

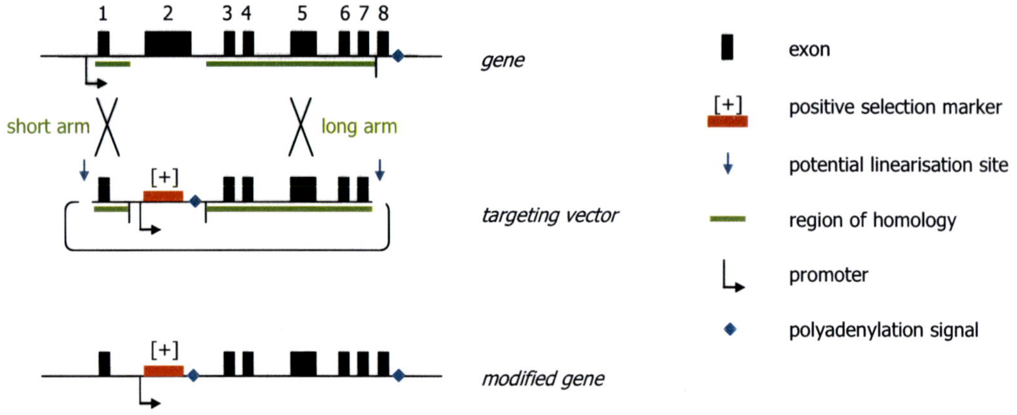

Figure 1. Homologous recombination using a replacement vector. Schematic representation of a hypothetical gene encompassing 8 exons. The right hand panel explains the symbols used in the left hand panel. A targeting vector is established which contains a positively selectable marker gene expression cassette (e.g. a neomycin-phospho-transferase coding sequence flanked by a ubiquitous promoter and a polyadenylation signal) flanked by two DNA segments homologous to the gene to be targeted. The targeting vector is linearised by digestion with a suitable restriction enzyme and transfected into embryonic stem cells. Cellular DNA repair enzymes mediate the integration of the selection marker gene into one allele of the gene of interest. The targeting event removes the second exon from the hypothetical gene and renders the encoded protein non-functional.

Replacement vectors are linearized at a unique restriction site located outside of the regions of homology and then electroporated into ES cells. A double-reciprocal recombination then results in the chromosomally located homologous regions plus intervening sequences being replaced by the vector derived homologous sequences, along with the positive selection marker and any other sequences they flank. Vector sequences not flanked by the homologous regions are lost. Replacement vectors are the tools of choice for generating a knockout allele, because in addition to the insertion of a selectable marker, they can also facilitate the deletion of all or an essential part of a target gene if it lies between the regions of homology [21, 22]. Replacement vectors are also useful for the generation of knock-in alleles, which are targeted alleles that have an introduced transgene under the control of an endogenously located gene [18]. To achieve this, the transgene to be knocked-in is incorporated into the replacement vector in between the regions of homology, upstream of the selectable marker (Figure 2). As discussed in more detail below (section 6.2.3) the selection marker is usually flanked with site-specific recombinase target sites to allow for its subsequent removal once it has fulfilled its function (Figure 2).

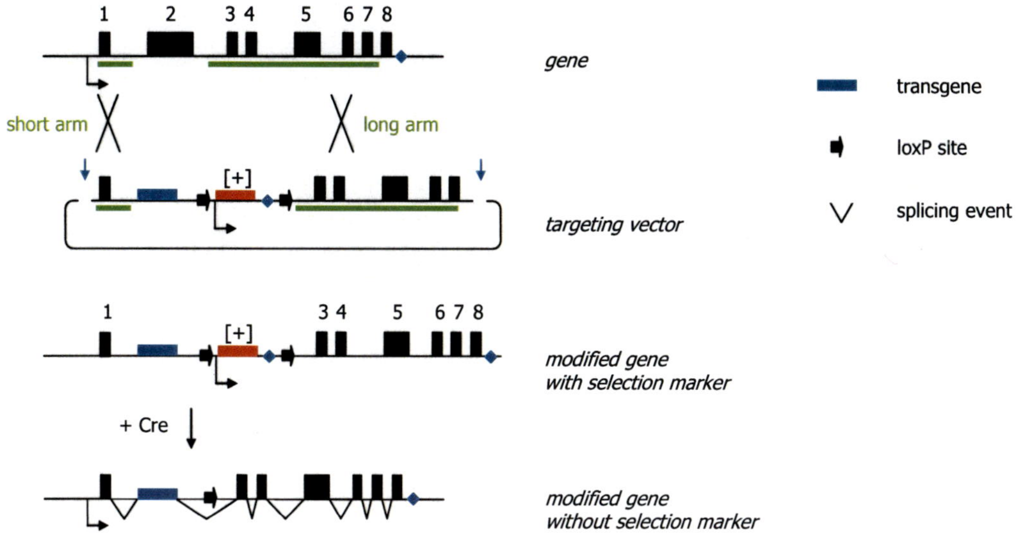

Figure 2. Homologous recombination as a means of integrating a transgene at a precise genomic site. The targeting vector contains a transgene of interest that replaces the second exon of the putative gene. The transgene coding region becomes part of a chimeric gene-transgene mRNA, which is expressed from the promoter of the endogenous gene. The selection marker gene is removed from the genome by Cre recombinase-mediated excision.

3.1.2. Insertion Vectors

Insertion vectors contain essentially the same components as a replacement vectors [18, 21]. However, in contrast to replacement vectors the positive selection marker can be located either within the homologous regions or in the vector backbone. Unlike replacement vectors, insertion vectors are linearised at a unique restriction site positioned inside the regions of homology prior to electroporation. These vectors undergo single-reciprocal recombination with the chromosomal homologous sequences, which results in the entire vector being inserted into the target site (Figure 3). Therefore, the modified allele contains a duplication of the homologous sequences, separated by the vector backbone (Figure 3). In most cases this modification will be sufficient to completely disrupt a genes function and therefore create a null allele. However, because none of the exons are actually deleted using this approach, in some cases a functional protein may still be produced (for a full discussion see ref [21]). Therefore, this approach is considered to be less reliable than one using a replacement vector for the generation a null allele. Nevertheless, insertion vectors have two advantages over replacement vectors: (1) they can give a 5-20 fold higher recombination frequency [23]; and (2) they can form the basis for the introduction of more subtle mutations (discussed in section 4.3.1).

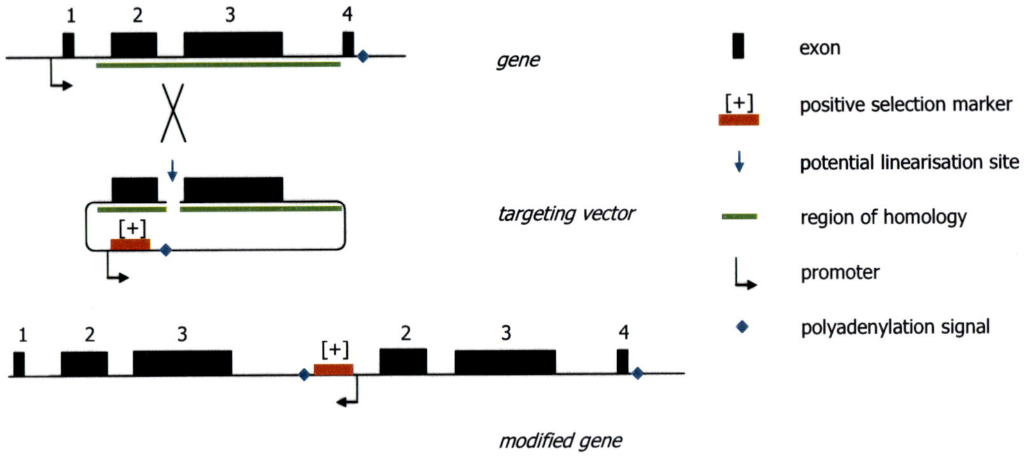

Figure 3. Homologous recombination using an insertion vector. Schematic representation of a hypothetical gene encompassing 4 exons. An insertion vector carrying regions of homology that encompass exons 2 and 3 and introns 2 and 3 is linearized within the region of homology. Insertion of the targeting vector into the genome leads to a partial duplication of the gene and functional inactivation of the encoded protein.

3.2. Selection Strategies

Homologous recombination is a low frequency event and targeted integration of the vector only occurs in a very small proportion of cells. Therefore a selection strategy is required [17]. A simple strategy can be used that selects all integrants, whether targeted or random, and these are then further screened by PCR or Southern blot to identify the homologous recombinants. However, because random integration occurs at a much higher frequency than homologous recombination-based targeted integration the majority of the clones that survive the selection are random integrants and this can necessitate the screening of large numbers of clones to identify a correctly target one [17]. Therefore, alternative more stringent selection strategies can be applied that specifically select for targeted integrants.

3.2.1. Simple Positive Selection

The simplest selection strategy is to configure the positive selection cassette, in the targeting vector, to contain all the necessary elements for expression, that is to say a full promoter and termination/polyadenylation signals (Figure 1). This strategy enables the selection of all stable integrants; these can then be screened by PCR (ideally) or Southern blot to identify those that are correctly targeted [21, 22]. We have used this strategy with several different targeting vectors and routinely achieve a targeting efficiency of 1 – 5 % (percentage of positively selected clones that are correctly targeted), which is ample given that the goal of most ES cell experiments is to isolate only a few targeted integrants, which can then be used as a basis for subsequent manipulations.

3.2.2. Promoter-Trap Positive Selection

A more stringent strategy utilises the promoter of the targeted gene to drive the expression of the positive selection marker [21]. In this case a promoterless selection marker is used in the targeting vector (Figure 4). Upon targeted insertion the endogenous promoter is linked to the promoterless selection marker, rendering targeted integrants resistant to the selection agent. In contrast, the resistance marker will remain promoterless in random integrants (unless it is fortuitously integrated adjacent to an active promoter) therefore they remain sensitive to the selection agent. This strategy can yield a 100-fold enrichment for targeted clones compared to the simple positive selection strategy [21]. One drawback to this approach is that the promoter of the targeted gene must be active in the cell type used for the experiment (typically ES cells).

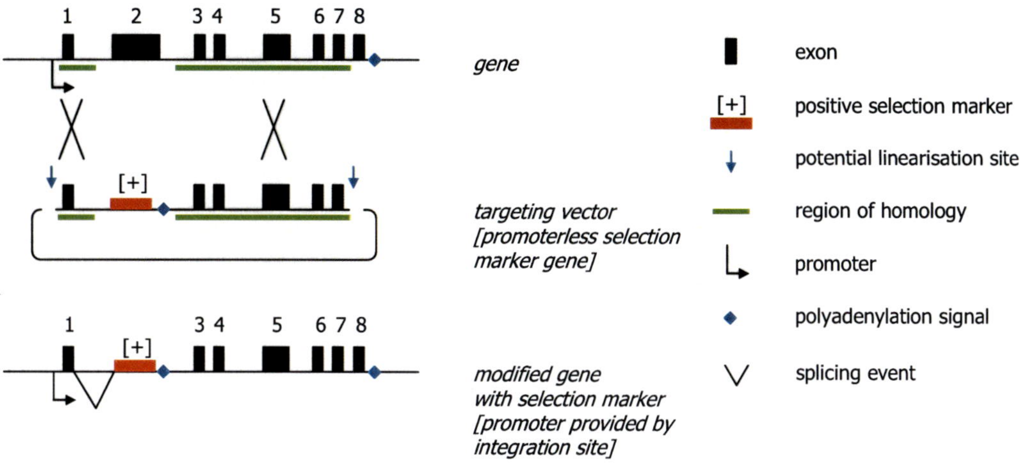

Figure 4. Strategies for the enrichment of cells carrying targeted genes. Promoter trap: the targeting construct contains a promoterless selection marker gene that is only activated if integrated adjacent to an active promoter element. Site-specific integration of the selection marker gene via homologous recombination links its coding region to the promoter of the targeted gene.

3.2.3. Polyadenylation-Trap Positive Selection

A second stringent enrichment strategy makes use of the termination/polyadenylation signals in the endogenous gene to regulate the introduced selection marker [21]. In this scenario the positive selection cassette in the targeting vector is configured to contain its own promoter but to lack the termination/polyadenylation signals necessary for the production of a correctly terminated stable transcript. Therefore, upon targeted integration, the incoming selection marker becomes linked to the endogenous termination/polyadenylation signals, which confers resistance to the positive selective agent. In contrast, random integrants produce an unstable transcript, which is rapidly degraded, and therefore remain sensitive. This strategy typically yields a 5 - 50-fold enrichment for targeted clones in comparison to the simple selection strategy [21]. The advantage this strategy has over the promoter-trap strategy is that it does not depend on the targeted gene being transcriptionally active in the cell type used for targeting.

3.2.4. Positive-Negative Selection

A further enrichment strategy that can be used with replacement vectors involves the use of both positive and negative selection markers [21]. For this approach a negative marker is situated in the plasmid backbone adjacent to one of the arms of homology in the targeting vector (Figure 5). After electroporation, cells are exposed to both the positive and negative selective agents. As the negative marker is outside the arms of homology it will be lost in targeted integrants and therefore they will be resistant to both negative and positive selective agents. However, random integrants will contain the entire targeting vector and although resistant to the positive selective agent they will be sensitive to the negative selective agent and will die. This strategy can yield a 20-fold enrichment for targeted clones in compared to a simple positive selection [21]. The advantage this and the simple selection strategy share compared to the promoter or polyadenylation-trap strategies is that they do not depend on any elements present in the target gene to select for targeted integrants.

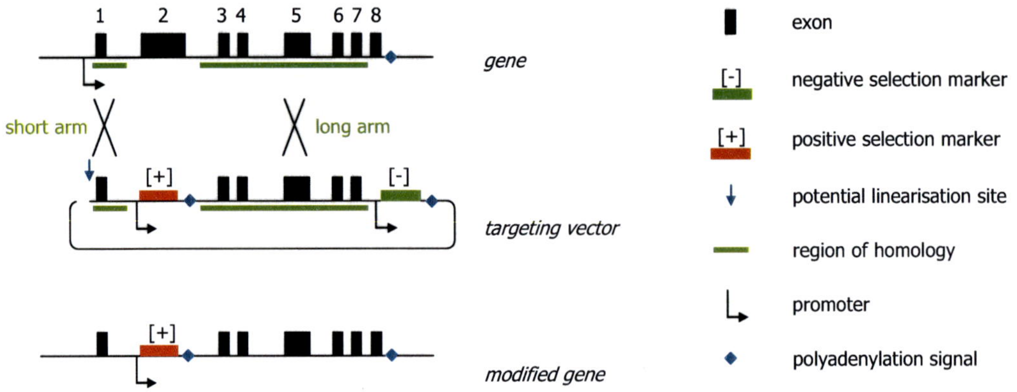

Figure 5. Strategies for the enrichment of cells carrying targeted genes. Positive-negative selection: the targeting construct contains a positive selection marker gene, which allows cell survival in the presence of a drug. In addition the targeting construct also contains a negative selection marker gene (e.g. thymidine kinase), which induces cell death in the presence of a corresponding drug (Gancyclovir). Integration of the targeting construct by homologous recombination ensures the retention of the positive selection marker and the loss of the negative selection marker.

3.2. Two-Step Strategies for the Introduction of Subtle Modifications

While a null mutation is a useful starting point, it is often desirable to introduce subtle changes into the coding or regulatory regions to fully appreciate the function of a gene. One requirement of this type of modification is that no selection marker cassette or bacterial vector backbone sequences should remain in the target locus after the subtle mutation has been introduced. This is because these sequences can potentially interfere with the expression of the targeted or neighbouring endogenous genes [24, 25]. Two types of targeting strategies requiring two rounds of homologous recombination have been used to achieve this [18, 19, 21].

3.3.1. 'Hit-and-Run' (or 'In-and-Out') Strategy

Hit-and-Run vectors are insertion-type vectors that contain both positive and negative selection markers in the vector backbone and the desired subtle mutation in the homologous sequences (Figure 6) [21, 23, 26]. In the first step of the strategy the targeting vector is introduced into the target gene, creating a duplication, and integrants are selected using a positive selection. A second round of spontaneous homologous recombination between the duplicate homologous sequences removes the vector sequences, selection markers and the unmodified copy of the duplicated homologous sequences. The resulting allele contains just the subtle modification and none of the vector sequences or selection markers. Since the negative selection marker is lost, these targeted clones can be identified by virtue of their resistance to the negative selection agent. Examples when this strategy has been used include the introduction of subtle modification into the *HPRT* [26], *Hox-2.6* [23] and β-amyloid precursor protein [27] loci.

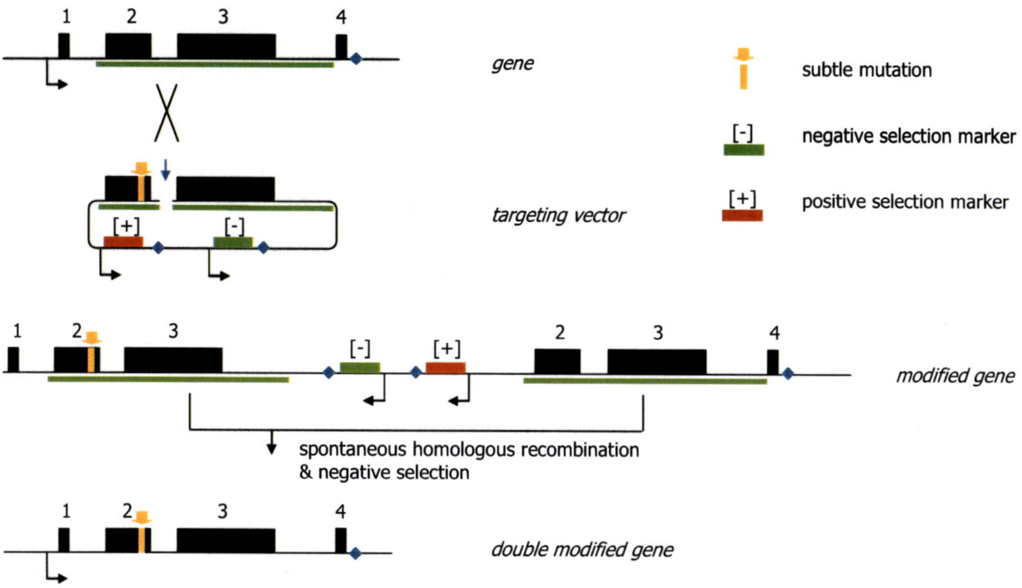

Figure 6. Introduction of subtle mutations. Hit & Run: the targeting construct is based on an insertion-vector design and contains both a positive and a negative selection marker gene. In addition the targeting vector also carries a subtle mutation in the second exon of the hypothetical gene. By selection for the positive marker gene, cells in which the targeting construct has been integrated by homologous recombination can be identified (among cell clones, in which integration has occurred at random). Due to the juxtaposition of homologous sequences at the target site, the intervening sequences can be removed via a spontaneous homologous recombination event. Cells in which this event has occurred can be isolated by selection for the absence of the negative selection marker expression cassette.

3.3.2. 'Tag-and-Exchange' (Double Replacement) Strategy

This strategy is achieved using a replacement type vector that contains both positive and negative selection markers that are located between the two regions of chromosomal homology [19, 28, 29]. The first step of this strategy (the 'tagging' step), involves the replacement of a portion or the entire targeted gene with the selectable markers by homologous recombination, with these targeted integrants being identified with a positive selection. In the second homologous recombination step (the 'exchange' step), the genomic locus is retargeted with a second replacement vector that contains the modified version of the endogenous gene. This results in the reconstruction of the original locus with the incorporated modification and the simultaneous loss of the selection marker cassettes. These targeted integrants can be identified with a negative selection because the negative selection marker has been lost. The advantage this strategy has over the hit-and-run strategy is that any modification can be introduced in the second step and, therefore, it is possible to generate a series of ES cell clones/transgenic mice each containing different mutations at the same genomic locus. An example of the use of this type of strategy includes the introduction of subtle mutations into the Huntingdon's disease homolog (*Hdh*) gene [30] and a prion protein gene [31].

3.4. Limitations

(a) The principal limitation of these strategies is that homologous recombination is generally only efficient in embryonic stem cells, which are only readily available for the mouse [17, 20]. Therefore, while it is a powerful way to site-specifically manipulate the mouse genome, its applicability to other mammalian species or somatic cell gene therapy is limited. However, despite this limitation it has been possible, although very laborious and technically demanding, to generate targeted transgenic animals in other species including pigs and sheep. This has been achieved by performing the homologous recombination event in somatic cells and then using these to generate transgenic animals by nuclear transfer [20].

(b) Even in mouse embryonic stem cells homologous recombination is a relative infrequent occurrence compared to random integration [17]. Therefore the use of strategies involving two homologous recombination steps to manipulate the mouse genome can be particularly time consuming.

(c) Only a limited size of DNA fragments can be conveniently handled in plasmid vectors. The introduction of specific alterations in large genes can therefore be complicated. In addition there may be limitations to the size of the DNA segment that can be inserted by homologous recombination.

4. Improved Homologous Recombination-Based Targeting Strategies Using Nuclease-Induced Double-Strand Breaks

One approach developed to overcome the low frequency of gene targeting obtained with the basic homologous recombination strategies described above is to introduce a double-strand break (DSB) into the target locus. This approach is based on the observation that a chromosomal double-strand break can stimulate homologous recombination frequencies by up to 1000-fold or more [32].

4.1. Introduction of DSBs Using the Endonuclease I-*SceI*

The most developed strategy for DSB-induced targeting involves the use of the endonuclease I-*SceI* from *Saccharomyces cerevisiae* [32]. I-*SceI* is an intron-encoded homing endonuclease, which is involved in the copying (or homing) of the intron from an intron-containing allele of the 21S ribosomal gene to an intronless allele of the same gene [33]. I-*SceI* is an extremely rare cutting enzyme that has an 18bp recognition sequence that is predicted to be absent from most mammalian-sized genomes [32]. This is important in the context of using I-*SceI* for the manipulation of mammalian genomes, because the restriction of any endogenous recognition sites could lead to undesirable consequences.

A generalised I-*SceI*-based gene targeting strategy consists of two steps (Figure 7) [32, 34, 35]. In the first step, positive and negative selectable markers flanked by an I-*SceI* site are introduced into the target locus by homologous recombination using a replacement vector and a positive selection. In the second step, the locus is retargeted by cotransfection of an I-*SceI* expressing plasmid and a second replacement vector. I-*SceI* introduces a DSB at the I-*SceI* site, which enhances homologous recombination between the target locus and the vector. No selection markers or I-*SecI* recognition sequences remain after the second step and targeted clones are identified using a negative selection. This strategy is similar in principle to the tag-and-exchange strategy (section 4.3.2.), but is much improved because the frequency of recombination achieved in the second step is up to 5000-fold higher than conventional homologous recombination [34, 35]. An I-*SceI* approach has also been shown to enhance the intrachromosomal homologous recombination step of a hit-and-run strategy by 120-fold [34].

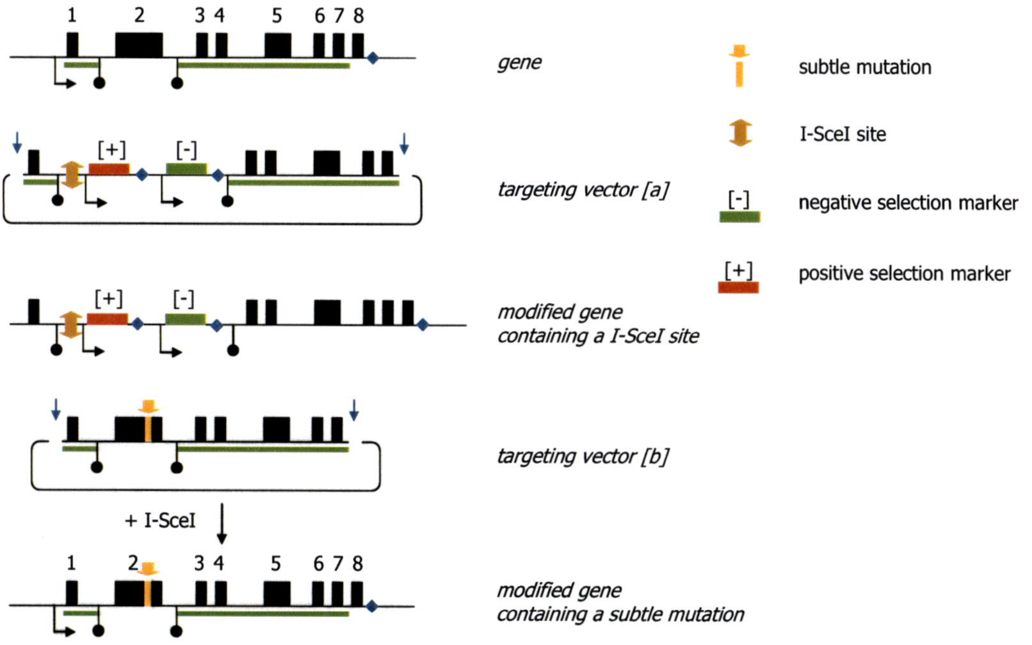

Figure 7. Genomic engineering using I-SceI induced double strand breaks. The targeting vector [a] contains a positive and a negative selection marker and a recognition site for the endonuclease I-SceI. These three features are incorporated into a specific genomic site by homologous recombination and targeted cell clones can be identified after selection for the positive marker gene. The modified gene locus can then be readily re-targeted by using a conventional targeting vector [b] devoid of any selection marker gene and a vector encoding I-SceI. Targeted cell clones can be identified after selection against the negative selection marker.

Recently it has also been shown that the introduction of chromosomal DSBs with I-*SceI* can be used to increase the frequency of homologous recombination between the single-stranded viral genome of AAV vectors and the chromosome. Therefore, combining AAV-based vectors with the generation of DSBs is another potentially useful gene targeting tool [36, 37].

4.2. Introduction of DSBs Using Designer Endonucleases

A major limitation to the I-*SceI* and similar endonuclease targeting strategies is that recognition sites for the enzyme have to first be inserted into the genome using a classical homologous recombination step, which is inefficient. Therefore, it would be very beneficial if endonucleases could be designed such that they recognise and site-specifically cleave unique natural sites in the genome. Two strategies have been used to test the feasibility of this approach.

The first strategy involves the generation of chimeric enzymes made up of a sequence-specific DNA binding domain fused to a non-specific nuclease domain. Initial attempts have used chimeric nucleases that consist of a three zinc finger DNA-binding domain linked to the non-specific cleavage domain of the type II restriction enzyme *FokI* [38]. Each zinc finger module recognises and binds a triplet within the target DNA sequence, and therefore a three-finger domain will bind a 9bp target sequence. Given that the nuclease domain must dimerize to be active, functional chimeric nuclease dimers will contain six zinc fingers in total and therefore will recognise an 18bp target sequence. The modular nature of zinc fingers should eventually allow the construction of binding domains, made up of an array of distinct zinc finger modules, each module being specific for a particular triplet, which are able to recognise any desired DNA sequence [39, 40]. A recent report has demonstrated the feasibility of using these zinc finger nucleases for gene targeting in mammalian cells. This report showed that chimeric nucleases could mediate gene targeting at target sites placed in a chromosome of human cells [41]. The efficiency of targeting was comparable to an equivalent I-*SceI* strategy and over 2000-fold higher than spontaneous homologous recombination, giving an absolute targeting efficiency of 0.4%. However, the continued expression of the nuclease was toxic possibly due to the non-specific cleavage of other sites. The future development of these approaches is now dependent on advances in the ability to engineer zinc finger combinations to specifically recognise a given target site.

The second strategy for engineering designer endonucleases is by recombining different domains from homing endonucleases. Two artificial endonucleases have been created by fusing domains of the homing endonucleases I-*DmoI* and I-*CreI* [42, 43]. These novel endonucleases have altered DNA specificity and cleave I-*DmoI*/I-*CreI* hybrid recognition sequences. Therefore, this strategy combined with directed protein evolution methods should also prove useful for the generation of novel endonucleases which specifically recognise unique natural target sequences in mammalian genomes.

4.3. Limitations

(a) I-*SceI* targeting strategies require the pre-introduction of I-*SceI* recognition sequences into the genome by a conventional homologous recombination step, which is inefficient. Therefore, they are essentially limited to the modification of the mouse genome. However, these strategies do improve the efficiency of the hit-and-run and tag-and-exchange strategies for the site-specific introduction of subtle modifications in mice.

(b) While designer endonuclease strategies show much promise for efficient site-specific genome modifications they are still in their infancy and currently the methods needed to engineer an enzyme to reliably and specifically recognise and cleave a given sequence in the genome is time consuming and far from perfected. However, in the future chimeric endonucleases should prove to be useful tools in situations where classical homologous recombination-based strategies are not feasible, including gene therapy applications and for the modification of non-murine mammalian genomes.

5. Site-Specific Recombinase-Based Targeting Strategies

Another approach to overcome the limitations of some of the classical homologous recombination-based gene targeting strategies is to use site-specific recombinases [15, 44]. Site-specific recombinases recognise and mediate the recombination between short (30-40bp or more), well-characterised DNA sequences resulting in the integration, excision or inversion of DNA fragments (Figure 8) [15]. Site-specific recombinases form two distinct families based on their sequence homology and biochemical properties [45]. The integrase family of recombinases, so-named because of their homology to λ integrase, use a conserved tyrosine catalytic residue. Other well-known members of this family include Cre recombinase from phage P1 and Flp invertase from *S. cerevisiae*. The second family is the invertase/resolvases family, so-called because of their homology to Tn3 resolvase, which use a conserved serine residue for catalysis. This family includes ΦC31 integrase from the *Streptomyces* ΦC31 phage. Members of both these families have been used to introduce site-specific modifications into the mammalian genome [15, 46], and here we focus on genome modification strategies involving the three most commonly used recombinases – Cre, Flp and ΦC31.

5.1. Basic Tools - Cre, Flp and ΦC31

5.1.1. Cre and Flp Recombinase Systems

The Cre and Flp systems are simple recombinase systems, each consisting of a single recombinase protein that recognises and mediates recombination between identical target recognition sequences. The Cre system is by far the most commonly used for mammalian genome modification, with the majority of reports describing its application in the mouse [15, 47]. Cre recognises and recombines target sites called loxP sites, which are 34bp in length and consist of a central 8bp spacer sequence flanked by two 13bp inverted repeats (Table 1). The central spacer is asymmetric, and this determines the orientation of the site and the outcome of the recombination reaction. Two Cre molecules, which each bind to one of the inverted repeats, cleave the DNA backbone and catalyse recombination in the central spacer region.

Flp recombinase recognises target sites called FRT [48, 49]. A full-length FRT site is 48bp in length and similar to loxP sites it consists of an asymmetric central 8bp spacer sequence, flanked by a pair of 13bp inverted repeats (Table 1). However, in contrast to loxP sites, it also contains a third 13bp direct repeat. Three Flp molecules, each bound to one of the repeats, cleave the DNA and mediate recombination in the central spacer region. Minimal FRT sites, which are 28 – 34bp in length and lack the third direct repeat, have been shown to effectively mediate the excision reaction but not integration [49, 50]. Flp recombinase is less active than Cre in mammalian cells, probably due to its lower thermostability [51]. This may partly explain why Flp is less frequently used to engineer genome modifications. Attempts to overcome this limitation have led to the creation of a mutant of Flp (Flpe) by cycling mutagenesis, which has enhanced thermostability and activity [52], and functions efficiently in mammalian cells [53]. However, in assays with chromosomally located FRT sites, Flpe still only shows 10% the recombination activity of Cre [54].

Table 1. target sites of Cre, Flp and fC31 recombinase. Inverted repeat sequences are shown in italics.

LoxP	*ATAACTTCGTATA*	ATGTATGC	TATACGAAGTTAT
	TATTGAAGCATAT	TACATACG	*ATATGCTTCAATA*
FRT	*GAAGTTCCTATTCCGAAGTTCCTATTC*	TCTAGAAA	GTATAGGAACTTC
	CTTCAAGGATAAGGCTTCAAGGATAAG	AGATCTTT	CA*TATCCTTGAAG*
attP	CCCCAACTGGGGTAACCT	TTG	A*GTTCT*C*T**CAGTTGGGGG*
	*GGGGTTGACC*CCAT*TGGA*	AAC	ACAAGAGAGTCAACCCCC
attB	GTGC*CAG*G*GC*G*T*G*CCC*	TTG	GGCTCCCCGGGCGCG
	CACGGTCCCGCACGGG	AAC	*CCGA*G*G*G*GCC*C*GCGC*

Box: Spacer/core sequence; Arrow: Cleavage point

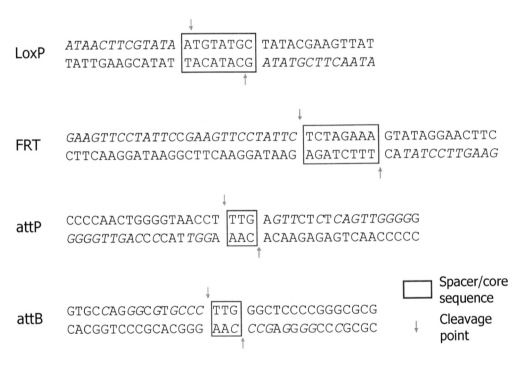

5.1.2. Limitation of Cre and Flp

One important consideration when using these recombinase systems for the integration of DNA into genome engineering is that the target site sequences for Cre and Flp are identical both before and after a recombination reaction. This is a problem because the integration of a plasmid into the genome creates two target sites in close proximity to each other (Figure 8), which then immediately become substrates for an excision reaction. Furthermore, the excision reaction is thermodynamically favoured over integration [55]. Therefore, the integrated DNA is highly unstable and will immediately be excised in the continued presence of the recombinase.

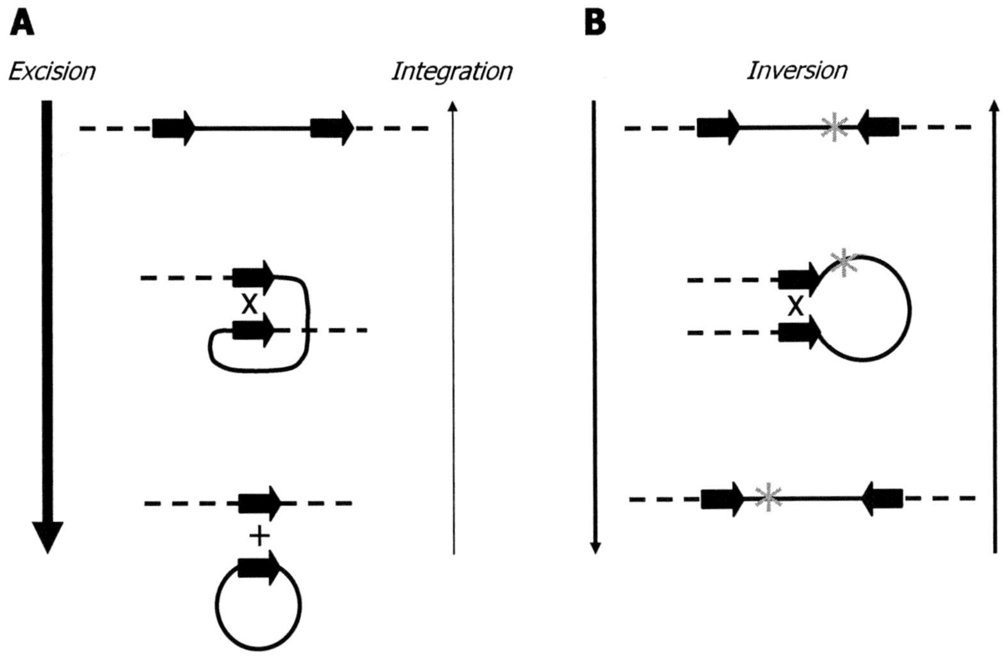

Figure 8. Reactions catalysed by "conservative" site-specific recombinases like Cre or FLP. Recombination target sites are identical before and after the recombination reaction. Recombination reactions mediated by these recombinases are therefore reversible.

5.1.3 ΦC31 Recombinase System

The ΦC31 recombinase system is more complex than the Cre and Flp systems [46, 56]. The biological role of the ΦC31 integrase is to mediate the integration of the ΦC31 phage into the *Streptomyces* genome by recombining target sites present in the phage and bacterial genomes, called attP (attachment site in phage genome) and attB (attachment site in bacterial genome), respectively [46]. Minimal functional attB and attP target sites are 39 and 34bp in length, respectively (Table 1) [57]. Although the two target sites are different, they both contain an identical 3bp central sequence, where the DNA is cleaved and the crossover occurs, flanked by imperfect inverted repeats. Recombination between attP and attB sites generates an integration product that is flanked by hybrid sites, called attL and attR, which are no longer substrates for the integrase in the absence of additional cofactors [58]. Therefore, unlike Cre and Flp, ΦC31 is a unidirectional integrase that only supports integration, which makes it an attractive tool for the integration of transgenes into the mammalian genome. Although wild type ΦC31 functions adequately in mammalian cells [57, 59, 60], it has a relatively low level of activity compared to Cre [54]. However, a modified version of the ΦC31 integrase that contains an introduced C-terminal nuclear localisation signal has a comparable level of activity [54]. Furthermore, attempts to directly evolve ΦC31 suggest that this may be a promising approach to further increase its efficiency [61].

5.2. Strategies for Recombinase-Mediated Deletion

The most common genome modification performed using site-specific recombinases is the deletion of DNA sequences. This is particularly important for the conditional inactivation or activation a gene at a certain developmental stage or tissue-specific manner, or the removal of selection markers from an integrated transgene cassette [15]. Since most of these strategies require the use of mouse ES cells they have typically only been performed in the mouse.

5.2.1. Gene Inactivation

The conditional inactivation of a gene is important for the study of genes, which are embryonic lethal if completely inactivated or, in some other way, prevent a precise analysis of its function in a particular tissue or stage of development [15]. The first step to achieve a conditional knockout using the Cre recombinase system is the generation of a transgenic mouse line in which all, or an essential part, of the gene to be inactivated is flanked by a tandem repeat of loxP sites (floxed) [15]. This is achieved by classical homologous recombination and the loxP sites are positioned in non-coding regions of the gene so that its function is not disrupted. The second step of the procedure involves delivering Cre recombinase at an appropriate developmental stage and/or to the appropriate tissue. This can be achieved using several approaches [15]. One approach involves the generation of a second line of transgenic mice, called the 'inducer line' that carries a Cre-encoding under the control of a tissue specific promoter or an inducible promoter. The inducer line is then bred with the mouse line containing the floxed allele, which results in the excision of the floxed DNA fragment from the genome, thereby inactivating the gene, in all cells that express the recombinase [62]. A second approach involves breeding mice containing the floxed allele with transgenic mice that contain the Cre recombinase open reading frame fused to the hormone-binding domain of a steroid receptor [63, 64]. In the absence of steroid hormone induction this Cre fusion protein remains in the cytoplasm. Upon hormone addition, which can be achieved either locally or systemically, Cre is transferred to nucleus whereupon it can mediate the excision reaction. A third approach for achieving the developmental stage and tissue-specific expression of Cre recombinase is to deliver the Cre-encoding transgene using viral vectors [65, 66].

5.2.2. Gene Activation

The conditional activation of a gene can be achieved using the same strategies as described for conditional gene inactivation (Figure 9) [15, 67, 68]. Except that in non-induced cells the gene to be activated is separated from its promoter by a floxed DNA fragment that contains a transcriptional stop signal. The induction of Cre activity results in the excision of the floxed stop signal and allows expression of the gene.

5.2.3. Selection Marker Removal

Another important application of recombinase-mediated DNA deletion is the removal of selection marker cassettes from an integrated transgene construct. One example already mentioned above (section 4.1.1) is the removal of the selection marker after a homologous recombination-based gene knock-in (Figure 2) [18]. In this example the selection marker is floxed. Once integrants have been identified using the appropriate selection agent, cells are then exposed to Cre recombinase and the selection marker is removed from the genome. This is important because selection marker cassettes may interfere with the expression of the co-integrated transgene and the targeted or neighbouring endogenous genes [15, 24, 25, 69, 70].

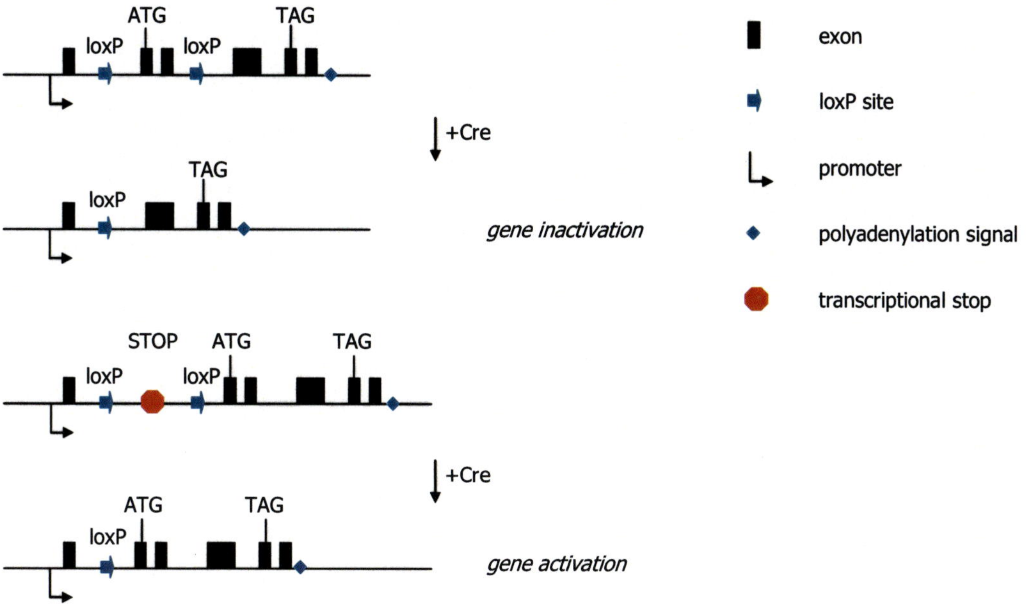

Figure 9. Cre-mediated excision of DNA fragments. Cre-mediated recombination can be utilised to activate or inactivate gene expression. Gene inactivation can be accomplished by deletion of essential gene sequences, which are flanked by identical direct repeats of loxP sites (i.e. floxed). Activation can be achieved by the deletion of a floxed transcriptional stop signal, which prevents transcription of the gene of interest.

5.3. Basic Strategies - Integration into a Single Target Site

5.3.1. Promoter-Trap Positive Selection

The simplest strategy to integrate a transgene into a target site pre-existing in the host genome by site-specific recombination is to use a plasmid containing the transgene and recombinase target sites together with an expression vector for the Cre or Flp recombinase. However, as discussed above (section 6.1.2) the problem with this approach is the integrated transgene will be excised immediately in the continued presence of the recombinase. Therefore, stable integration is a rare event. Nevertheless this problem can be overcome by the use of a stringent selection strategy. One such strategy using the Cre recombinase system involved the insertion of a promoter flanked by a loxP site into the genome using a classical homologous recombination strategy (Figure 10) [71]. Cells were then co-transfected with a plasmid containing a promoterless selection marker flanked by two directly orientated loxP sites, and a Cre-expressing plasmid. Cre recombinase mediates the excision of the floxed selectable marker from the plasmid backbone and its integration into the chromosomally located loxP target site. This links the pre-integrated promoter to the promoterless selection marker, which renders the targeted clones resistant to the selection agent, whereas clones that have randomly integrated the plasmid remain sensitive.

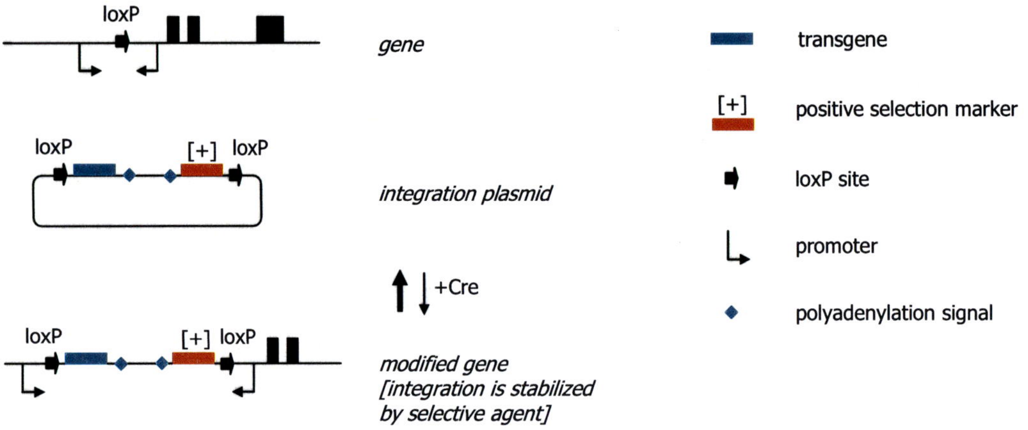

Figure 10. Cre-mediated integration of DNA fragments. Site-specific integration of transgene into a loxP site pre-existing in a genome. The loxP site is flanked by a promoter element, which can activate an incoming promoterless positive selection marker gene. Cells carrying the desired integration can be isolated after incubation in the appropriate selective agent. Note that in the continued presence of Cre and in the absence of the selective agent the integration reaction is readily reversed.

5.3.2. Mutated Lox Half SITES

An alternative to strategies that employ a stringent selection are approaches which favour the integration of a transgene over its excision. One such strategy using the Cre recombinase system involves the use of mutated loxP half sites (Figure 11) [72, 73]. These half sites contain mutations in one of their inverted repeats, which significantly reduces the binding affinity between Cre and that repeat. However, the mutated half site still remains a substrate for Cre because the binding of two Cre molecules to a loxP site is cooperative, so the Cre molecule bound to the unmodified repeat facilities the loading of the second Cre molecule onto the mutated inverted repeat. The first step of this strategy involved the random integration into the genome of a mutated half site (lox71) that contains alterations in the left repeat [72]. The second step involved the co-transfection of a plasmid containing a selectable marker flanked by a different half site (lox66) that has alterations in right repeat, and a Cre-expressing plasmid. Site-specific recombination between the two half sites resulted in the integration of the whole plasmid. This genomically integrated plasmid is flanked by one wild-type loxP site and a site (lox72) which has mutations in both inverted repeats. lox72 is a poor substrate for Cre recombinase and this prevents the excision of the integrated plasmid, thereby increasing the frequency of stable integration. This strategy could therefore be used with a simple positive selection, which resulted in up to 16% of resistant clones containing the desired modification. In this scenario Cre behaves in much the same way as the unidirectional ΦC31 integrase.

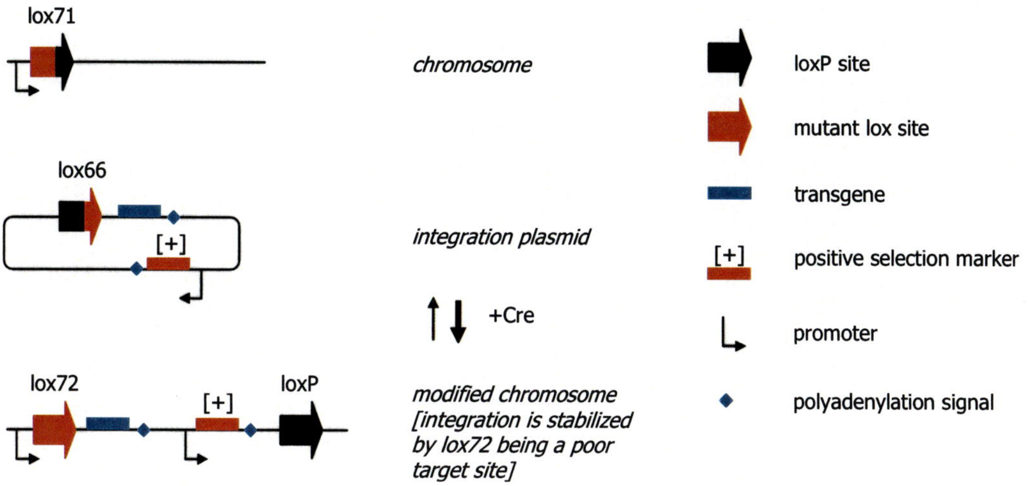

Figure 11. Cre-mediated integration of DNA fragments using mutant lox sites. A chromosomal target is established by integration of one mutant lox site (lox71). In a site-specific recombination event using a second mutant lox site (lox66) a transgene is integrated into the pre-defined site. Recombination of lox71 with lox66 results in the formation of a lox72 site and a loxP site. As lox72 is a poor target for Cre-recombinase the integration reaction is not readily reversed.

5.3.3. Unidirectional Recombinases

An obvious alternative strategy that overcomes the problem of the instability of the integrated transgene is to use a unidirectional recombinase such as the ΦC31 integrase. A ΦC31 integrase strategy has recently been tested in both human and mouse cells (Figure 12) [59]. The first step of this strategy involved the random integration of an attP site into the genome. In the second step the cells were co-transfected with a plasmid containing a selection marker cassette flanked by an attB site, and a ΦC31-expressing plasmid. A simple positive selection was used to identify clones that contained a site-specifically integrated plasmid in the genomic attP site. An analysis of resistant clones from human cell experiments revealed that 15% of clones contained the desired site-specific modification. Interestingly, in the majority of the other resistant clones the plasmid was found to have integrated into pseudo attP sites, which are native sites that have partial sequence identity to attP sites. None of the clones analysed contained multiple integrations. Further analysis revealed that a plasmid bearing an attB site could be integrated into 31 and 57 different pseudo sites in unmodified human and mouse cells, respectively. The use of a more stringent selection strategy which rendered targeted integrants resistant to the selection agents, but random or pseudo attP integrants sensitive, resulted in nearly 100% of resistant clones containing the desired integration at the inserted attP site [59].

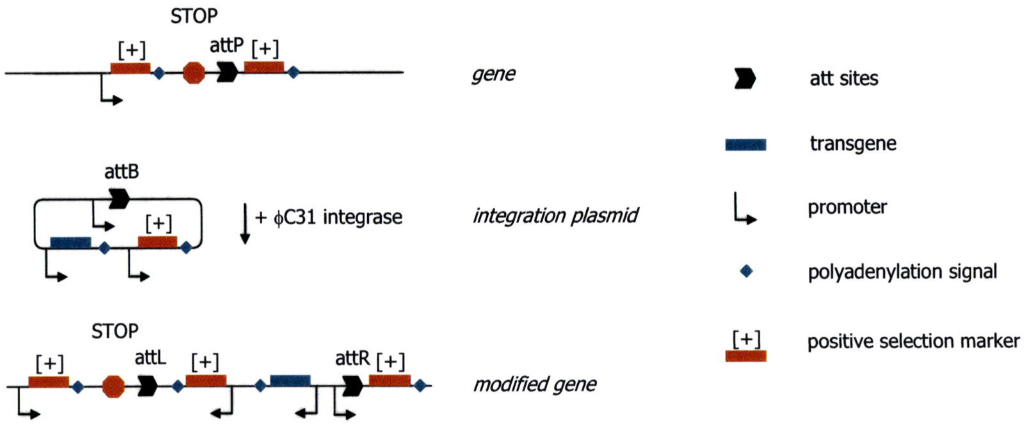

Figure 12. DNA integration mediated by the ΦC31 recombinase (adapted from [59]). A recombination target site (attP-attachment site in the ΦC31 phage genome) flanking a promoterless positive selection marker is placed into the host genome (using a second transcriptionally active positive selection marker). An incoming plasmid carrying the complementary attB site (bacterial attachment site) adjacent to a promoter element is site specifically inserted into the genomic location tagged by attP. The recombination reaction links the promoter element to the promoterless selection marker and thereby renders the cells resistant to the corresponding drug. The presence of a positive selection marker cassette on the incoming plasmid also allows for a simple positive selection to be performed. The reaction also generates two sites (attL and attR) which are no longer recognized by the ΦC31 recombinase in the absence of other co-factors. Therefore the recombination reaction is irreversible. Note that the entire incoming plasmid is incorporated into the host genome.The potential applications of the ΦC31 integrases ability to mediate transgene integration into native pseudo attP sites have started to be explored. One report has described the stable ΦC31 integrase-mediated integration of human factor IX (hFIX) into the genome of mice [74]. A plasmid containing an hFIX expression cassette flanked by an attB site and a ΦC31-expressing plasmid were co-injected into mice using the high-pressure tail vein injection method. The hFIX cassette was site-specifically integrated into liver cells at two pseudo attP sites and this resulted in long-term therapeutically useful hFIX serum levels [74]. Several studies have shown the potential of ΦC31 integrase-mediated transgene integration for the *ex vivo* correction of genetic human skin disease [75-77]. In the first proof-of-principle study a correct version of the human type VII collagen gene was integrated into pseudo attP sites in isolated human keratinocytes mutant for this gene [75]. Defects in this gene cause a lethal childhood skin disease called recessive dystrophic epidermolysis bullosa (RDEB). The grafting of these corrected cells onto immune-deficient mice resulted in the regeneration of human skin tissue that exhibited stable correction of the RDEB phenotype [75]. Collectively these studies show the utility of ΦC31 integrase for both gene therapy and animal transgenesis applications.

5.4. Improved Strategies - Recombinase-Mediated Cassette Exchange (RMCE)

Although very useful for DNA integration, these strategies are limited by the fact that they result in the co-integration of at least one selectable marker, and, in most cases, bacterial sequences from the plasmid backbone. These are known to have adverse effects on the expression of the co-integrated transgenes [69, 70]. One way to overcome these limitations is to site-specifically integrate transgenes using a technique called recombinase-mediated cassette exchange (RMCE). RMCE involves the exchange of a chromosomally placed DNA cassette for a cassette located on an incoming plasmid [49, 55]. Four types of strategy have been developed that achieve this.

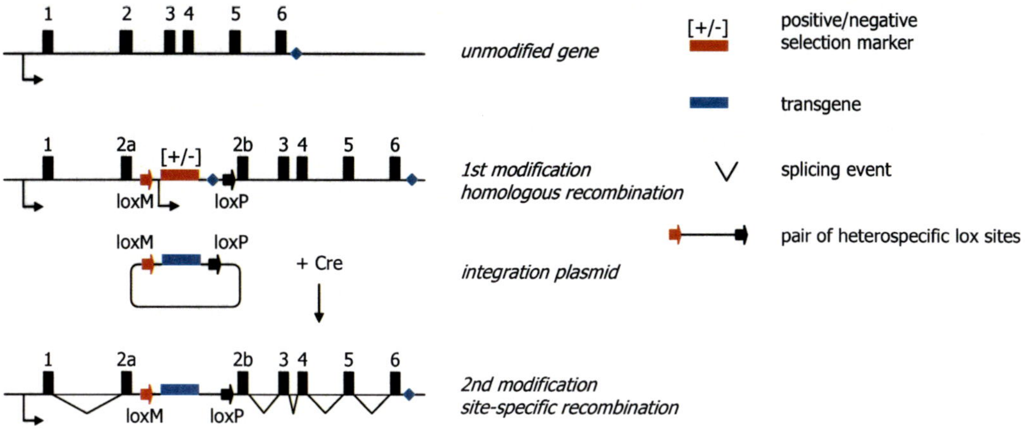

Figure 13. Recombinase mediated cassette exchange (RMCE) using Cre recombinase (adapted from [84]). A hypothetical gene is first targeted using conventional homologous recombination to insert a pair of heterospecific (i.e. incompatible) directly repeated lox sites. In this process a positive/negative selection marker gene (e.g. hypoxanthine-phospho-ribosyl-transferase, HPRT) is inserted into the genome (and cells carrying the modification can be identified after selection in the corresponding drug). By using Cre-mediated recombination the selection marker is subsequently exchanged for a transgene, which is flanked by an identical pair of heterospecific lox sites. Cells, which have successfully undergone site-specific recombination can be isolated after negative selection against the positive/negative selection marker gene. The cassette exchange is thermodynamically favoured as the incoming integration plasmid is in significant molar excess over the selection marker cassette present in the host genome.

5.4.1. Incompatible Target Sites

Strategies based on the use of incompatible (heterospecific) target sites can be used with either the Cre or Flp recombinase systems (Figure 13) [78-84]. The first step of the strategies involves the integration of a DNA cassette that is flanked by two incompatible target sites in the same orientation, one wild-type and one that has a spacer mutation, into the host genome. In the second step cells are co-transfected with a plasmid that contains a transgene cassette flanked by the same pair of incompatible sites and a recombinase-expressing plasmid. Since the two sites on each cassette are incompatible they can only recombine with the identical site present on the other cassette. This results in the genomic cassette being exchanged for the incoming cassette via a double-reciprocal crossover (Figure 13). The integrated cassette is stable because the incompatibility of the target sites prevents it from being excised and the transfection of a vast excess of the incoming plasmid prevents the replaced cassette from being exchanged back into the genome. Importantly, because the only part of the incoming plasmid to be integrated is the transgene cassette, no bacterial plasmid backbone sequences are being transferred. Moreover, if a positive/negative selection marker gene is incorporated into the cassette that is pre-inserted into the genome, clones that have undergone a cassette exchange can be identified using a negative selection and no selection marker will remain in the genome.

To date, the most efficient application of this strategy has been achieved using Cre recombinase and DNA cassettes flanked by directly orientated loxP and lox2272 sites [84]. lox2272 sites contain two point mutations in their central 8bp spacer sequence, which makes them incompatible with loxP sites [84, 85]. RMCE experiments in ES cells using a simple negative selection resulted in over 90% of selected clones having the desired targeted modification [84]. One attractive application of mammalian transgenesis is the production of useful recombinant proteins in the milk [86]. This loxP/lox2272 RMCE strategy has been shown to mediate the efficient insertion of a foreign gene into the murine β-casein gene (a highly expressed gene in the lactating mammary gland) in mouse ES cells [84]. This demonstrates the potential of this and similar strategies for the expression of foreign proteins in the milk of transgenic animals.

5.4.2. Inverted Target Sites

In a second strategy used to achieve RMCE the DNA cassettes to be exchanged are flanked with a pair of inverted loxP sites (Figure 14) [82]. In this situation any recombination that occurs between the loxP sites flanking the integrated cassette results in an inversion and not a deletion. This has the disadvantage that additional screening may be needed to identify clones that contain the integrated cassette in the desired orientation; however, this can be advantageous in situations that require transgene expression to be evaluated in both orientations [87]. The use of this strategy with wild-type loxP sites in murine erythroleukemia cells using a negative selection, resulted in almost 100% of selected having the desired modification [82]. However, the same strategy in mouse ES cells only result in 10-50% of selected clones having been correctly targeted [82]. In both experiments each orientation was found in approximately half of the targeted clones. The use of this strategy in erythroleukemia cells without any selection resulted in 4-16% of transfected clones undergoing a stable cassette exchange [82].

5.4.3. Combination of Recombinases

A third strategy to achieve RMCE uses both the Cre and Flp recombinases [88] . For this approach a DNA cassette flanked by both a loxP and an FRT site (froxing) is integrated into the genome at random or at a predetermined site by homologous recombination. In the second step cells are co-transfected with a plasmid bearing a froxed cassette and a Cre/Flpe-expressing plasmid. Incoming cassettes are stably integrated because loxP and FRT sites share no sequence homology and are therefore incompatible and cannot support an excision reaction. The use of this strategy in ES cells with a promoter-trap positive selection resulted in 61-78% of resistant clones having the desired targeted integration [88]. However, it was not tested with a negative selection only, and such a selection would be expected to be less efficient than the promoter-trap positive selection. Therefore, this strategy is less efficient than a loxP/lox2272 approach [84]. Some clones were identified that had only undergone recombination between the loxP sites [88]. This was most likely due to the lower activity of Flpe compared to Cre in mammalian cells and may in part explain the reduced efficiency of this strategy [54].

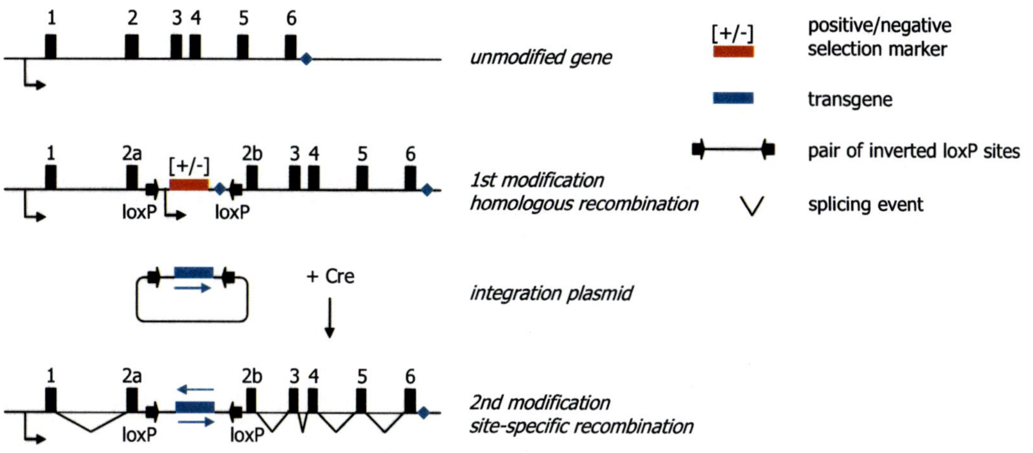

Figure 14. Recombinase mediated cassette exchange using Cre recombinase and a pair of inverted loxP sites. A hypothetical gene is first targeted using conventional homologous recombination to insert a pair of inverted loxP sites. In this process a positive/negative selection marker gene (e.g. hypoxanthine-phospho-ribosyl-transferase, HPRT) is inserted into the genome. Cre catalyses the inversion of DNA segments flanked by inverted lox sites. As the incoming integration plasmid is in significant molar excess over the selection marker cassette in the host genome, the insertion of the transgene is thermodynamically favoured. Note that the inserted transgene can be integrated in both orientations. However, only one orientation will lead to transgene expression. Therefore only 50% of the cells thus modified will express the gene.

5.4.4. RMCE with Unidirectional Recombinases

A fourth strategy recently described to achieve RMCE uses the unidirectional ϕC31 recombinase [60]. In this strategy a DNA cassette containing ΦC31 integrase flanked by attP was randomly integrated into the genome of ES cells (Figure 15). The expression of ΦC31 integrase was driven from a promoter positioned outside of the attP-flanked region in the integrated construct. These cells were transfected with a plasmid containing an attB-flanked promoterless selection marker. Upon targeted integration of the incoming cassette the pre-integrated promoter is linked with the promoterless selection marker which renders cells resistant to the selective agent. With this stringent promoter-trap selection up to 89% of the resistant clones were found to have undergone a stable site specific recombination reaction, however, only 33% of these had undergone a complete cassette exchange. The other site-specific integrants were generated by a single reciprocal recombination between one of the attP and attB sites, which resulted in the integration of the entire incoming plasmid. This failure of the majority of clones to recombine at both sets of sites is most likely due to the poor activity of wild-type ΦC31 in mammalian cells [54]. Although attempts to achieve selection-free cassette exchange failed, no attempts were made to evaluate the use of a simple negative selection. Such a selection would be expected to be less efficient than a stringent promoter-trap selection and is therefore less efficient than a loxP/lox2272 site strategy [84].

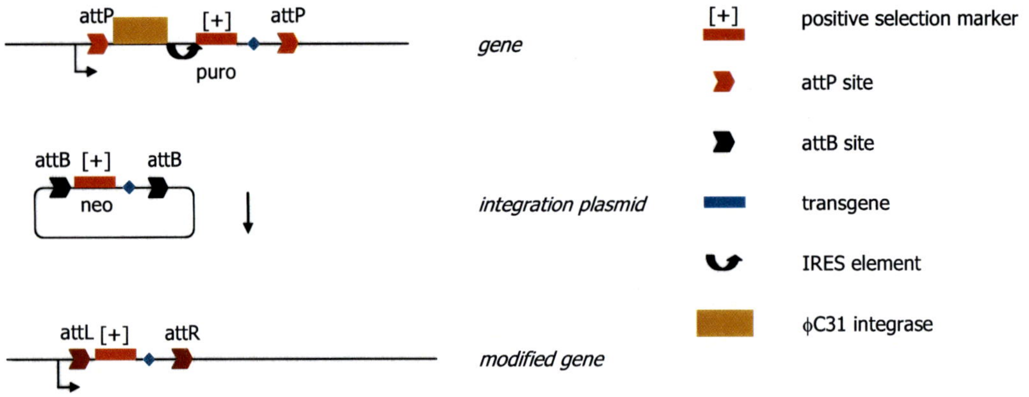

Figure 15. Cassette exchange using the ΦC31 recombinase (adapted from [60]). The ΦC31 recombinase gene and a positive selection marker expression cassette (a puromycin-resistance gene linked via an internal ribosomal entry site, IRES) flanked by two attP sites is integrated into the host genome. The promoter driving the expression of the two genes lies outside the attP sites. Subsequently the attP-flanked cassette is exchanged for a second promoterless selection marker gene (a neomycin-resistance gene), which is flanked by two attB sites. The second marker gene can only be activated by integration adjacent to the promoter element. A transgene of interest could theoretically be linked to the second selection marker gene via an IRES element.

5.5. Strategies Using Designer Recombinases

The limitation of almost all of the recombinase strategies described so far for the site-specific modifications of the genome is that a recombinase target site has to be first inserted into the genome using a classical homologous recombination step, which is inefficient. Therefore several approaches have been used to assess the feasibility of engineering designer recombinases that are able to recognise predetermined unique natural chromosomal sites.

The first approach involves the directed evolution of recombinases using multiple cycles of DNA shuffling/mutagenesis and selection [89]. The potential of this approach has been demonstrated by the generation of new variants of Cre and Flp that have an altered sequence recognition specificity [90-92], and a ΦC31 variant that favours the integration of a transgene into a native pseudo attP site on human chromosome 8 [61]. The use of an appropriate screen is important for the outcome of this approach. The application of a positive screen only, i.e. one that only identifies recombinase variants that recognise a new target site, tends to result in the identification of variants that have a relaxation of target-site specificity and can recognise both the new and wild-type target sites [90]. Whereas a combination of positive and negative screening, i.e. a screen for variants that bind the new site but not the wild-type one, will result in variants with an altered specificity [91].

A second more radical approach for creating designer recombinases involves changing the site specificity of the enzyme by replacing its DNA binding domain with another binding domain that recognises a new target sequence [93]; this is similar in principle to the strategy for creating designer endonucleases discussed above (section 5.2). The feasibility of this approach has been tested using Tn3 resolvase, a member of the serine family of recombinases [93]. This recombinase was selected for several reasons. Firstly, the crystal structure of the closely related E. coli γ/δ resolvase is known [94]. Secondly, Tn3 recombinase mutants that recognize a short 28bp target site (instead of the usual 120bp "res" recognition site) are available. Finally, as a serine-recombinase the DNA-binding domain and catalytic domain of Tn3 resolvase are structurally and spatially distinct and therefore the DNA-binding domain can be replaced with minimal effect on the catalytic domain (Figure 16) [93, 94]. This is in contrast to Cre and Flp, which have catalytic and DNA-binding domains that are inseparable [95]. Several chimeric Tn3 resolvases, called Z-resolvases, were created by fusing the catalytic domain from a hyperactive mutant Tn3 resolvase with the three zinc finger DNA-binding domain from the mouse transcription factor Zif268 using short linker peptides (Figure 16) [93]. Z-resolvase dimers were able to mediate efficient recombination at synthetic target sites, called Z-sites, which contained two 9bp Zif268 target sites (Figure 16). Given the potential for the customisation of zinc finger DNA-binding domains (see discussion in section 5.2) these results pave the way to generating designer recombinases that act at a chosen native target sequence.

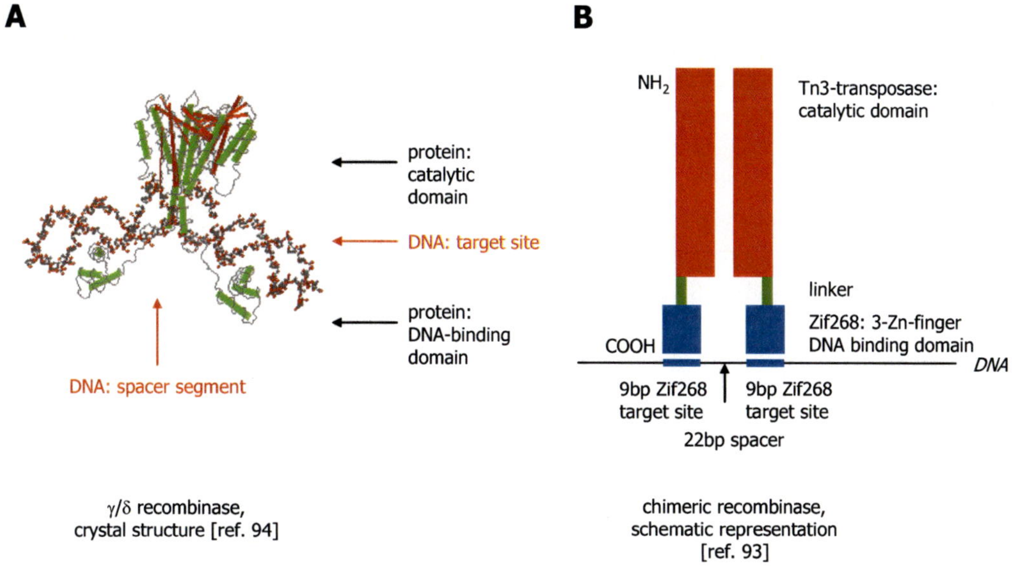

Figure 16. Chimeric recombinases. Panel A: Serine-recombinases (like the γ/δ recombinase shown) have a DNA binding domain that is physically separated from the catalytic domain. Panel B: The natural DNA binding domain of the resolvase-type recombinases can therefore be exchanged for other domains which recognize DNA targets. The mouse Zn-finger transcription factor Zif268 can be evolved in vitro to recognize a DNA sequence of choice. Therefore recombinases can theoretically be engineered to catalyse site-specific integration into defined genomic sites.

5.6. Limitations

(a) Most of the strategies for recombinase-mediated deletion, integration into a single target site and RMCE require the pre-integration of recombinase target sites into the genome by homologous recombination, which is inefficient and limits their applicability to the modification of mammals other than mice or gene therapy. This could potentially be overcome by the use of ΦC31-mediated integration into pseudo attP sites or the use of designer recombinases engineered to recognise a chosen native target site.

(b) Strategies involving recombinase-mediated integration of a transgene into a single target site are limited by the co-integration of selection marker and bacterial vector sequences which can have an adverse effect on the expression of the transgene. This limitation can be overcome using RMCE.

(c) While designer recombinase strategies show much promise, they are still at an early stage of development and, as discussed above for the designer endonucleases, the methods needed to engineer these proteins are time consuming and far from perfected.

6. Retroviral-Based Targeting Strategies

A further approach to achieve site-specific integration into the mammalian genome has involved attempts to target retroviral integration by fusing DNA-binding domains to retroviral integrases, the proteins responsible for integrating the cDNA copy of the virus into the host chromosomes [96]. DNA-binding domains that have been tested in such strategies include those of the phage λ repressor [97], *E.coli* LexA repressor [97, 98] and the mouse transcription factor Zif268 [99], and a synthetic domain consisting of six zinc fingers called E2C [100]. These integrase fusion proteins were shown to mediate retroviral integration into specific sites in optimised reactions *in vitro*. However, attempts to introduce these fusions into the retroviral genome have proved problematic and the feasibility of using this strategy to achieve efficient site-specific integration into the mammalian genome remains to be demonstrated [96, 98, 99].

7. Conclusions

These site-specific modification strategies are key tools for the precise alteration of mammalian genomes and have broad applications in basic research, biomedicine and biotechnology. They enable the insertion of a single copy of a transgene or therapeutic gene into a predefined chromosomal locus that is known to be permissive for achieving a stable level of expression over an extended period of time. The big limitation of the majority of these strategies is that they depend on at least one step of classical homologous recombination, which is inefficient. Therefore, while they work well in mice via the use of ES cells, they are very difficult to extend to more commercially useful mammals and are inappropriate for somatic cell gene therapy. One exception is strategies involving ΦC31 integrase-mediated transgene integration into native pseudo attP sites, which bypass the need for homologous recombination. Therefore, ΦC31 strategies show much promise for both gene therapy and animal transgenesis applications [46]. Attractive future strategies to overcome the constraints imposed by classical homologous recombination will involve the use of chimeric endonucleases, recombinases and viral integrases that have been engineered to act at chosen native sequences within mammalian chromosomes [41-43, 93, 96].

References

[1] Niidome, T. and L. Huang, Gene therapy progress and prospects: nonviral vectors. *Gene Ther*, 2002. 9(24): p. 1647-52.

[2] Colosimo, A., et al., Transfer and expression of foreign genes in mammalian cells. *Biotechniques*, 2000. 29(2): p. 314-331.

[3] Nishikawa, M. and L. Huang, Nonviral vectors in the new millennium: delivery barriers in gene transfer. *Hum Gene Ther*, 2001. 12(8): p. 861-70.

[4] Lund, A.H., M. Duch, and F.S. Pedersen, Transcriptional Silencing of Retroviral Vectors. *J Biomed Sci*, 1996. 3(6): p. 365-378.

[5] Pannell, D. and J. Ellis, Silencing of gene expression: implications for design of retrovirus vectors. *Rev Med Virol*, 2001. 11(4): p. 205-17.

[6] Pfeifer, A., et al., Transgenesis by lentiviral vectors: lack of gene silencing in mammalian embryonic stem cells and preimplantation embryos. *Proc Natl Acad Sci U S A*, 2002. 99(4): p. 2140-5.

[7] Hofmann, A., et al., Efficient transgenesis in farm animals by lentiviral vectors. *EMBO Rep*, 2003. 4(11): p. 1054-60.

[8] Dutheil, N., et al., Adeno-associated virus site-specifically integrates into a muscle-specific DNA region. *Proc Natl Acad Sci U S A*, 2000. 97(9): p. 4862-6.

[9] Nakai, H., et al., Extrachromosomal recombinant adeno-associated virus vector genomes are primarily responsible for stable liver transduction in vivo. *J Virol*, 2001. 75(15): p. 6969-76.

[10] Nakai, H., et al., AAV serotype 2 vectors preferentially integrate into active genes in mice. *Nat Genet,* 2003. 34(3): p. 297-302.

[11] Huttner, N.A., et al., Analysis of site-specific transgene integration following cotransduction with recombinant adeno-associated virus and a rep encoding plasmid. *J Gene Med*, 2003. 5(2): p. 120-9.

[12] Izsvak, Z. and Z. Ivics, Sleeping Beauty Transposition: Biology and Applications for Molecular Therapy. *Molecular Therapy*, 2004. 9(2): p. 147-156.

[13] Clark, A.J., et al., Chromosomal position effects and the modulation of transgene expression. *Reprod Fertil Dev*, 1994. 6(5): p. 589-98.

[14] Baum, C., et al., Chance or necessity? Insertional Mutagenesis in Gene Therapy and Its Consequences. *Molecular Therapy*, 2004. 9(1): p. 5-13.

[15] Kolb, A.F., Genome engineering using site-specific recombinases. *Cloning Stem Cells*, 2002. 4(1): p. 65-80.

[16] Portlock, J.L. and M.P. Calos, Site-specific genomic strategies for gene therapy. Current Opinion in *Molecular Therapeutics*, 2003. 5(4): p. 376-382.

[17] Vasquez, K.M., et al., Manipulating the mammalian genome by homologous recombination. *Proceedings of the National Academy of Sciences of the United States of America*, 2001. 98(15): p. 8403-8410.

[18] van der Weyden, L., D.J. Adams, and A. Bradley, Tools for targeted manipulation of the mouse genome. *Physiol Genomics*, 2002. 11(3): p. 133-64.

[19] Muller, U., Ten years of gene targeting: targeted mouse mutants, from vector design to phenotype analysis. *Mech Dev*, 1999. 82(1-2): p. 3-21.

[20] Clark, J. and B. Whitelaw, A future for transgenic livestock. *Nature Reviews Genetics*, 2003. 4(10): p. 825-833.

[21] Hasty, P. and A. Bradley, *Gene targeting vectors for mammalian cells*, in Gene Targeting: A Practical Approach, A.L. Joyner, Editor. 1993, IRL Press: Oxford. p. 1-31.

[22] Cheah, S.S. and R.R. Behringer, Contemporary gene targeting strategies for the novice. *Mol Biotechnol*, 2001. 19(3): p. 297-304.

[23] Hasty, P., et al., Introduction of a subtle mutation into the Hox-2.6 locus in embryonic stem cells. *Nature*, 1991. 350(6315): p. 243-6.

[24] Hug, B.A., et al., Analysis of mice containing a targeted deletion of beta-globin locus control region 5' hypersensitive site 3. *Mol Cell Biol*, 1996. 16(6): p. 2906-12.

[25] Pham, C.T., et al., Long-range disruption of gene expression by a selectable marker cassette. *Proc Natl Acad Sci U S A,* 1996. 93(23): p. 13090-5.

[26] Valancius, V. and O. Smithies, Testing an "in-out" targeting procedure for making subtle genomic modifications in mouse embryonic stem cells. *Mol Cell Biol*, 1991. 11(3): p. 1402-8.

[27] Gschwind, M. and G. Huber, Introduction of hereditary disease-associated mutations into the beta-amyloid precursor protein gene of mouse embryonic stem cells: a comparison of homologous recombination methods. *Mol Cell Biol,* 1998.18(8):p.4651-8.

[28] Askew, G.R., T. Doetschman, and J.B. Lingrel, Site-directed point mutations in embryonic stem cells: a gene-targeting tag-and-exchange strategy. *Mol Cell Biol*, 1993. 13(7): p. 4115-24.

[29] Stacey, A., et al., Use of double-replacement gene targeting to replace the murine alpha-lactalbumin gene with its human counterpart in embryonic stem cells and mice. *Mol Cell Biol*, 1994. 14(2): p. 1009-16.

[30] Cearley, J.A. and P.J. Detloff, Efficient repetitive alteration of the mouse Huntington's disease gene by management of background in the tag and exchange gene targeting strategy. *Transgenic Res*, 2001. 10(6): p. 479-88.

[31] Moore, R.C., et al., Double replacement gene targeting for the production of a series of mouse strains with different prion protein gene alterations. *Biotechnology* (N Y), 1995. 13(9): p. 999-1004.

[32] Jasin, M., Genetic manipulation of genomes with rare-cutting endonucleases. *Trends in Genetics,* 1996. 12(6): p. 224.

[33] Dujon, B., Group I introns as mobile genetic elements: facts and mechanistic speculations--a review. *Gene*, 1989. 82(1): p. 91-114.

[34] Donoho, G., M. Jasin, and P. Berg, Analysis of gene targeting and intrachromosomal homologous recombination stimulated by genomic double-strand breaks in mouse embryonic stem cells. *Molecular and Cellular Biology*, 1998. 18(7): p. 4070-4078.

[35] Cohen-Tannoudji, M., et al., I-SceI-induced gene replacement at a natural locus in embryonic stem cells. *Molecular and Cellular Biology*, 1998. 18(3): p. 1444-1448.

[36] Miller, D.G., L.M. Petek, and D.W. Russell, Human Gene Targeting by Adeno-Associated Virus Vectors Is Enhanced by DNA Double-Strand Breaks. *Mol. Cell. Biol.*, 2003. 23(10): p. 3550-3557.

[37] Porteus, M.H., et al., Efficient gene targeting mediated by adeno-associated virus and DNA double-strand breaks. *Mol Cell Biol*, 2003. 23(10): p. 3558-65.

[38] Chandrasegaran, S. and J. Smith, Chimeric restriction enzymes: what is next? *Biol Chem*, 1999. 380(7-8): p. 841-8.
[39] Choo, Y. and M. Isalan, Advances in zinc finger engineering. *Curr Opin Struct Biol*, 2000. 10(4): p. 411-6.
[40] Jantz, D., et al., The design of functional DNA-binding proteins based on zinc finger domains. *Chem Rev,* 2004. 104(2): p. 789-99.
[41] Porteus, M.H. and D. Baltimore, Chimeric Nucleases Stimulate Gene Targeting in Human Cells. *Science*, 2003. 300(5620): p. 763-.
[42] Chevalier, B.S., et al., Design, activity, and structure of a highly specific artificial endonuclease. *Mol Cell*, 2002. 10(4): p. 895-905.
[43] Epinat, J.C., et al., A novel engineered meganuclease induces homologous recombination in yeast and mammalian cells. *Nucleic Acids Res*, 2003. 31(11): p. 2952-62.
[44] Sorrell, D.A. and A.F. Kolb, Targeted integration of transgenes into the mammalian genome using site-specific recombinases: Tools and strategies, in Recent research developments in analytical biochemistry, S.G. Pandalai, Editor. 2003, Transworld Research Network: *Trivandrum*. p. 133-153.
[45] Stark, W.M., M.R. Boocock, and D.J. Sherratt, Catalysis by site-specific recombinases. *Trends Genet*, 1992. 8(12): p. 432-9.
[46] Groth, A.C. and M.P. Calos, Phage integrases: biology and applications. *J Mol Biol*, 2004. 335(3): p. 667-78.
[47] Nagy, A., Cre recombinase: the universal reagent for genome tailoring. *Genesis*, 2000. 26(2): p. 99-109.
[48] Kilby, N.J., M.R. Snaith, and J.A. Murray, Site-specific recombinases: tools for genome engineering. *Trends Genet*, 1993. 9(12): p. 413-21.
[49] Bode, J., et al., The transgeneticist's toolbox: novel methods for the targeted modification of eukaryotic genomes. *Biol Chem*, 2000. 381(9-10): p. 801-13.
[50] Senecoff, J.F., R.C. Bruckner, and M.M. Cox, The FLP recombinase of the yeast 2-micron plasmid: characterization of its recombination site. *Proc Natl Acad Sci U S A*, 1985. 82(21): p. 7270-4.
[51] Buchholz, F., et al., Different thermostabilities of FLP and Cre recombinases: implications for applied site-specific recombination. *Nucleic Acids Res*, 1996. 24(21): p. 4256-62.
[52] Buchholz, F., P.O. Angrand, and A.F. Stewart, Improved properties of FLP recombinase evolved by cycling mutagenesis. *Nat Biotechnol*, 1998. 16(7): p. 657-62.
[53] Rodriguez, C.I., et al., High-efficiency deleter mice show that FLPe is an alternative to Cre-loxP. *Nat Genet*, 2000. 25(2): p. 139-40.
[54] Andreas, S., et al., Enhanced efficiency through nuclear localization signal fusion on phage phi C31-integrase: activity comparison with Cre and FLPe recombinase in mammalian cells. *Nucleic Acids Research*, 2002. 30(11): p. 2299-2306.
[55] Baer, A. and J. Bode, Coping with kinetic and thermodynamic barriers: RMCE, an efficient strategy for the targeted integration of transgenes. *Curr Opin Biotechnol*, 2001. 12(5): p. 473-80.
[56] Smith, M.C. and H.M. Thorpe, Diversity in the serine recombinases. *Mol Microbiol*, 2002. 44(2): p. 299-307.

[57] Groth, A.C., et al., A phage integrase directs efficient site-specific integration in human cells. *Proc Natl Acad Sci* U S A, 2000. 97(11): p. 5995-6000.

[58] Thorpe, H.M. and M.C. Smith, In vitro site-specific integration of bacteriophage DNA catalyzed by a recombinase of the resolvase/invertase *family. Proc Natl Acad Sci U S A*, 1998. 95(10): p. 5505-10.

[59] Thyagarajan, B., et al., Site-specific genomic integration in mammalian cells mediated by phage phiC31 integrase. *Mol Cell Biol*, 2001. 21(12): p. 3926-34.

[60] Belteki, G., et al., Site-specific cassette exchange and germline transmission with mouse ES cells expressing phi C31 integrase. *Nature Biotechnology*, 2003. 21(3): p. 321-324.

[61] Sclimenti, C.R., B. Thyagarajan, and M.P. Calos, Directed evolution of a recombinase for improved genomic integration at a native human sequence. *Nucleic Acids Res,* 2001. 29(24): p. 5044-51.

[62] Kulkarni, R.N., et al., Tissue-specific knockout of the insulin receptor in pancreatic beta cells creates an insulin secretory defect similar to that in type 2 diabetes. *Cell,* 1999. 96(3): p. 329-39.

[63] Feil, R., et al., Ligand-activated site-specific recombination in mice. *Proc Natl Acad Sci U S A*, 1996. 93(20): p. 10887-90.

[64] Feil, R., et al., Regulation of Cre recombinase activity by mutated estrogen receptor ligand-binding domains. *Biochem Biophys Res Commun*, 1997. 237(3): p. 752-7.

[65] Chang, B.H., et al., Liver-specific inactivation of the abetalipoproteinemia gene completely abrogates very low density lipoprotein/low density lipoprotein production in a viable conditional knockout mouse. *J Biol Chem*, 1999. 274(10): p. 6051-5.

[66] Rinaldi, A., K.R. Marshall, and C.M. Preston, A non-cytotoxic herpes simplex virus vector which expresses Cre recombinase directs efficient site specific recombination. *Virus Res*, 1999. 65(1): p. 11-20.

[67] Lakso, M., et al., Targeted oncogene activation by site-specific recombination in transgenic mice. *Proc Natl Acad Sci* U S A, 1992. 89(14): p. 6232-6.

[68] Grieshammer, U., et al., Muscle-specific cell ablation conditional upon Cre-mediated DNA recombination in transgenic mice leads to massive spinal and cranial motoneuron loss. *Dev Biol*, 1998. 197(2): p. 234-47.

[69] Jaenisch, R., Transgenic animals. Science, 1988. 240(4858): p. 1468-74.

[70] Clark, A.J., G. Harold, and F.E. Yull, Mammalian cDNA and prokaryotic reporter sequences silence adjacent transgenes in transgenic mice. *Nucleic Acids Res*, 1997. 25(5): p. 1009-14.

[71] Kolb, A.F., et al., Insertion of a foreign gene into the beta-casein locus by Cre-mediated site-specific recombination. *Gene*, 1999. 227(1): p. 21-31.

[72] Araki, K., M. Araki, and K. Yamamura, Targeted integration of DNA using mutant lox sites in embryonic stem cells. *Nucleic Acids Res*, 1997. 25(4): p. 868-72.

[73] Albert, H., et al., Site-specific integration of DNA into wild-type and mutant lox sites placed in the plant genome. *Plant J,* 1995. 7(4): p. 649-59.

[74] Olivares, E.C., et al., Site-specific genomic integration produces therapeutic Factor IX levels in mice. *Nature Biotechnology*, 2002. 20(11): p. 1124-1128.

[75] Ortiz-Urda, S., et al., Stable nonviral genetic correction of inherited human skin disease. *Nature Medicine*, 2002. 8(10): p. 1166-1170.

[76] Ortiz-Urda, S., et al., Injection of genetically engineered fibroblasts corrects regenerated human epidermolysis bullosa skin tissue. *J Clin Invest*, 2003. 111(2): p. 251-5.
[77] Ortiz-Urda, S., et al., PhiC31 integrase-mediated nonviral genetic correction of junctional epidermolysis bullosa. *Hum Gene Ther*, 2003. 14(9): p. 923-8.
[78] Schlake, T. and J. Bode, Use of mutated FLP recognition target (FRT) sites for the exchange of expression cassettes at defined chromosomal loci. *Biochemistry*, 1994. 33(43): p. 12746-51.
[79] Seibler, J. and J. Bode, Double-reciprocal crossover mediated by FLP-recombinase: a concept and an assay. *Biochemistry*, 1997. 36(7): p. 1740-7.
[80] Seibler, J., et al., DNA cassette exchange in ES cells mediated by Flp recombinase: an efficient strategy for repeated modification of tagged loci by marker-free constructs. *Biochemistry*, 1998. 37(18): p. 6229-34.
[81] Bouhassira, E.E., K. Westerman, and P. Leboulch, Transcriptional behavior of LCR enhancer elements integrated at the same chromosomal locus by recombinase-mediated cassette exchange. *Blood*, 1997. 90(9): p. 3332-44.
[82] Feng, Y.Q., et al., Site-specific chromosomal integration in mammalian cells: Highly efficient CRE recombinase-mediated cassette exchange. *Journal of Molecular Biology*, 1999. 292(4): p. 779-785.
[83] Lauth, M., et al., Characterization of Cre-mediated cassette exchange after plasmid microinjection in fertilized mouse oocytes. *Genesis*, 2000. 27(4): p. 153-8.
[84] Kolb, A.F., Selection-marker-free modification of the murine beta-casein gene using a lox2722 site. *Analytical Biochemistry*, 2001. 290(2): p. 260-271.
[85] Lee, G. and I. Saito, Role of nucleotide sequences of loxP spacer region in Cre-mediated recombination. *Gene*, 1998. 216(1): p. 55-65.
[86] Houdebine, L.M., Transgenic animal bioreactors. *Transgenic Res*, 2000. 9(4-5): p. 305-20.
[87] Feng, Y.Q., et al., Position effects are influenced by the orientation of a transgene with respect to flanking chromatin. *Molecular and Cellular Biology*, 2001. 21(1): p. 298-309.
[88] Lauth, M., et al., Stable and efficient cassette exchange under non-selectable conditions by combined use of two site-specific recombinases. *Nucleic Acids Research*, 2002. 30(21): p. art. no.-e115.
[89] Collins, C.H., et al., Engineering proteins that bind, move, make and break DNA. *Curr Opin Biotechnol*, 2003. 14(4): p. 371-8.
[90] Buchholz, F. and A.F. Stewart, Alteration of Cre recombinase site specificity by substrate-linked protein evolution. *Nat Biotechnol*, 2001. 19(11): p. 1047-52.
[91] Santoro, S.W. and P.G. Schultz, Directed evolution of the site specificity of Cre recombinase. *Proc Natl Acad Sci U S A*, 2002. 99(7): p. 4185-90.
[92] Voziyanov, Y., et al., Stepwise Manipulation of DNA Specificity in Flp Recombinase: Progressively Adapting Flp to Individual and Combinatorial Mutations in its Target Site. *Journal of Molecular Biology*, 2003. 326(1): p. 65-76.
[93] Akopian, A., et al., Chimeric recombinases with designed DNA sequence recognition. *PNAS*, 2003. 100(15): p. 8688-8691.
[94] Yang, W. and T.A. Steitz, Crystal structure of the site-specific recombinase gamma delta resolvase complexed with a 34 bp cleavage site. *Cell*, 1995. 82(2): p. 193-207.

[95] Guo, F., D.N. Gopaul, and G.D. van Duyne, Structure of Cre recombinase complexed with DNA in a site-specific recombination synapse. *Nature*, 1997. 389(6646): p. 40-6.

[96] Bushman, F., Targeting retroviral integration? *Molecular Therapy*, 2002. 6(5): p. 570-571.

[97] Bushman, F.D., Tethering human immunodeficiency virus 1 integrase to a DNA site directs integration to nearby sequences. *Proc Natl Acad Sci U S A*, 1994. 91(20): p. 9233-7.

[98] Katz, R.A., G. Merkel, and A.M. Skalka, Targeting of retroviral integrase by fusion to a heterologous DNA binding domain: in vitro activities and incorporation of a fusion protein into viral particles. *Virology*, 1996. 217(1): p. 178-90.

[99] Bushman, F.D. and M.D. Miller, Tethering human immunodeficiency virus type 1 preintegration complexes to target DNA promotes integration at nearby sites. *J Virol*, 1997. 71(1): p. 458-64.

[100] Tan, W., et al., Fusion proteins consisting of human immunodeficiency virus type 1 integrase and the designed polydactyl zinc finger protein E2C direct integration of viral DNA into specific sites. *J Virol,* 2004. 78(3): p. 1301-13.

In: Trends in Genome Research
Editor: Clyde R. Williams, pp. 119-138
ISBN 1-60021-027-9

Chapter 4

Dynamic Transcription: Genome-Wide Identification and Analyses of the Transcriptional Start Sites and Adjacent Promoter Regions of Human Genes

Yutaka Suzuki [*] ***and Sumio Sugano***
Laboratory of Functional Genomics, Department of Medical Genome Sciences, Graduate School of Frontier Sciences, the University of Tokyo: 4-6-1 Shirokanedai, Minatoku, Tokyo 108-8639, Japan

Abstract

Large-scale compilation of the 5'-end data of human full-length cDNAs enabled us for the first time to identify the precise locations of the transcriptional start sites (TSSs) on a genome-wide scale. The information obtained on the TSSs was further utilized to retrieve the adjacent promoter regions from the recently completed human genomic sequence. Now, with the massively compiled information about the TSSs and promoters, analyses are underway to obtain a comprehensive view of the regulatory mechanisms of the transcriptional regulation. Detailed analysis of the positional information of the TSSs revealed that the TSS(s) of a gene are generally scattered over a 50-bp region on average and the patterns of the distribution of the TSSs differ significantly depending on the promoter, possibly reflecting the dynamics of the interaction between the promoters and the transcriptional machineries. A catalogue of representative promoter sequences was generated and provides a database that will serve as a foundation for further network-level studies of human transcriptional regulation. Moreover, recent advances in genome sequencing in other organisms, such as mouse, rat and dog, made it possible to study the molecular evolution of the promoters. Interestingly, intensive comparative studies of the human and mouse promoters suggested that quite a few promoter motifs seemed not to be conserved between human and mouse. Constant evolutional

[*] E-mail address: ysuzuki@hgc.jp, TEL: 81 4 7136 3607, FAX: 81 4 7136 3607

generation and loss of transcriptional regulatory modules may help to explain the molecular basis of speciation.

Introduction

One of the most important steps in the regulation of gene expression is thought to be the transcription initiation step. According to the widely accepted model, the transcriptional initiation of eukaryotic mRNAs is preceded by the formation of a multi-subunit pre-initiation complex consisting of RNA polymerase II and additional protein components. The component molecules are assembled at the future transcriptional start site (TSS) in a stepwise manner, with the binding of each factor promoting the association of the next. The DNA sequence of the region proximal to or overlapping with the TSS plays a pivotal role in determining the efficiency of the assembly of the complex. This region is called the promoter, and several sequence elements which are recognized by various protein factors, namely, general transcription factors (GTFs) or other transcription regulatory factors (TFs), are embedded therein(1-3).

Our current understanding of the regulation of the transcription initiation mechanism, especially knowledge about the numerous components of RNA polymerase II, GTFs and their interactions with DNA elements embedded in the promoters, has mainly been achieved using *in vitro* cell-free systems(4). The power of these systems is that purified components can be used in a strictly controlled combinatorial manner, which is extremely advantageous for analyzing highly complex machinery such as the RNA polymerase II complex. Actually, many of the basic protein factors, including numerous protein components of the RNA polymerase II complex, GTFs, other TFs and their interacting DNA elements, have been identified and characterized using these systems. However, for *in vitro* systems, promoters with very strong promoter activities, such as housekeeping gene promoters or even viral promoters, which may have many rather extreme characteristics, have usually been used as model cases(3). It still remains mostly unclear exactly where and how RNA polymerase II, GTFs and TFs are assembled and what is actually occurring during the transcriptional initiation events on the human genome *in vivo* in general.

In this review, we summarize how the recent progress in genome research has been applied to shed light on the genome-wide features of the transcriptional initiation events of average human genes. The accumulation of genomic sequence data as well as large-scale full-length cDNA informational resources have enabled us for the first time to precisely determine the genomic positions of the TSSs and adjacent promoter regions. Taking advantage of the unprecedented amount of compiled TSS and promoter data, attempts have been initiated to gain a comprehensive view of the transcriptional regulatory networks in humans.

Development of Full-Length cDNA Library Construction Methods and Generation of Full-Length cDNA Collections

Until the middle 90s, when cDNA libraries were constructed by conventional methods, it was usually necessary to collect hundreds of cDNAs per gene until a full-length cDNA could finally be obtained. In addition, it could not be guaranteed that the longest available cDNA really corresponded to the desired "full-length" cDNA without additional 5'RACE experiments(5), which required several rounds of intensive work for every gene. Although such procedures are frequently used for research on individual genes, it is impractical to scale them up for use with tens of thousands of genes in research aiming to cover the major part of all human genes. Therefore, the cDNA information accumulated in the past was generally incomplete and somewhat confusing. It is true that, by the mid 90s, millions of partially sequenced cDNA sequences were registered as ESTs(6). However, it was almost always uncertain whether a given cDNA sequence really corresponded to that of the full-length cDNA, with its 5'-end representing a real TSS. Sometimes it was even difficult to determine whether two cDNAs with different sequences were derived from distinct transcripts or from different parts of the same transcript.

In order to overcome these problems, novel methods were developed in the late 90s to construct a so-called full-length cDNA library, in which most of the cDNA clones correspond to full-length cDNAs. In these methods, a cap-targeting procedure is performed before the library construction. Figure 1 shows three representative methods for the cap targeting, namely, oligo-capping(7), cap trapper(8) and Smart/G-capping (9, 10)(the last one is not a cap-targeting method in a strict sense, but is practically useful for constructing a full-length cDNA library; for further details, see the reference; Suzuki and Sugano, Current Genomic, in press). These methods either enzymatically (oligo-capping, Smart/G-capping) or chemically (cap trapper) mark the cap structure of the mRNA, which is a characteristic structure at the 5'-end of full-length transcripts transcribed by RNA polymerase II. In other words, these cap-targeting methods introduce "a tag" to the nucleotide to which the cap structure is attached (note this is equivalent to identifying the very nucleotide from which the transcription is initiated *in vivo*. Also see the sections below). Since the termination sites of the transcripts are explicitly defined by polyA, full-length cDNAs could be selectively cloned between the two defined ends. The core principles of how the cap is marked in these methods are illustrated in Figure 1. For further details of the experimental protocols, see the corresponding references or related review article (Suzuki and Sugano, Current Genomics, in press).

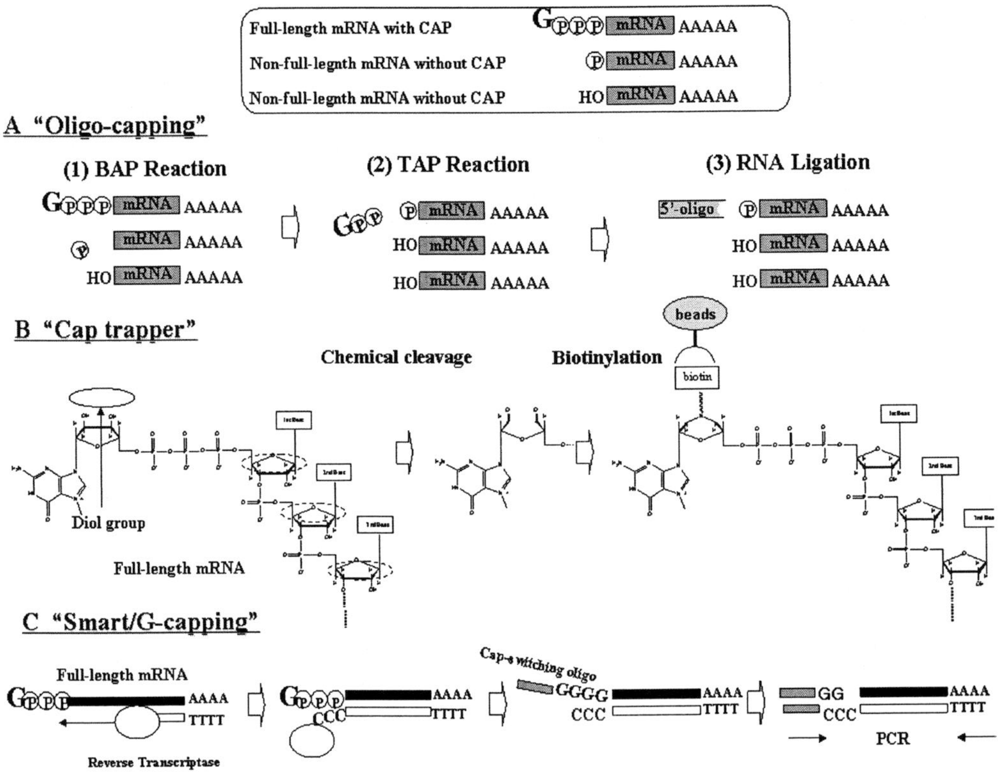

Figure 1. Scheme of representative cap targeting methods. (A) Oligo-capping. This method consists of three steps of enzymatic reactions: (1): Bacterial alkaline phosphatase (BAP) hydrolyzes the phosphate from the 5'-ends of truncated mRNAs that are non-capped, while the cap structure on full-length mRNAs remains intact; (2) Tobacco acid pyrophosphatase (TAP) hydrolyzes the cap structure, leaving a phosphate at the 5'-ends of mRNAs; (3) T4 RNA ligase selectively ligates a synthetic oligoribonucleotide to the phosphate at the 5'-end. As a result, the oligoribonucleotide is introduced selectively at the 5'-ends of mRNAs that originally had the cap structure. (B) Cap trapper. This method chemically introduces a biotin group into the diol group of the cap structure. The chemical reaction to cleave the cap structure is shown in the inset. The carbon-carbon bond between the diol structure indicated by a solid circle is cleaved by NaIO4 treatment, so that the biotin group can be introduced to this site. Note that the diol structure exists only at the position indicated by a solid circle and not at broken circles. For selection of the full-length mRNAs, the biotin residue introduced at the cap sites is trapped using streptavidin-coated magnetic beads. (C) Smart/G-capping. This method makes use of the oligo-G sequence which is occasionally attached to the 5'-end of the mRNA when reverse transcriptase reaches the 5'-ends of mRNA without having fallen off in the middle. By hybridizing a "switching oligo" with the oligo-G, the 5'-end sequence tag is introduced as in the case of oligo-capping. However, note that the fact that reverse transcriptase reached the end of the transcript does not necessarily mean that the product is a full-length cDNA. Therefore, the quality of the library (frequency of the full-length cDNAs) is strongly dependent on the quality (intactness) of the starting mRNAs.

Introduction of the full-length cDNA library methods has made collection of the full-length cDNAs technically far easier. On the other hand, as the human genome sequencing project proceeded, it gradually became clear that finding genes in the genomic sequences based solely on computational methods would be very difficult(11). The importance of supportive information from experimentally isolated transcripts, preferably full-length transcripts, came to be well recognized. As a result, several large-scale cDNA collection projects aiming to generate a collection of full-length cDNAs covering most, if not all, of the protein-coding genes in humans and mice were launched around 2000(12-15). Full-length cDNA libraries were constructed from hundreds of kinds of tissues and cultured cells, and intensive sequence analyses of them were carried out. Now millions of one-pass sequences and nearly one hundred thousand complete sequences of cDNAs from those full-length cDNA libraries have been registered in public sequence databases (Genbank: http://www.ncbi.nlm.nih.gov/Genbank/index.html; EMBL: http://www.ebi.ac.uk/embl/; DDBJ: http://www.ddbj.nig.ac.jp/Welcome-e.html).

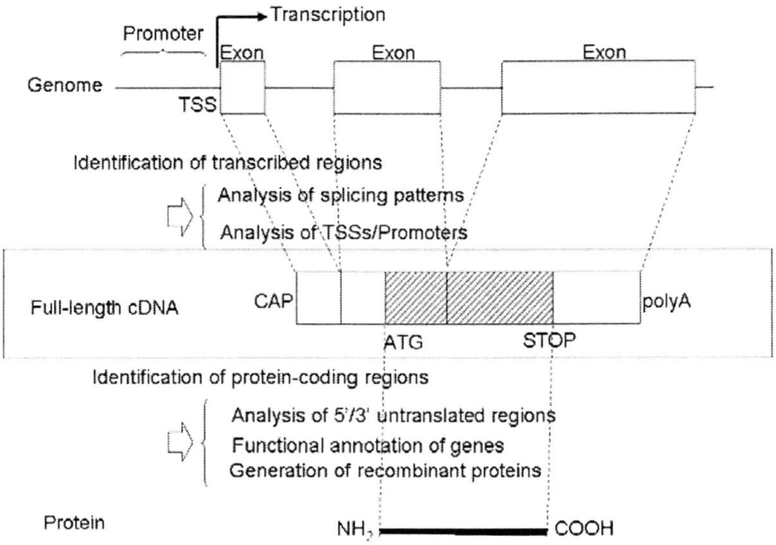

Figure 2. Use of full-length cDNAs for interpretation of the functions of human genes.

The generated full-length cDNA collections were extremely helpful for interpreting the codes in the genomic sequences in various ways (Figure 2). By computational mapping of the full-length cDNAs onto the genomic sequences, it was possible to identify the precise location and genomic organization (exon-intron structures) of the transcripts for the major part of the entire set of human genes. As described below, this information was useful for genome-wide identification of the precise positions of the TSSs. Also, detailed analyses of the differential usage of the exons allowed the identification of thousands of alternative transcript variants in human genes (on this topic, see the reference(16)). Moreover, full-length cDNAs were highly useful not only as informational data resources, but also as physical clone resources for assigning further biological meaning to the genomic sequence data. Since the full-length cDNAs contain complete protein coding sequences not split by introns, they can be directly used as templates to produce recombinant proteins. Various approaches have utilized such physical full-length cDNA resources for experimental characterization of the biological functions of newly discovered genes and novel biological functions of previously discovered genes in a high-throughput manner(17, 18). The concurrent analyses, which are collectively called "functional genomics", are reviewed elsewhere (Suzuki and Sugano; submitted). Because of these multi-faceted uses of the full-length cDNA resources, the full-length cDNA collection and analysis projects are being carried out in parallel with the corresponding genome sequencing projects in various organisms. Now, integrated information about the full-length cDNAs together with the corresponding genomic data is also presented in a user-friendly manner in Ensembl (http://www.ensembl.org/), NCBI MapViewer (http://www.ncbi.nlm.nih.gov/mapview/), UCSC genome browser (http://genome.ucsc.edu/), and H-invitational database (http://www.jbirc.aist.go.jp/hinv/index.jsp).

Mapping of the 5'-Ends of Full-length cDNAs onto the Genomic Sequences for Large-Scale Identification of the TSSs

One especially powerful use of the full-length cDNA data, which had been either fully sequenced or partially sequenced from the 5'-ends, was the massive identification of the 5'-end boundaries of the first exons corresponding to cDNAs that. As mentioned above, as the 5'-end sequences of the full-length cDNAs correspond to the exact nucleotides where the transcription is initiated, these ends were mapped onto the genomic sequences to identify the genomic positions of the TSSs. As a result, in humans, the exact positions of the TSSs were determined for over 15,000 previously annotated protein-coding genes. Dozens of 5'-end sequences of full-length cDNAs were usually found per gene, each of which represents a TSS. Recent statistical data analysis showed that the base composition of the exact TSSs was 51%, 25%, 17% and 7% for A, G, C and T, respectively (Figure 3; Kimuta et al., submitted).

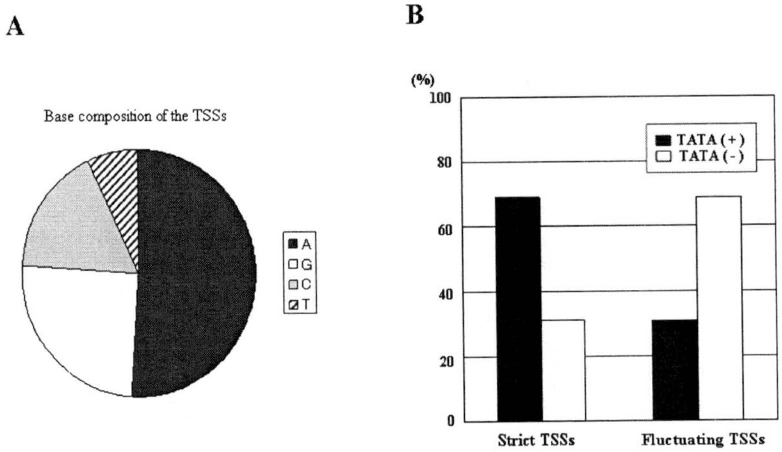

Figure 3. Detailed Analysis of the TSSs. (A) Base composition of the exact nucleotide from which transcription is initiated in human genes. (B) Relation between the distribution manner of the TSSs and the presence of the TATA boxes in the promoters. The proportion of TATA-containing promoters in the "Promoters with strict TSS (standard deviation of the TSS distribution <5; left columns) and the "Promoters with fluctuating TSS" (standard deviation of the TSS distribution ≥ 5; right columns) is shown(19).

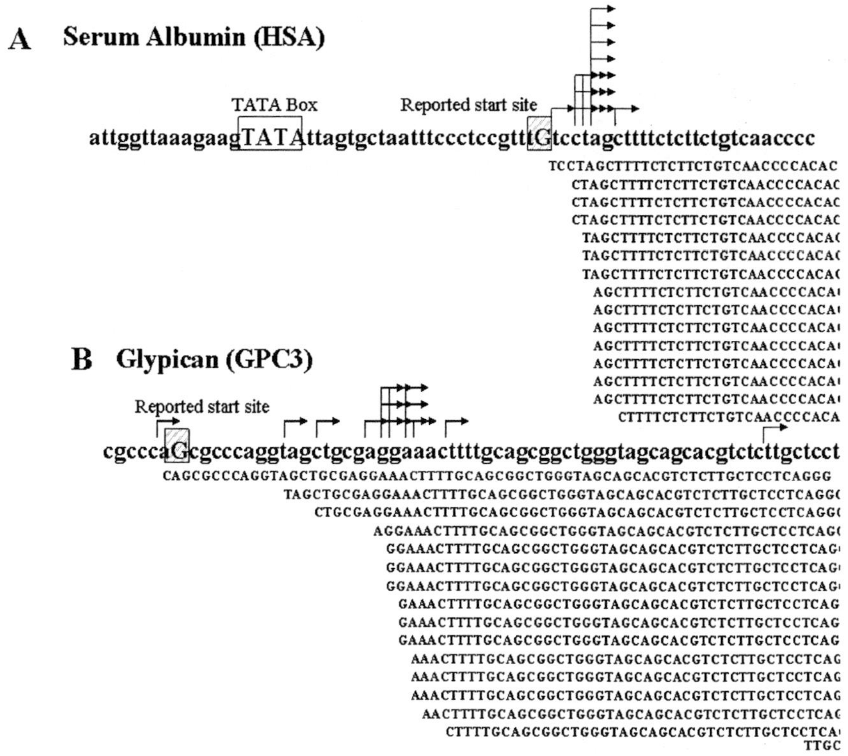

Figure 4. Distribution of the TSSs. Sequence alignment of the 5'-ends of the full-length cDNAs and the mapped TSSs in the human serum albumin gene (HSA) gene (A) and the human glypican (GPC3) gene (B). An arrow shows the mapped position of the 5'-end of each full-length cDNA. The TSSs which had been identified previously by conventional methods are shown by upper case letters and shaded boxes.

Interestingly, detailed analysis of the TSSs revealed that there were almost no genes for which all the TSSs redundantly identified for multiple full-length cDNAs mapped to a single nucleotide at precisely the same position(19). As exemplified in Figure 4A, it was usually the case that there were multiple transcription-starting nucleotides which were scattered over 50 bp on average. In total, gross analysis of the data for millions of full-length cDNAs enabled identification of about 250,000 independent positions of TSSs, corresponding to 15,000 RefSeq (http://www.ncbi.nlm.nih.gov/RefSeq/) genes, indicating that there are 17 independent TSSs in a single human gene on average (Kimura et al., submitted; also see http://dbtss.hgc.jp). This is somewhat opposed to the previously common view that transcription is initiated from a single or at most a few particular nucleotides. What is nearer to the fact is the notion that there is a transcription initiation "area" from which transcription is initiated, possibly following a probabilistic or stochastic model.

Indeed, even the data obtained using the conventional methods in the pre-genomic era implied general fluctuations in the positions of TSSs. However, such fluctuations were overlooked in most cases, by usually selecting the TSS that was located furthest upstream as a representative. For example, as shown in Figures 4B and 4C, for the human HAS gene and the human GPC3 gene, the start sites identified at the most upstream positions seem to have been registered, although they were demonstrated to be accompanied by many minor start sites in subsequent studies. This may be due to the indirect nature of the conventional methods, which rely on the principle that the 5'-end of the longest cDNA should be considered as the start site (5, 20, 21). Since the full-length cDNA methods allowed us to identify the position of the cap structure of the mRNA directly (7), the accuracy, reliability, and above all, the resolution of the TSS detection are much improved compared with those of the conventional methods.

Identification and Characterization of the Fluctuation of the TSSs

As represented in Figure 4, the distribution patterns of the TSSs differed from gene to gene despite the fact that all of the transcripts are transcribed by RNA polymerase II (note the full-length cDNA libraries were constructed by cap selection methods, and thus the mRNAs originally contained cap structures, which is characteristic of the transcripts transcribed by the RNA polymerase II system). RNA polymerase II itself does not have the property of sequence-specific binding; instead, its promoter recognition and orientation depend on additional factors. Therefore, it was supposed that there should be *trans*-acting protein factors which determine the distribution patterns of the TSSs and that the *cis*-acting DNA elements corresponding to their binding sites should be found in the promoter regions.

The analysis of the relationship between the presence of a particular sequence element in the promoters and how the TSSs are scattered over genomic regions revealed that TATA boxes are significantly enriched in the population of genes with tightly clustered TSSs(19)(Figure 5). The TATA box is a recognition site of TBP, a component of one of the GTFs, TFIID. The TATA box is regarded as one of the most important sequence elements for transcriptional initiation among the many elements thus far identified in promoters. Indeed, the criterion of whether the promoter is TATA-containing or not is often employed for initial characterization of promoters(3)(also see the section below for further discussion on the genome-wide prevalence of the TATA boxes). The crystal structure of the ternary complex of TFIIB (another GTF)-TBP-TATA box has shown that the DNA backbone is bent by 90 degrees when TBP is recruited to the TATA box (22). This structural change may cause the DNA to be anchored rigidly to the polymerase active site of RNA polymerase II. Once such a rigid structure if formed, the position of the TSS relative to the active site should be strictly determined. In contrast, if there is no TATA box in the promoter, the active site may remain unstable on the promoter. Without the anchoring effect of the TATA box, the active site may slide over the promoter, which results in transcriptional initiation from widely distributed positions. Such a hypothesis from a molecular dynamics viewpoint may explain why TSSs are tightly clustered in TATA-containing promoters. More generally, the distribution patterns of the TSSs might reflect the flexibility of the interaction between TFs, RNA polymerase II and promoter DNA. Currently, crystal structures of many of the TFs (either alone or co-crystallized with their interacting promoters) and biophysical data on the interactions between single molecules are becoming available (http://www.rcsb.org/pdb/strucgen.html). Integrative analyses of the patterns of the TSSs, each of which reflects an independent transcriptional initiation event in vivo, together with the analysis of the molecular dynamics of the interacting components will eventually clarify the molecular mechanisms underlying the transcription initiation events.

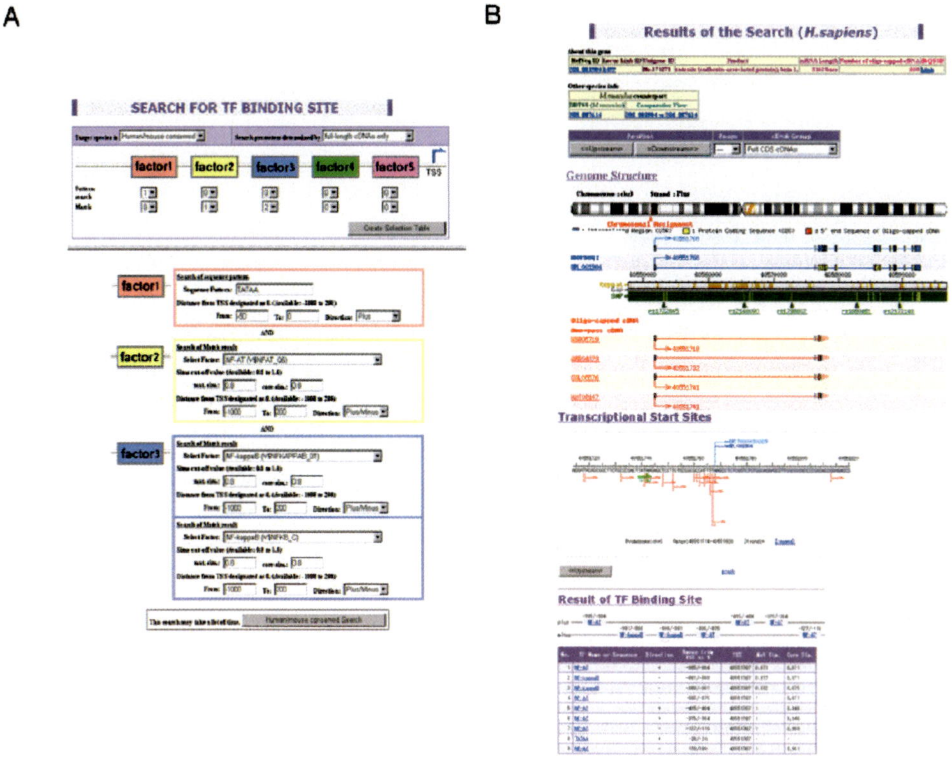

Figure 5. Search for putative TF binding sites in the generated promoter dataset. A search for possible TF target sites using DBTSS. (A) Forms that are used for search by queries, by putative TF binding sites and their combinations are illustrated. The fields to specify the TF binding sites are represented by red, yellow and blue boxes (Factor 1-3). For each of the boxes, users can choose the search method, choosing between exact sequence match and matrix search, using position weight matrices. As exemplified for the case of "Factor 3", users can also specify TF binding sites, any of which should be contained in the targets, by creating additional boxes. This search can be done for either human or mouse promoters individually or for the promoter elements conserved between human and mouse. Results of the search are displayed as shown in (B).

Genome-Wide Identification and Analysis of Promoter Sequences

The availability of the massively accumulated precise positional information about TSSs allowed us to retrieve the adjacent promoter sequences from large volumes of genomic sequence data as well. In order to obtain clues about which TFs are involved in the transcriptional modulation of genes, the retrieved promoter sequences were subjected to searches to determine whether they contained corresponding binding sites. For this purpose, DNA sequences ranging up to 1kp upstream from the TSSs were catalogued as putative promoter regions and presented as a database, DataBase of Transcriptional Start Sites (DBTSS; http://dbtss.hgc.jp)(23). This region was used for the initial search, since about 82 % of the previously characterized TF binding sites were located within this range. (As the TSSs are usually scattered over genomic regions at least to some extent, the representative

TSS positions subjected to the analysis were the most frequently used TSSs; also see Figure 1). In DBTSS, the so-far accumulated promoter sequences of 15,000 human genes are registered and are freely accessible for public users.

Using the generated data set of the representative promoter sequences, our ability to analyze transcriptional modulation has been greatly expanded. In addition to conventional approaches for characterizing promoters, which examine the presence or absence of the binding consensus sequences of the TFs gene by gene, now it is possible to comprehensively investigate how many and what kinds of genes contain binding target sequences of particular TFs in the human genes as a whole. For example, one can retrieve a complete list of human genes containing "TATA-containing promoters with NF-kB binding site(s) and with either NF-AT site(s) or AP-1 site(s)" in order to search for genes possibly involved in inflammatory responses (24, 25). The results of a search by putative TF binding sites can be viewed as shown in Figure 5.

Also, the compilation of the promoter data shed light on the general organization of the regulatory sequence motifs in the promoters for the first time. As described above, at one time TATA boxes were thought to be commonly observed in the promoters of human genes, playing an indispensable role. However, a recent survey of TATA boxes in the vicinity of the TSSs in human promoters showed that genes with so-called TATA-containing promoters are far less common than previously thought, comprising no more than 10- 20% of human genes(26). The false notion that the TATA boxes play "indispensable" roles for most, even not all, human gene promoters might have arisen from the fact that conventional studies mainly employed exceptionally strong promoters containing TATA boxes as models and that the numerous fundamental discoveries made about transcriptional regulation were made through the analyses of these strong promoters. Some other motifs are even more commonly observed. For example, GC-box-like GC-rich stretches were observed in almost all of the promoters. CpG islands are present in about 60 % of promoters. It should also be noted that these two motifs are now considered to be the most important factors for computational predictions of promoters (also see below)(27).

Attempts to correlate motifs in the promoters with the expression profile data, which reflect the eventual output levels of the transcription, have also been started. For example, studies on the correlation between the presence of the CpG islands and the tissue-specificity of the expression patterns showed that genes lacking CpG islands in the promoters tend to be expressed with a higher degree of tissue specificity(28). Among such attempts, the most challenging may be the gross comparison of the promoter data with the expression data generated from microarray and other high-throughput methods. One approach now being taken to interpret the massively accumulated expression data is analysis of the consensus binding sequences whose occurrence is significantly enriched in genes whose mRNA levels are altered in response to a particular conditional perturbation. Although such approaches are still at the preliminary level due to the inaccuracy of both the expression data (29)and the TF binding site prediction methods (also see below)(30), the integrated analyses of the black box of the transcriptional regulation from both the upstream (promoter) and downstream (mRNA) sides would further enrich our understanding of transcriptional regulation at the network level.

Lastly, it is worth mentioning that efforts are also being made towards *ab initio* computational prediction of the promoters by utilizing the accumulated promoter data as an educational dataset for the machine learning in various ways(30). The promoter predictions are also expected to be complementarily used with previously developed gene prediction programs, which are basically unable to predict the 5'-end terminal exons. Many factors are considered, such as the presence of CpG islands, and the presence or possible enrichment of specific promoter motifs, such as TATA boxes and consensus binding sites of other TFs. These statistical properties are evaluated against the universal genomic sequences using neural networks, linear and quadratic discriminant analyses, Relevance Vector Machine, interpolated Markov model or a combination of these. In general, current promoter prediction programs show better performance for G+C-rich CpG-island-related promoters. However, unfortunately, at the current stage, none of the developed programs has reached a level with sufficient sensitivity and selectivity (e.g. >65%) to predict candidate promoters for further experimental validation. A recent evaluation of representative promoter prediction programs also showed that previous estimations of the performances of the promoter prediction programs deduced from a limited number of chromosomes or smaller data sets did not hold true when re-evaluation was performed at the level of the whole genome, with especially serious inaccuracy of the predictions for non-CpG-island-related promoters(27). However, promoter data are being rapidly accumulated for a number of other mammals, which would be helpful for further tuning-up of the programs. The development of better programs taking evolutional conservation into consideration can be expected in the very near future.

Large-scale Comparative Studies of Promoters

Full-length cDNA data together with genomic sequence data are rapidly being accumulated for non-human mammals as well as humans. Using other organisms' data as references, comparative studies of the promoters are now possible. In particular, remarkable progress has been made in the full-length cDNA project FANTOM(31) in mice and the compilation of the TSS and promoter information is at the same level as in humans.

It is well recognized that sequence comparison among organisms is a powerful method to reduce the rate of dubious predictions of TF binding sites. As many of the TF binding sites are short (6- 12 bp) and their consensus sequences are often degenerate, discriminating the genuine TF binding sites, which have biological significance *in vivo*, from insignificant sequences that occur randomly and very frequently in the large volumes of human genomic sequences is an intricate problem. In searches for possible TF targets such as the one exemplified in Figure x, it is always a concern that not all of the obtained matches are true positives (32). However, by taking into consideration whether the detected sites are evolutionarily conserved or not, it is possible to select biologically meaningful hits from a vast number of dubious hits. It is expected that the predicted TF binding sites of functional relevance are evolutionarily conserved and could thereby be discriminated from non-conserved ones, which are supposed to be under weaker or no functional constraints (33, 34). For example, using the promoter alignment data as a filter for selecting conserved TF binding sites, the hits obtained in the search represented in Figure x can be narrowed down to 22,794 hits conserved between human and mouse(35). Such a procedure should be extremely helpful for expediting experimental validation of the TF binding sites in a cost- and labor-effective manner.

In addition to the relatively simple application for evaluating whether a given individual TF binding site seems to warrant further validation, large-scale comparative data of the promoters also enabled us to analyze how the transcriptional regulatory modules have taken their current forms as a consequence of long-term molecular evolution. A recent study of the sequence alignment of representative promoters between 3,324 human and putative orthologous mouse counterpart genes revealed that the sequence conservation did not extend further on average than 500 bp upstream of the TSSs in about one-third of the genes. This discontinuous manner of sequence conservation suggests that the promoter sequences have been conserved in a "block" manner rather than as a mere accumulation of single nucleotide substitutions. Consistently, G+C content and CpG frequency were significantly different inside versus outside the "blocks", suggesting a qualitative difference in the manner of sequence conservation between the sides of the border. Since in about half of the "blocks" the 5'-ends were bound by interspersed repetitive elements, it was also suggested that genomic rearrangements nucleated by them might have been responsible for generating the discontinuity. Interestingly, about 10 % of the previously characterized TF binding sites were located outside of those "blocks", and thus were not conserved between humans and mice (36). Also, there are reports showing that the transcriptional regulation of many genes is significantly divergent between humans and mice (37, 38). Different combinations of the TFs might be used to regulate target genes as long as the basic requirements are met as a whole, and the flexibility of transcriptional modulation appears to be greater than used to be thought.

Finding the above-described evolutional conservation in the promoters immediately suggests certain mutually contradictory aspects of comparative studies. That is, in order to discriminate false-positives, it is helpful to focus on the "conserved" elements. On the other hand, non-conserved sequence motifs should not be automatically overlooked since the possibility always remains that some of them really have biological relevance. It should be kept in mind that there are significant differences between humans and mice at the organismal level, at least. Those elements which are involved in species-specific transcriptional regulation would never be identified without intensive analyses of the non-conserved elements. Indeed, it has long been supposed that the genetic basis for various anatomical and physiological similarities/differences between humans and other organisms lies in alterations in the expression of genes rather than changes in the functions of their encoded protein products (39). It seems reasonable to assume that unique fine adjustments of the transcriptional regulation are responsible for the acquisition of species-specific tuning of the transcriptome(40, 41). There has been no clear demonstration as yet of the truth of this assumption. However, the speed of the generation of genomic sequence data is continuing to accelerate and the release of the draft sequences of more than a dozen mammalian genomes is expected within the next couple of years. Also, newly developed methods combining full-length cDNA and SAGE methods (42-44)will enable more efficient accumulation of TSS data. Data about both the genomic sequences and TSSs from many other organisms, such as primates, cattle, dogs and cats, have laid or will shortly lay the foundation for a more precise understanding of which sequences play a leading role (e.g., serving as direct binding sites for TFs), and which play a supporting role in transcriptional regulation.

Alternative Promoters of Human Genes

Alternative usage of promoters has been reported to lead to functional diversification for particular genes. One of the well-known examples is the human Src proto-oncogene gene.

This gene has two alternative promoters: one drives ubiquitous expression, while the other, located 1kb upstream, contains a binding site of a tissue-specific TF, HNF-1, and is involved in tissue-specific expression of this gene, though the encoded protein sequence does not differ between the two promoters(45). In addition to the diversification of the transcriptional regulation, several examples have also been reported in which alterations in the promoter usage followed by alternative uses of the first exons produce alterations in the encoded amino acids around the N-terminus. Some of them result in changes of the protein motifs or subcellular localization signals located at the N-terminus, such as secretory signal peptides and mitochondria targeting signals, and thus have significant biologically explicit functional relevance to the diversification of the protein functions themselves, too(46). However, in spite of the potential importance, very little is understood about the usage of alternative promoters in a genome-wide manner. Until very recently, it was not even clear how many and what kind of genes are subject to regulation via alternative promoters, mainly because of the general lack of precise TSS data(46).

As a result of recent analyses of the TSS data, it is gradually becoming clear that an unexpectedly large population of human genes possess multiple clusters of TSSs (each consisting of multiple TSSs), each of which seems to be regulated by distinct alternative promoters (Figure 6). Recent statistical analyses suggested that 20- 50% of the examined human genes had multiple clusters of TSSs, which are separated form each other by significant intervals and thus are regulated by distinct alternative promoters (Kimura et al., submitted). Essentially the same results were also obtained in mice and other organisms(47). However, when the massively identified alternative promoters were compared between species, it also became clear that the large part of them seem not to be evolutionarily conserved (Tsuritani et al., in preparation). Assuming that functionally relevant products are conserved because of functional constraints (also with the same caveat described in the above), many non-conserved products may be biologically meaningless.

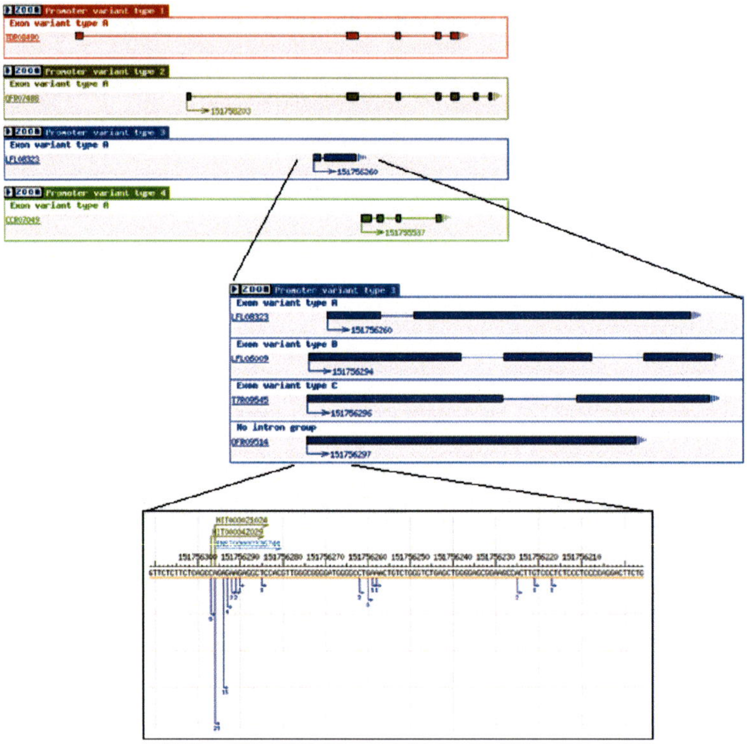

Figure 6. Alternative promoters in human genes. Alternative use of promoters in human gene is exemplified by the case of the human Shc gene. Alternative promoter groups are represented by different colors. The middle and lower panels are magnifications of the indicated regions. Also note that within the transcript belonging to the same promoter group, several variations in the exon types are observed.

This brings to mind a recently discovered novel class of transcripts, so-called TUFs (Transcripts of Unknown Function; formerly called simply noncoding RNAs, "ncRNAs"). The TUFs show clear traces of splicing, which ensures that they are not originated from erroneous cloning of contaminating genomic DNA but are real transcripts, although these transcripts seem not to encode any proteins. There are several known types of transcripts that function as RNA without being used as templates for translation, such as rRNAs, tRNAs and many kinds of miRNAs. However, these ncRNAs are mostly transcribed by RNA polymerase I or III, and examples of ncRNAs transcribed by RNA polymerase II were limited in the past. The TUFs were identified in cDNA libraries constructed using cap-targeting methods (also see Figure 1), and thus presumably were transcribed by RNA polymerase II. TUFs were named separately from the other classes of ncRNAs to reflect this fact. Recently, thousands of kinds of TUFs were identified from both human and mouse transcriptomes by full-length cDNA projects; however, like alternative promoters, they are mostly non-conserved between organismal lineages. Wang et al. also suggested that the TUFs identified in mouse full-length cDNA collections seem simply to be subject to evolutional drift with a rate which accords well with neutral evolution theory (48). The biological relevance of those TUFs is now a subject of heated discussion. It seems likely that most of the tens of thousands of kinds of

TUFs or alternative promoters exist without any *raison d'etre* rather than that each of them has species-specific role(s). Interestingly, our recent experimental analysis demonstrated that universal non-gene-related genomic DNAs come to occasionally acquire potential transcription activation activities comparable to those of canonical promoters (Sakakibara et al., submitted). The massively discovered alternative promoters and TUFs might be originated from such sporadically occurring promoter activities. Consistently, recent genome-wide chip-on-chip analysis targeted for possible binding sites of RNA polymerase II showed that RNA polymerase II interacts with an unexpectedly large number of genomic DNA sites, either within or outside of genic regions(49). Although it is too early to speculate further without additional experimental validation, it might be hypothesized that those binding sites which are present in genic regions should be recognized as "alternative promoters", while those which are present outside should drive the transcription of TUFs. Since the cDNA projects have intensively explored transcripts of "novel" genes as part of the analysis of the transcriptome, these "non-orthodox" transcripts, whose expression levels should be low, have begun to be identified.

Conclusions

In this review, we described how the recent progress in genome research made possible the genome-wide identification of TSSs and the characterization of the adjacent promoter regions. As surveyed above, we have begun to grasp the general features of transcriptional initiation and its regulation, which seems far more dynamic than previously thought with regards to molecular dynamics and molecular evolution. Such dynamism could not have been revealed by prolonged conventional analyses based on a static and pre-deterministic transcription initiation model and performed using a limited number of promoters under somewhat artificial experimental conditions. It will now be of great interest to examine to what extent the events posited in the current model of transcriptional regulation correspond to those actually occurring in the cell in general.

It is especially intriguing that transcription of no explicit biological relevance seems to be occasionally initiated from unexpectedly numerous genomic regions, possibly accounting for the identification of TUFs and alternative promoters. This is somewhat similar to what happens in alternative splicing. As a result of intensive analysis of the accumulated EST data, it was also shown that about half of human genes produce at least four alternatively spliced variants, but a majority of them seem not to be conserved between human and mouse(50). A report describing translation of unorthodox proteins from noncanonical reading frames has also been published(51). Indeed, in cells, a number of RNA and protein products seem to be synthesized just to be discarded. The genome systems in higher eukaryotes might be noise- and byproduct-permissive as long as there are no deleterious effects. As an evolving genome becomes larger, harboring a larger number of genes, tight control of the entire system becomes much more costly than permitting the occasional generation of totally useless products. At least, the role of such products as material for the evolutional invention of novel molecules should not be a bad trade against the disadvantage of the loss of the energy consumed to produce molecules with no biological function. Alternatively, the development of a tightly designed system producing no waste and the production of a system with sufficient robustness may have been mutually exclusive. A lack of strict rationality (purpose-oriented-ness) has been inevitable as genes emerged from the changing genomic DNA sequence during uncounted rounds of scrap-and-build trials during evolution. Without any play (or buffer), slight perturbations of the system invoked by various types of extra-cellular stimuli could easily cause catastrophic consequences.

Understanding of such a byproduct- or noise-permissive system would never be achieved by simple compilation of individual pieces of information. Instead, the only way to tackle the system may be through theoretical deductions from the comprehensive knowledge of the entire system. Such inherent difficulties are already being confronted by the recently launched large-scale post-genome project, ENCODE(49). ENCODE aims eventually to comprehensively identify and characterize all of the genomic elements. However, the natures of the transcriptome and proteome worlds are so dynamic that the approaches which were useful to analyze the static genome systems are of no use. The cellular contexts defining the status of each of the transcripts and proteins are innumerable, producing many products which do not themselves deserve "functional" characterization. Therefore the completion of the functional analyses of the "elements" would never be accomplished simply by one-by-one specific descriptions of the elements. For these ends, system-level analysis of the entire gene network, which seems to be a great detour at first glance, might be the only way(52). "Comprehensive analyses" would be first completed in a strict sense as a consequence of theoretical deductions from the knowledge of the systems. With the launch of ENCODE, we may inevitably face a paradigm shift of genome sciences in which genome science changes from a descriptive data collection phase to an interpretation and information deduction phase. Although still far from complete, the accumulation of information about each of the genes seems to have reached a level making it possible to initiate system-level analyses of the human gene network.

Acknowledgements

We are grateful to the members of the IMSUT sequencing team for having laid the groundwork for the full-length cDNA projects and successive proteome studies described here. DBTSS was developed and maintained by K. Nakai and R. Yamashita. We thank J. M. Sugano, K. Kimura and T. Isogai for helpful discussions and suggestions, H. Hata, K. and K. Abe for excellent sequencing work and E. Sekimori and H. Wakaguri for technical support. We are also thankful to E. Nakajima for critical reading of the manuscript.

This work was supported by a Grant-in-Aid for Scientific Research on Priority Areas from the Ministry of Education, Science, Sports and Culture of Japan.

References

[1] Novina, C., D. and Roy, A., L. (1996) *Trends Genet* 12, p.351-356.

[2] Roeder, R., G. (1996) *Trends Biochem Sci* 21, p.327-362.

[3] Smale, S., T. (1997) *Biochim Biophys Acta* 1351, p.73-161.

[4] Mitchell, P., J. and Tjian, R. (1989) *Science* 245, p.371-379.

[5] Schaefer, B., C. (1995) *Anal Biochem* 227, p.255-328.

[6] Boguski, M., S. (1995) *Trends Biochem Sci* 20, p.295-301.

[7] Suzuki, Y. and Sugano, S. (2003) *Methods Mol Biol* 221, p.73-164.

[8] Carninci, P. and Hayashizaki, Y. (1999) *Methods Enzymol* 303, p.19-63.

[9] Matz, M., V.; Alieva, N., O.; Chenchik, A. and Lukyanov, S. (2003) *Methods Mol Biol* 221, p.41-50.

[10] Kato, S.; Sekine, S.; Oh, S., W.; Kim, N., S.; Umezawa, Y.; Abe, N.; Yokoyama-Kobayashi, M. and Aoki, T. (1994) *Gene* 150, p.243-293.

[11] Makarov, V. (2002) *Brief Bioinform* 3, p.195-204.

[12] Wiemann, S.; Weil, B.; Wellenreuther, R.; Gassenhuber, J.; Glassl, S.; Ansorge, W.; Bocher, M.; Blocker, H.; Bauersachs, S.; Blum, H.; Lauber, J.; Dusterhoft, A.; Beyer, A.; Kohrer, K.; Strack, N.; Mewes, H., W.; Ottenwalder, B.; Obermaier, B.; Tampe, J.; Heubner, D.; Wambutt, R.; Korn, B.; Klein, M. and Poustka, A. (2001) *Genome Res* 11, p.422-457.

[13] Zhang, Q., H.; Ye, M.; Wu, X., Y.; Ren, S., X.; Zhao, M.; Zhao, C., J.; Fu, G.; Shen, Y.; Fan, H., Y.; Lu, G.; Zhong, M.; Xu, X., R.; Han, Z., G.; Zhang, J., W.; Tao, J.; Huang, Q., H.; Zhou, J.; Hu, G., X.; Gu, J.; Chen, S., J. and Chen, Z. (2000) *Genome Res* 10, p.1546-1606.

[14] Ota, T.; Suzuki, Y.; Nishikawa, T.; Otsuki, T.; Sugiyama, T.; Irie, R.; Wakamatsu, A.; Hayashi, K.; Sato, H.; Nagai, K.; Kimura, K.; Makita, H.; Sekine, M.; Obayashi, M.; Nishi, T.; Shibahara, T.; Tanaka, T.; Ishii, S.; Yamamoto, J.; Saito, K.; Kawai, Y.; Isono, Y.; Nakamura, Y.; Nagahari, K.; Murakami, K.; Yasuda, T.; Iwayanagi, T.; Wagatsuma, M.; Shiratori, A.; Sudo, H.; Hosoiri, T.; Kaku, Y.; Kodaira, H.; Kondo, H.; Sugawara, M.; Takahashi, M.; Kanda, K.; Yokoi, T.; Furuya, T.; Kikkawa, E.; Omura, Y.; Abe, K.; Kamihara, K.; Katsuta, N.; Sato, K.; Tanikawa, M.; Yamazaki, M.; Ninomiya, K.; Ishibashi, T.; Yamashita, H.; Murakawa, K.; Fujimori, K.; Tanai, H.; Kimata, M.; Watanabe, M.; Hiraoka, S.; Chiba, Y.; Ishida, S.; Ono, Y.; Takiguchi, S.; Watanabe, S.; Yosida, M.; Hotuta, T.; Kusano, J.; Kanehori, K.; Takahashi-Fujii, A.; Hara, H.; Tanase, T., O.; Nomura, Y.; Togiya, S.; Komai, F.; Hara, R.; Takeuchi, K.; Arita, M.; Imose, N.; Musashino, K.; Yuuki, H.; Oshima, A.; Sasaki, N.; Aotsuka, S.; Yoshikawa, Y.; Matsunawa, H.; Ichihara, T.; Shiohata, N.; Sano, S.; Moriya, S.; Momiyama, H.; Satoh, N.; Takami, S.; Terashima, Y.; Suzuki, O.; Nakagawa, S.; Senoh, A.; Mizoguchi, H.; Goto, Y.; Shimizu, F.; Wakebe, H.; Hishigaki, H.; Watanabe, T.; Sugiyama, A.; Takemoto, M.; Kawakami, B.; Yamazaki, M.; Watanabe, K.; Kumagai, A.; Itakura, S.; Fukuzumi, Y.; Fujimori, Y.; Komiyama, M.; Tashiro, H.; Tanigami, A.; Fujiwara, T.; Ono, T.; Yamada, K.; Fujii, Y.; Ozaki, K.; Hirao, M.; Ohmori, Y.; Kawabata, A.; Hikiji, T.; Kobatake, N.; Inagaki, H.; Ikema, Y.; Okamoto, S.; Okitani, R.; Kawakami, T.; Noguchi, S.; Itoh, T.; Shigeta, K.; Senba, T.; Matsumura, K.; Nakajima, Y.; Mizuno, T.; Morinaga, M.; Sasaki, M.; Togashi, T.;

Oyama, M.; Hata, H.; Watanabe, M.; Komatsu, T.; Mizushima-Sugano, J.; Satoh, T.; Shirai, Y.; Takahashi, Y.; Nakagawa, K.; Okumura, K.; Nagase, T.; Nomura, N.; Kikuchi, H.; Masuho, Y.; Yamashita, R.; Nakai, K.; Yada, T.; Nakamura, Y.; Ohara, O.; Isogai, T.; Sugano, S. (2004) *Nat Genet* 36, p.40-45.

[15] Strausberg, R., L.; Feingold, E., A.; Grouse, L., H.; Derge, J., G.; Klausner, R., D.; Collins, F., S.; Wagner, L.; Shenmen, C., M.; Schuler, G., D.; Altschul, S., F.; Zeeberg, B.; Buetow, K., H.; Schaefer, C., F.; Bhat, N., K.; Hopkins, R., F.; Jordan, H.; Moore, T.; Max, S., I.; Wang, J.; Hsieh, F.; Diatchenko, L.; Marusina, K.; Farmer, A., A.; Rubin, G., M.; Hong, L.; Stapleton, M.; Soares, M., B.; Bonaldo, M., F.; Casavant, T., L.; Scheetz, T., E.; Brownstein, M., J.; Usdin, T., B.; Toshiyuki, S.; Carninci, P.; Prange, C.; Raha, S., S.; Loquellano, N., A.; Peters, G., J.; Abramson, R., D.; Mullahy, S., J.; Bosak, S., A.; McEwan, P., J.; McKernan, K., J.; Malek, J., A.; Gunaratne, P., H.; Richards, S.; Worley, K., C.; Hale, S.; Garcia, A., M.; Gay, L., J.; Hulyk, S., W.; Villalon, D., K.; Muzny, D., M.; Sodergren, E., J.; Lu, X.; Gibbs, R., A.; Fahey, J.; Helton, E.; Ketteman, M.; Madan, A.; Rodrigues, S.; Sanchez, A.; Whiting, M.; Madan, A.; Young, A., C.; Shevchenko, Y.; Bouffard, G., G.; Blakesley, R., W.; Touchman, J., W.; Green, E., D.; Dickson, M., C.; Rodriguez, A., C.; Grimwood, J.; Schmutz, J.; Myers, R., M.; Butterfield, Y., S.; Krzywinski, M., I.; Skalska, U.; Smailus, D., E.; Schnerch, A.; Schein, J., E.; Jones, S., J.; Marra, M., A. (2002) *Proc Natl Acad Sci U S* A 99, p.16899-17802.

[16] Modrek, B. and Lee, C. (2002) Nat Genet 30, p.13-22.

[17] Wiemann, S.; Arlt, D.; Huber, W.; Wellenreuther, R.; Schleeger, S.; Mehrle, A.; Bechtel, S.; Sauermann, M.; Korf, U.; Pepperkok, R.; Sultmann, H. and Poustka, A. (2004) *Genome Res* 14, p.2136-2180.

[18] Brasch, M. A.; Hartley, J. L. and Vidal, M. (2004) Genome Res 14, p.2001-2010.

[19] Suzuki, Y.; Taira, H.; Tsunoda, T.; Mizushima-Sugano, J.; Sese, J.; Hata, H.; Ota, T.; Isogai, T.; Tanaka, T.; Morishita, S.; Okubo, K.; Sakaki, Y.; Nakamura, Y.; Suyama, A. and Sugano, S. (2001) *EMBO Rep* 2, p.388-481.

[20] Berk, A. J. and Sharp, P. A. (1977) *Cell* 12, p.721-753.

[21] McKnight, S. L. and Kingsbury, R. (1982) *Science* 217, p.316-340.

[22] Nikolov, D. B. : Chen, H.; Halay, E. D.; Usheva, A. A.; Hisatake, K.; Lee, D. K.; Roeder, R. G. and Burley, S. K. (1995) *Nature* 377, p.119-147.

[23] Suzuki, Y.; Yamashita, R.; Sugano, S. and Nakai, K. (2004) Nucleic Acids Res 32 Database issue, Dp.78-159.

[24] Baeuerle, P. A. and Baltimore, D. (1996) *Cell* 87, p.13-33.

[25] Ho, I. C. and Glimcher, L. H. (2002) *Cell* 109 Suppl, Sp.109-129.

[26] Suzuki, Y.; Tsunoda, T.; Sese, J.; Taira, H.; Mizushima-Sugano, J.; Hata, H.; Ota, T.; Isogai, T.; Tanaka, T.; Nakamura, Y.; Suyama, A.; Sakaki, Y.; Morishita, S.; Okubo, K. and Sugano, S. (2001) *Genome Res* 11, p.677-761.

[27] Bajic, V. B.; Tan, S. L.; Suzuki, Y. and Sugano, S. (2004) *Nat Biotechnol* 22, p.1467-1540.

[28] Yamashita, R.; Suzuki, Y.; Sugano, S. and Nakai, K. (2005) Gene 350, p.129-265.

[29] Larkin, J. E.; Frank, B. C.; Gavras, H.; Sultana, R. and Quackenbush, J. (2005) *Nat Methods* 2, p.337-381.

[30] Fickett, J. W. and Wasserman, W. W. (2000) *Curr Opin Biotechnol* 11, p.19-43.

[31] Okazaki, Y.; Furuno, M.; Kasukawa, T.; Adachi, J.; Bono, H.; Kondo, S.; Nikaido, I.; Osato, N.; Saito, R.; Suzuki, H.; Yamanaka, I.; Kiyosawa, H.; Yagi, K .; Tomaru, Y.; Hasegawa, Y.; Nogami, A.; Schonbach, C.; Gojobori, T.; Baldarelli, R.; Hill, D.P.; Bult, C.; Hume, D.A.; Quackenbush, J.; Schriml, L.M.; Kanapin, A.; Matsuda, H.; Batalov, S.; Beisel, K.W.; Blake, J.A.; Bradt, D.; Brusic, V.; Chothia, C.; Corbani, L.E.; Cousins, S.; Dalla, E.; Dragani, T.A.; Fletcher, C.F.; Forrest, A.; Frazer, K.S.; Gaasterland, T.; Gariboldi, M.; Gissi, C.; Godzik, A.; Gough, J.; Grimmond, S.; Gustincich, S.; Hirokawa, N.; Jackson, I.J.; Jarvis, E.D.; Kanai, A.; Kawaji, H.; Kawasawa, Y.; Kedzierski, R.M.; King, B.L.; Konagaya, A.; Kurochkin, I.V.; Lee, Y.; Lenhard, B.; Lyons, P.A.; Maglott, D.R.; Maltais, L; Marchionni, L.; McKenzie, L.; Miki, H.; Nagashima, T.; Numata, K.; Okido, T.; Pavan, W.J.; Pertea, G.; Pesole, G.; Petrovsky, N.; Pillai, R.; Pontius, J.U.; Qi, D.; Ramachandran, S.; Ravasi, T.; Reed, J.C.; Reed, D.J.; Reid, J.; Ring, B.Z.; Ringwald, M.; Sandelin, A.; Schneider, C.; Semple, C.A.; Setou, M.; Shimada, K.; Sultana, R.; Takenaka, Y.; Taylor, M.S.; Teasdale, R.D.; Tomita, M.; Verardo, R.; Wagner, L.; Wahlestedt, C.; Wang, Y.; Watanabe, Y.; Wells, C.; Wilming, L.G.; Wynshaw-Boris, A.; Yanagisawa, M.; Yang, I; Yang, L.; Yuan, Z.; Zavolan, M.; Zhu, Y.; Zimmer, A.; Carninci, P.; Hayatsu, N.; Hirozane-Kishikawa, T.; Konno, H.; Nakamura, M.; Sakazume, N.; Sato, K.; Shiraki, T.; Waki, K.; Kawai, J.; Aizawa, K.; Arakawa, T.; Fukuda, S.; Hara, A.; Hashizume, W.; Imotani, K.; Ishii, Y.; Itoh, M.; Kagawa, I.; Miyazaki, A.; Sakai, K.; Sasaki, D.; Shibata, K.; Shinagawa, A .; Yasunishi, A.; Yoshino, M.; Waterston, R.; Lander, E.S.; Rogers, J.; Birney, E.; Hayashizaki, Y. (2002) *Nature* 420, p.563-636.

[32] Kel, A. E.; Gossling, E.; Reuter, I.; Cheremushkin, E.; Kel-Margoulis, O. V. and Wingender, E. (2003) *Nucleic Acids Res* 31, p.3576-3585.

[33] Hardison, R. C. (2000) *Trends Genet* 16, p.369-441.

[34] Boguski, M. S. (2002) *Nature* 420, p.515-521.

[35] Suzuki, Y.; Yamashita, R.; Shirota, M.; Sakakibara, Y.; Chiba, J.; Mizushima-Sugano, J.; Kel, A. E.; Arakawa, T.; Carninci, P.; Kawai, J.; Hayashizaki, Y.; Takagi, T.; Nakai, K. and Sugano, S. (2004) *In Silico Biol* 4, p.429-473.

[36] Suzuki, Y.; Yamashita, R.; Shirota, M.; Sakakibara, Y.; Chiba, J.; Mizushima-Sugano, J.; Nakai, K. and Sugano, S. (2004) *Genome Res* 14, p.1711-1719.

[37] Levy, S. and Hannenhalli, S. (2002) *Mamm Genome* 13, p.510-514.

[38] Rockman, M. V. and Wray, G. A. (2002) *Mol Biol Evol* 19, p.1991-3995.

[39] King, M. C. and Wilson, A. C. (1975) *Science* 188, p.107-123.

[40] Enard, W.; Khaitovich, P.; Klose, J.; Zollner, S.; Heissig, F.; Giavalisco, P.; Nieselt-Struwe, K.; Muchmore, E.; Varki, A., Ravid, R.; Doxiadis, G. M.; Bontrop, R. E. and Paabo, S. (2002) *Science* 296, p.340-343.

[41] Tautz, D. (2000) *Curr Opin Genet Dev* 10, p.575-584.

[42] Wei, C. L.; Ng, P.; Chiu, K. P.; Wong, C. H.; Ang, C. C.; Lipovich, L.; Liu, E. T. and Ruan, Y. (2004) *Proc Natl Acad Sci U S A* 101, p.11701-11707.

[43] Hashimoto, S.; Suzuki, Y.; Kasai, Y.; Morohoshi, K.; Yamada, T.; Sese, J.; Morishita, S.; Sugano, S. and Matsushima, K. (2004) *Nat Biotechnol* 22, p.1146-1155.

[44] Shiraki, T.; Kondo, S.; Katayama, S.; Waki, K.; Kasukawa, T.; Kawaji, H.; Kodzius, R.; Watahiki, A.; Nakamura, M.; Arakawa, T.; Fukuda, S.; Sasaki, D.; Podhajska, A.;

Harbers, M.; Kawai, J.; Carninci, P. and Hayashizaki, Y. (2003) *Proc Natl Acad Sci U S A* 100, p.15776-15857.

[45] Bonham, K.; Ritchie, S., A.; Dehm, S., M.; Snyder, K., and Boyd, F., M. (2000) *J Biol Chem* 275, p.37604-37615.

[46] Landry, J., R.; Mager, D, L. and Wilhelm, B. T. (2003) *Trends Genet* 19, p.640-648.

[47] Zavolan, M.; Kondo, S.; Schonbach, C.; Adachi, J.; Hume, D. A.; Hayashizaki, Y. and Gaasterland, T. (2003) *Genome Res* 13, p.1290-1590.

[48] Wang, J.; Zhang, J.; Zheng, H.; Li, J.; Liu, D.; Li, H.; Samudrala, R.; Yu, J. and Wong, G. K. (2004) *Nature* 431, 1 p following 757; discussion following 757.

[49] (2004) *Science* 306, p.636-676.

[50] Modrek, B. and Lee, C. J. (2003) *Nat Genet* 34, p.177-257.

[51] Oyama, M.; Itagaki, C.; Hata, H.; Suzuki, Y.; Izumi, T.; Natsume, T.; Isobe, T. and Sugano, S. (2004) *Genome Res* 14, p.2048-2100.

[52] Kitano, H. (2002) *Nature* 420, p.206-216.

In: Trends in Genome Research
Editor: Clyde R. Williams, pp. 139–153
ISBN 1-60021-027-9

Chapter 5

Flexible Statistical Methods for Array-based Comparative Genomic Hybridization Analysis

Jeffrey C. Sklar *
Department of Statistics, California Polytechnic State University,
San Luis Obispo, CA 93407, USA,

Wendy Meiring† **and *Yuedong Wang***‡
Department of Statistics and Applied Probability,
University of California, Santa Barbara CA 93106, USA.

Abstract

Array-based comparative genomic hybridization (array CGH) enables simultaneous genome-wide screening for regions of genomic alterations in a test genomic sample relative to a reference sample. Genomic alterations may be identified by region-specific copy number gains or losses. Identification of these specific regions of copy number change may aid identification of genomic alterations associated with specific diseases, such as tumorigenisis. The detection of genomic alterations using array CGH requires careful statistical analysis to account for many sources of variation, such as spatial correlation along each chromosome, and heterogeneity of variances. The hybrid adaptive spline (HAS) method has been previously applied to array CGH data to deal with spatial inhomogeneity, by modeling copy numbers in terms of an adaptively selected set of basis functions. The traditional HAS procedure uses a fixed inflated

*E-mail address: jsklar@calpoly.edu
†E-mail address: meiring@pstat.ucsb.edu
‡E-mail address: yuedong@pstat.ucsb.edu

degrees of freedom (IDF) to account for the increased cost of adaptive basis function selection. However, we demonstrate that a fixed selection cost may lead to HAS selecting too many basis functions in the final model. To overcome this problem, we propose a data-driven measure of the IDF based on the concept of the generalized degrees of freedom (GDF). Our extended hybrid adaptive spline procedure based on this estimated IDF is more adaptive to different data sets and basis functions. We use a bootstrap method to compute p-values, which does not require a Gaussian assumption. We also use the False Discovery Rate (FDR) to circumvent the problem of multiple comparisons. We use a well known BAC array data set to illustrate our methods.

Keywords: bootstrap, false discovery rate, forward stepwise selection, generalized cross-validation, generalized degrees of freedom, hybrid adaptive spline, inflated degrees of freedom, statistical method

1 Introduction

CGH was developed as a molecular cytogenetic technique to overcome shortcomings of conventional cytogenetics and fluorescence *in situ* hybridization (FISH) analysis (Kallioniemi, Kallioniemi, Sudar, Rutovitz, Gray, Waldman and Pinkel 1992). It is a powerful technique that allows whole-genome screening for copy-number changes in chromosomes associated with tumorigenesis.

With CGH, specific genomic regions with copy number gains or losses can be identified, without apriori specification of regions of interest. The application of CGH analyses have unmasked numerous recurrent copy-number changes or alterations in cancer that had not been detected previously by other means. Characterization of these alterations is important in the diagnosis of, and prognosis assessment in cancer, and in the delineation of molecular genetic mechanisms that underly tumorigenesis.

However, CGH has two disadvantages: the low throughput (Veltman, Schoenmakers, Eussen, Janssen, Merkx, van Cleef, van Ravenswaaij, Brunner, Smeets and van Kessel 2002, Wessendorf, Fritz, Wrobel, Nessling, Lampel, Goettel, Kuepper, Joos, Hopman, Kokocinski, Dohner, Bentz, Schwaenen and Licher 2002) and the limited resolution, typically 5-10 Mb for deletions and 2 Mb for amplifications (Bentz, Plesch, Stilgenbauer, Dohner and Lichter 1998, Kirchhoff, Gerdes, Maahr, Rose, Bentz, Dohner and Lundsteen 1999). The array CGH, or matrix-based CGH as it is sometimes called, overcomes these limitations (Solinas-Toldo, Lampel, Stilgenbauer, Nickolenko, Benner, Dohner, Cremer and Lichter 1997, Pinkel, Segraves, Sudar, Clark, Poole, Kowbel, Collins, Kuo, Chen, Zhai, Dairkee, Ljung, Gray and Albertson 1998, Pollack, Perou, Alizadeh, Eisen, Pergamenschikov, Williams, Jeffrey, Botstein and Brown 1999, Snijders, Nowak, Segraves, Brown, Conroy, Hamilton, Hindle, Huey, Kimura, Law, Myambo, Palmer, Ylstra, Yue, Gray, Jain, Pinkel and Albertson 2001). Array CGH has been shown to be more accurate than conventional CGH in detecting genomic alterations (Yano, Matsuyama, Matsuda, Matsumoto, Yoshihiro and Naito 2004), is increasingly becoming the method of choice for high-throughput, high-resolution screening of genomic alterations, and has been hailed as "a revolutionary platform" (Mantripragada, Buckley, de Stahl and Dumanski 2004).

The purpose of an array CGH is to detect and map chromosomal aberrations on a genomic scale. In a typical array CGH experiment, genomic DNAs isolated from test and reference samples are labeled respectively with red (Cy5) and green (Cy3) fluorescent dyes. The differentially labeled samples are hybridized onto an array containing genomic clones. Digital images are captured from each of the fluorescent dyes. The ratios of red and green fluorescent signals in paired samples are measured for each gene/clone. These ratios are indicative of copy-number differences between the test and the reference samples (after normalization to account for dye-differences, and other biases, which we do not discuss here).

For illustration, we downloaded a BAC array data set, GM01524, from the website *http://www.nature.com/ng/journal/v29/n3/suppinfo/ng754_S1.html.* The data result from an experiment aimed at measuring copy number changes for the cell strain GM01524 (test sample) against a normal male reference DNA (reference), which were co-hybridized on a CGH array containing 2,460 BAC and P1 clones in triplicate (7,380 spots) and with an average resolution of $\sim$ 1.4 Mb (Snijders et al. 2001). We will focus on chromosome 6. Figure 1 shows the profile of $\log_2$ fluorescent ratios plotted against the physical position of the corresponding BACs on the genome. Our goal is to detect and map locations (genes/clones) on the profile which are significantly different from zero, since a $\log_2$ ratio of zero would correspond to equal copy numbers in both the test and reference samples.

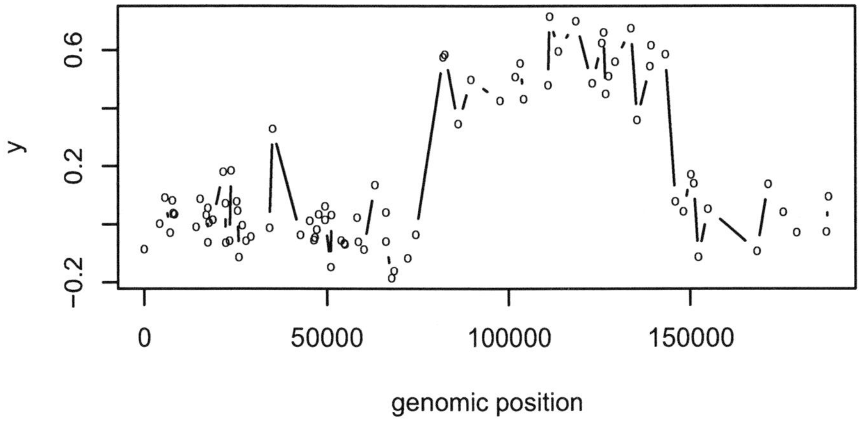

Figure 1: Profile of $\log_2$ fluorescent ratios (vertical axis) for chromosome 6.

From a statistical standpoint, the identification of genomic alterations with array CGH appears to be more challenging than the identification of differentially expressed genes in cDNA microarrays, since, in addition to all the data normalization issues and the need to account for various sources of variations, the former may also need to take account of spatial correlations along each chromosome, which could be safely ignored in the latter. This spatial information also is important in mapping where the genomic alterations are, in addition to the characterization of the alterations (e.g. loss or gain). Some statistical methods have already been proposed to address this challenge. Carothers (1997) accounted for the spatial correlations by assuming a fixed-width window with the same distance-dependent correlation. However a distance based correlation may be too rigid since, first, correlations may vary with chromosomal structures and thus locations, and, second, the size of genomic alterations may vary. The specification of the width of correlation in Carothers (1997) is somewhat arbitrary. We take an alternative approach, through extending a spatially adaptive flexible method based on the hybrid adaptive spline (HAS) procedure (Luo and Wahba 1997, Wang and Guo 2004), by improving the method of accounting for adaptive model selection costs. The HAS procedure has already proved valuable for the identification of genomic alterations in the endometrium of patients with endometriosis (Wang and Guo 2004, Guo, Wu, Strawn, Basir, Wang, Halverson, Montgomery and Kajdacsy-Balla 2004).

Since alterations typically occur in local regions, the expectation of a $\log_2$ ratio profile equals zero except in each region where alterations occur. High-resolution mapping of specific regions is of crucial importance for the subsequent discovery of the disease-associated clones and thus the genes they harbor. In the ideal situation, the profile is a block (step) function, with abrupt step changes at the beginning and ends of regions of genetic alteration or copy number changes. In this situation the problem is equivalent to detecting the number and locations of change points. Several methods have been proposed for change point detection in array CGH data (Autio, Hautaniemi, Kauraniemi, Yli-Harja, Astola, Wolf and Kallioniemi 2003, Jong, Marchiori, Meijer, Van Der Vaart and Ylstra 2004, Wang, Kim, Pollack, Narasimhan and Tibshirani 2005, Picard, Robin, Lavielle, Vaisse and Daudin 2005). In this article, we extend the HAS procedure to detect the number and locations of change points, while adjusting for the cost of adaptive model selection.

2 Introduction to the HAS Procedure with Fixed IDF

We will assume the following model

$$y_i = f(x_i) + \varepsilon_i, \quad i = 1, \cdots, n, \tag{1}$$

where y_i are $\log_2$ ratios (normalized when necessary), f is a function of the physical position x_i along the chromosome, and ε_i's are random errors with mean zero and variance σ^2. For simplicity we transformed the location variable x into the interval $[0,1]$. We assume that f is a block function and our goal is to detect locations or regions where $f(x) \neq 0$. Since a block function has discontinuous points and is spatially inhomogeneous, common nonparametric regression methods such as smoothing splines do not provide good estimates for f, leading us to consider the spatially adaptive method of HAS.

Since f is a block function, instead of representing the function f in (1) using cubic spline basis functions as used by Luo and Wahba (1997) in a different application area, we will use the following $(n+1)$ block basis functions: $\phi_1(x) = 1$ and $\{\xi_i(x) = I(x > x_i) : i = 1, \ldots, n\}$ where each basis function is expressed in terms of $x \in [0,1]$, and where $I(x > x_i) = 1$ if $x > x_i$ and $I(x > x_i) = 0$ otherwise. We will estimate f by a linear combination of an adaptively selected subset of these basis functions.

The HAS procedure with fixed IDF

1. *initialization*: set the maximum number of basis functions $q \geq 1$ that will initially be selected to represent f in (1). Also fix the IDF in an attempt to account for model selection costs. Start with $k = 1$ and one basis function $\phi_1(x)$ in the initial model;

2. *forward stepwise selection*: for $k = 2, \cdots, q$, choose the kth basis function $\xi_{i_k}(x)$ from those not yet selected, to maximize the reduction in the residual sum of squares when this additional basis function is included in the model;

3. *optimal number of basis functions*: choose $1 \leq k \leq q$ as the minimizer of the generalized cross-validation (GCV) score

$$GCV(k) = RSS(k)/(n - (1 + (k-1) \times IDF))^2, \tag{2}$$

where RSS(k) is the residual sum of squares at step $k \in \{2, \cdots, q\}$;

4. *backward elimination*: perform backward elimination to the selected basis functions. Decide the final number of basis functions by the Akaike Information Criteria (AIC);

5. *fit*: fit a standard or ridge regression model to the final selected basis functions.

We have modified the original HAS programs for cubic splines to allow any form of basis functions. The key to spatial adaptiveness is to select basis functions adaptively based on data. The IDF is used to account for the added flexibility in adaptively selected basis functions. Luo and Wahba (1997) suggested to use a fixed IDF=1.2. For array CGH data, we found that this choice of IDF often leads to selection of too many basis functions and overfitting. The backward elimination step is thus added as an option to the original HAS procedure. Nevertheless, the final model with the backward elimination option still often selects too many basis functions.

3 Generalized Degrees of Freedom

In the HAS procedure, the IDF was introduced to account for the cost of basis function selection (Luo and Wahba 1997). During the forward stepwise selection procedure (step 2 of the algorithm in section 2), each additional basis function actually costs more than one degree of freedom. The need to adjust for model selection costs is not unique to HAS. Usually a fixed selection cost is used in practice: Luo and Wahba (1997) used IDF=1.2 while Friedman recommended IDF=3 for his MARS procedure (Friedman 1991). However, we have found that the true cost of basis function selection depends on many factors such as the properties of the basis functions and the true function. It is not surprising that Friedman (1991) and Luo and Wahba (1997) recommended different IDF's because they used quite different basis functions. We have also found that the cost of selecting each basis function depends on which basis functions have already been selected. Since the true function is never known and there is no clear rule for deciding the IDF, we propose to estimate the IDF using the generalized degrees of freedom (GDF) at each step of the selection.

We now review the concept of GDF for a modeling procedure. Consider a response vector $y = (y_1, \cdots, y_n)^T \sim N(\mu, \sigma^2 I)$, where $\mu = (\mu_1, \cdots, \mu_n)^T$. A modeling procedure (selection and estimation) is a map $\mathcal{M} : y \to \hat{\mu}$. Ye (1998) defined the generalized degrees of freedom (GDF) of $\mathcal{M}$ as

$$GDF(\mathcal{M}) = \sum_{i=1}^{n} h_i(\mu), \tag{3}$$

where $h_i(\mu) = \partial E(\hat{\mu}_i(y))/\partial \mu_i$. See also Efron (2004). The GDF is a natural extension of the standard degrees of freedom. To estimate $GDF(\mathcal{M})$, Ye (1998) suggested the following Monte Carlo approach:

The GDF procedure

1. Draw an n-dimensional sample $\delta \sim N(0, \tau^2 I)$, apply the modeling procedure $\mathcal{M}$ to the perturbed sample $y + \delta$ to get estimates $\hat{\mu}(y + \delta)$.

2. T repetitions of step 1 gives $\delta_t = (\delta_{t1} \cdots, \delta_{tn})^T$ and $\hat{\mu}(y + \delta_t) \triangleq (z_{t1}, \cdots, z_{tn})^T$, for $t \in \{1, \cdots, T\}$.

3. For each $i \in \{1, \cdots, n\}$, fit the following linear model

$$z_{ti} = \alpha + h_i \delta_{ti} + \eta_{ti}, \quad t = 1, \cdots, T,$$

   using least squares, where the η_{ti} are random errors. Denote the resulting slope estimates by $\{\hat{h}_i : i = 1, \ldots, n\}$.

4. Estimate $GDF(\mathcal{M})$ by $\sum_{i=1}^{n} \hat{h}_i$.

Ye (1998) suggests that choosing $\tau \in [.5\sigma, \sigma]$ is generally a good choice. The results are usually insensitive to the choice of τ when it is in this range. When σ^2 is unknown, we use the estimator $\hat{\sigma}^2 = \sum_{i=1}^{n-1} (y_{i+1} - y_i)^2 / (2(n-1))$ (Rice 1984). An alternative estimator of $\hat{\sigma}^2$ is given by Tong and Wang (2005).

4 Extended HAS Procedure

The GDF provides a general approach to account for the cost involved in a complicated selection process. In the HAS procedure, at each step of the forward selection process, a basis function is selected from those basis functions that have not yet been selected. For each value of k in the HAS procedure with a fixed IDF, the quantity $1 + (k-1) \times IDF$ in (2) estimated the total degrees of freedom (say D_k), for selecting $k-1$ basis functions $\{\xi_{i_2}(x), \cdots, \xi_{i_k}(x)\}$ from $\{\xi_2(x), \cdots, \xi_n(x)\}$, and for fitting the model $\mathcal{M}_k = \text{span}\{\phi_1(x), \xi_{i_2}(x), \cdots, \xi_{i_k}(x)\}$. We improve on this estimate by estimating D_k for each k using the GDF procedure described in Section 3, since our experience indicates that the GDF depends on many factors such as the nature of the basis functions, the property of the true function f in (1), and the basis functions that have already been selected. After estimating the GDF, we then modify the GCV criterion to account for the cost of adaptive model selection.

Specifically, for any fixed k, we apply forward selection (analogous to steps 1 and 2 in the HAS procedure) to get the model $\mathcal{M}_k = \text{span}\{\phi_1(x), \xi_{i_2}(x), \cdots, \xi_{i_k}(x)\}$. We then fit this model using step 5 in the HAS procedure to get the fits $\hat{f}_k = (\hat{f}_k(x_1), \cdots, \hat{f}_k(x_n))^T$. Letting $\hat{\mu} = \hat{f}_k$, we then estimate the GDF of $\mathcal{M}_k$ using the Monte Carlo method for this value of k. We denote the resulting estimate of the GDF as $\hat{D}_k$. We compute $\hat{D}_k$ for each $k \in \{2, \ldots, q\}$ where q is our maximal number of basis functions selected in the extended HAS procedure. By replacing $1 + (k-1) \times IDF$ in (2) by $\hat{D}_k$, we obtain a new GCV criterion for selecting the final model. Putting all steps together, we have the following extended HAS (EHAS) procedure.

The EHAS Procedure

1. *initialization*: set the maximum number of basis functions q $(q \geq 1)$. Start with $k = 1$ and one basis function $\phi_1(x)$ in the model;

2. *forward stepwise selection*: for $k = 2, \cdots, q$, choose the kth basis $\xi_{i_k}(x)$ from those not yet selected, to maximize the reduction in the residual sum of squares when this additional basis function is included in the model. Estimate the GDF $\hat{D}_k$ as described in the previous paragraph;

3. *optimal number of basis functions*: choose $k \geq 1$ as the minimizer of the generalized cross-validation (GCV) score

$$GCV(k) = RSS(k)/(n - \hat{D}_k)^2,$$

   for $k \in \{1, \ldots, q\}$;

4. *fit*: fit a standard or ridge regression model to the final selected basis functions.

Our preliminary experience indicates that the backward elimination step in the HAS procedure is not necessary in EHAS.

5 Inference

We use the following bootstrap procedure to calculate p-values. Denote the HAS or EHAS estimates of f and σ as $\hat{f}$ and $\hat{\sigma}$ respectively. Let $e_i = y_i - \hat{f}(x_i)$ for $i = 1, \ldots, n$. Let B denote the number of bootstrap samples we will use in our uncertainty assessment. For each $b \in \{1, \ldots, B\}$, let $\{e^*_{b1}, \ldots, e^*_{bn}\}$ be a sample of size n taken with replacement from $\{e_1, \ldots, e_n\}$. Let

$$y^*_{ib} = \hat{f}(x_i) + e^*_{ib}, \quad i = 1, \cdots, n,$$

be the bth bootstrapped sample. Run HAS or EHAS to estimate f and σ based on each bootstrapped sample, and denote the resulting estimates by $\hat{f}^*_b$ and $\hat{\sigma}^*_b$ respectively. Let $D^*_i(b) = (\hat{f}^*_b(x_i) - \hat{f}(x_i))/\hat{\sigma}^*_b$. Let the p-value for clone i be calculated as

$$p_i = \#\{b : |D^*_i(b)| > |\hat{f}(x_i)|/\hat{\sigma}\}/B.$$

Then clones with $p_i \leq \alpha$ are significantly different from zero at pointwise significance level α. The false discovery rate (FDR) can be used to circumvent the problem of multiple comparisons (Wang and Guo 2004). We can also construct bootstrap confidence intervals based on $\{\hat{f}_b^* : b = 1, \ldots, B\}$ (Wang and Wahba 1995).

6 Application

We apply the HAS and EHAS procedures to the GM01524 data described in Section 1. Figure 2 shows HAS and EHAS fits with 95% bootstrap confidence intervals. Figure 3 shows p-values and locations with significant changes in copy numbers between the test and reference samples. Both HAS and EHAS procedures identified the same region as Snijders et al. (2001) and Wang et al. (2005). It is interesting to note that the HAS procedure also identified an isolated gain in the 6p region, but EHAS did not. This could be a false positive, but it is also possible that the gain, due to its apparently small size, may be too small to be detected by standard cytogenetic karyotyping methods.

To take a closer look at the performance of the HAS and EHAS procedures, we plot $\hat{D}_k$ for the first 50 iterations in the top panel of Figure 4. It is above the diagonal line which means that the total degrees of freedom at iteration k is greater than k. We estimate the IDF at iteration k ($k \geq 2$) as $(\hat{D}_k - 1)/(k-1)$, and our estimates are plotted in the lower panel of Figure 4. It is obvious that the IDF is not a constant and could be quite different from 1.2. The first two basis functions are easy to choose (corresponding to two locations of estimated change-points in the fitted function f). Therefore, they incur negligible extra expenses and the estimated IDF for each of these two basis functions is close to one. The estimated IDFs are greater than two when $4 \leq k \leq 30$, doubling the usual degrees of freedom due to the extra cost for selecting basis functions at these iterations. This indicates that the selection of these additional basis functions is less obvious than the previous two. The estimated IDF gradually decreases back to one.

We plot the GCV scores for the HAS (top panel) and EHAS (lower panel) procedures in Figure 5. The GCV scores from the HAS procedure keep decreasing even until the 50th iteration. Therefore, HAS selects a large number of basis functions. The GCV scores from the EHAS procedure reach a clear minimum at $k = 3$.

7 Conclusion

Many human health problems are the result of abnormalities or alterations in the number of copies of segments of genomic DNA. CGH was developed to measure alterations in DNA sequences throughout the entire genome in a single experiment. Array-based CGH further improved the resolution of these experiments, with great potential for uncovering genes involved in specific diseases. However, the high-throughput and high-resolution array CGH poses challenges to many existing statistical methods.

In this article we extend the spatially adaptive HAS method to EHAS, to address the challenges raised by spatial inhomogeneity in the copy number profile. EHAS is a fully data-driven approach, that accounts for adaptive model selection costs at each stage through

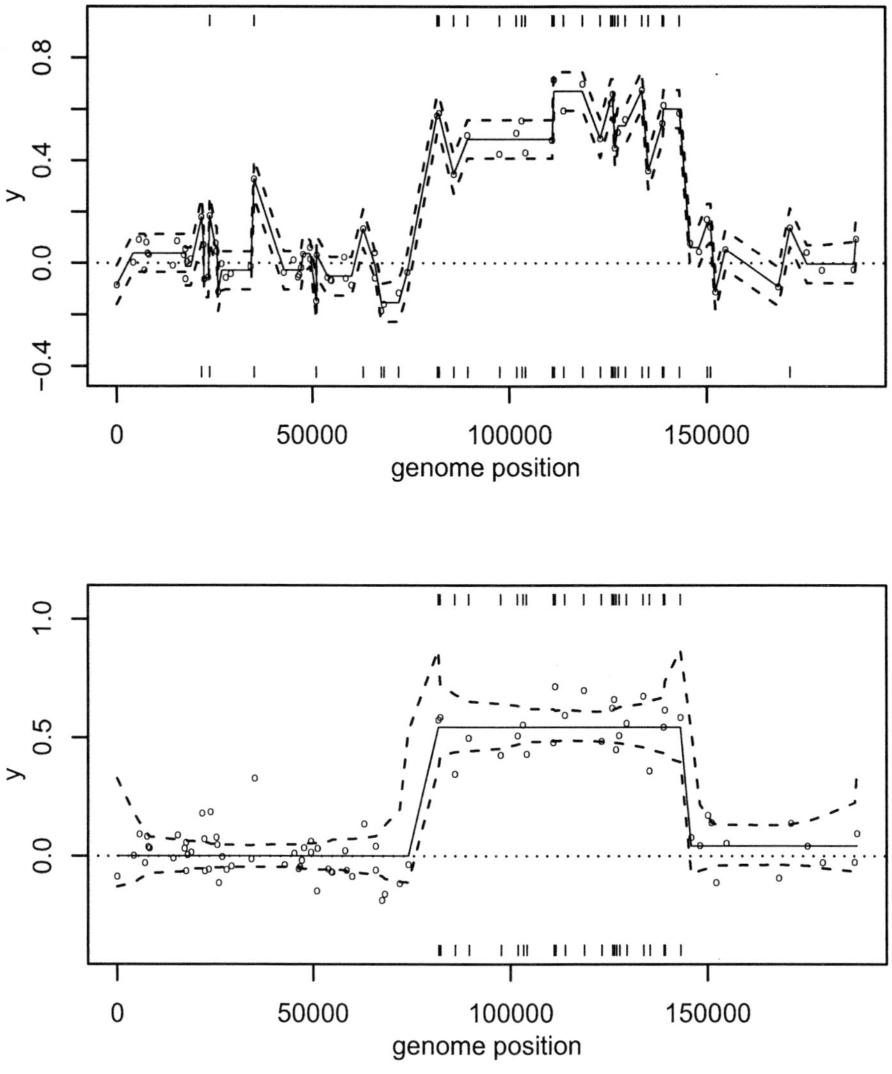

Figure 2: HAS fits (above) and EHAS fits (below) with 95% bootstrap confidence intervals (dashed lines). Locations with significant changes in copy numbers at the 5% level based on bootstrap p-values with $B = 10000$ are marked at the bottom of the plot. Locations with significant change at $FDR \leq .05$ level are marked at the top of the plot. The observations at the observation locations (x_i) are the same in both plots, shown as open circles.

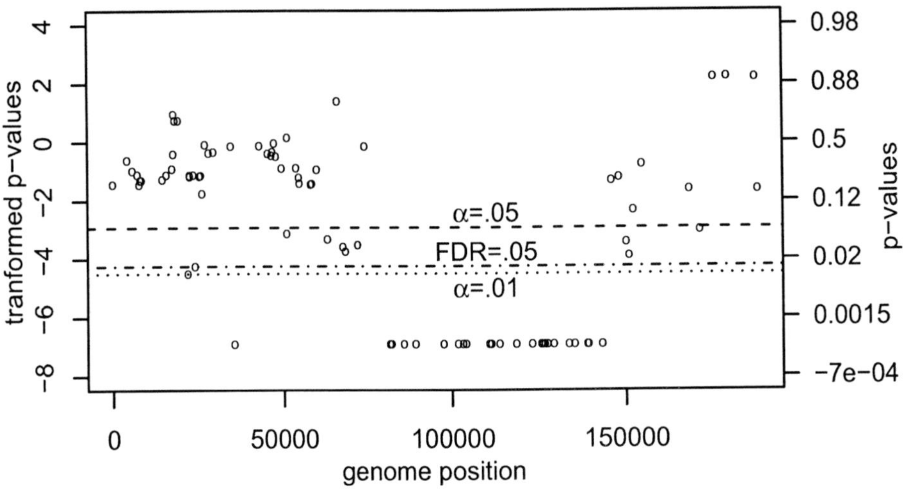

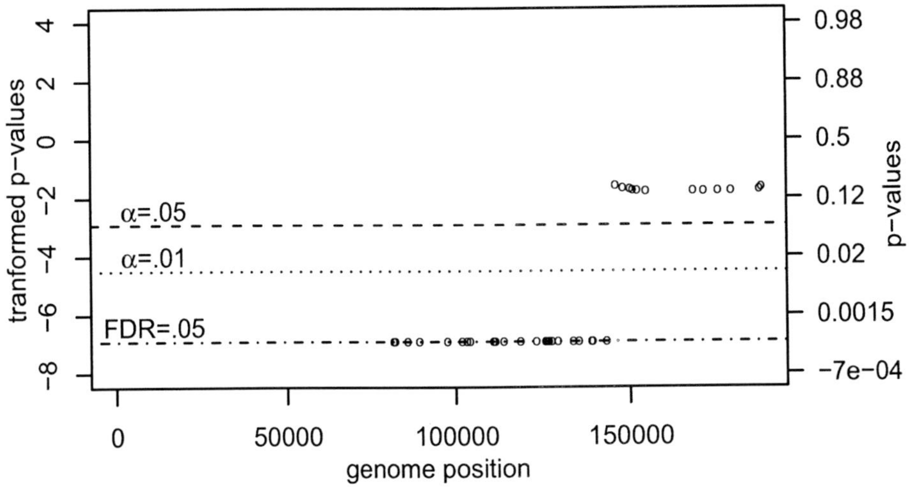

Figure 3: Transformed bootstrap p-values, $\log((p+a)/(1-p+a))$ with $a = 0.001$, are plotted as circles for the HAS procedure (above) and the EHAS procedure (below) respectively. Regions below the three dotted lines represent rejection regions with $\alpha = .01$ and $\alpha = .05$ and $FDR \leq .05$ respectively. In the lower plot, some p-values in the left of the region are greater than 0.98, and are not shown due to non-uniform increments of the non-linear transformation near $p = 1$.

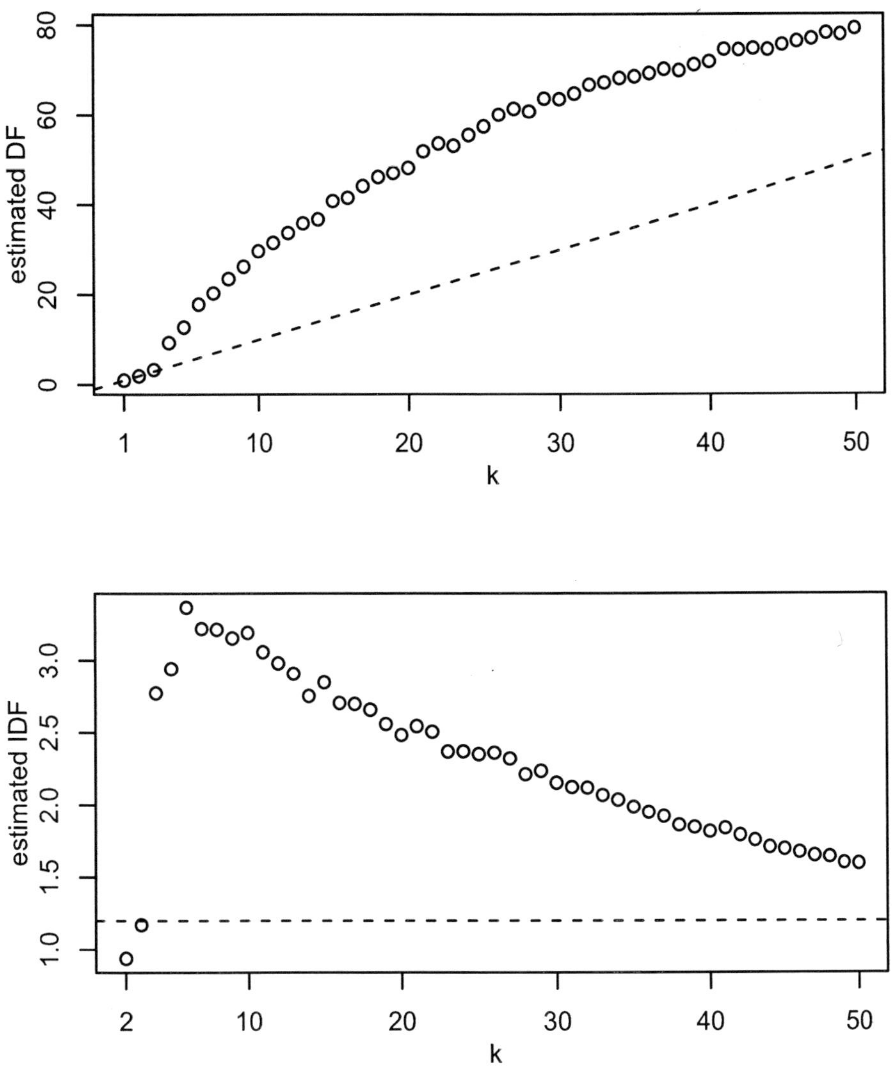

Figure 4: Top panel: plot of $\hat{D}_k$ for $k = 1,\ldots,50$. The dashed line is the diagonal line. Lower panel: plot of the estimated IDF defined as $(\hat{D}_k - 1)/(k-1)$, for $k = 2,\ldots,50$. The dashed line represents the constant 1.2, which was previously used as the IDF by Luo and Wahba (1997).

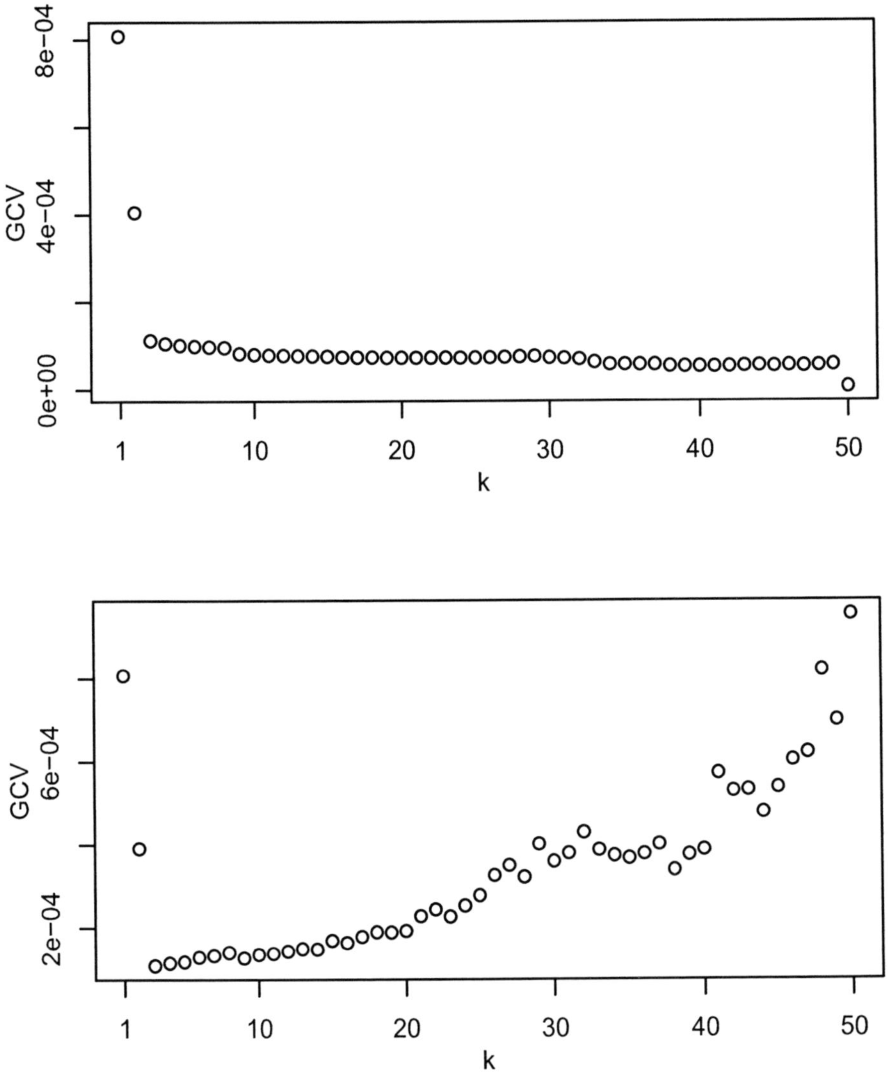

Figure 5: Top panel: plot of the GCV scores from the HAS procedure with IDF = 1.2. Lower panel: plot of the GCV scores from the EHAS procedure, illustrating a clear minimum at $k = 3$.

an estimated IDF based on the generalized degrees of freedom concept. The EHAS procedure handles nicely the inhomogeneous "curvature"/jumps of the ratio profiles along the genome. While the GDF estimation requires normality, our bootstrap-based inference procedure does not require the normality assumption. Further research is necessary to systematically evaluate the performance of the EHAS procedure and compare its performance with other existing methods.

Acknowledgments

This work was supported by an NIH Grant R01 GM58533 (YW).

References

Autio, R., Hautaniemi, S., Kauraniemi, P., Yli-Harja, O., Astola, J., Wolf, M. and Kallioniemi, A. (2003). CGH-Plotter: MATLAB toolbox for CGH-data analysis, *Bioinformatics* **19**: 1714–1715.

Bentz, M., Plesch, A., Stilgenbauer, S., Dohner, H. and Lichter, P. (1998). Minimal sizes of deletions detected by comparative genomic hybridization, *Genes, Chromosomes and Cancer* **21**: 172–175.

Carothers, A. D. (1997). A likelihood-based approach to the estimation of relative DNA copy number by comparative genomic hybridization, *Biometrics* **53**: 848–856.

Efron, B. (2004). The estimation of prediction error: Covariance penalties and cross-validation (with discussion), *Journal of the American Statistical Association* **99**: 619–632.

Friedman, J. H. (1991). Multivariate adaptive regression splines (with discussion), *Annals of Statistics* **19**: 1–67.

Guo, S. W., Wu, Y., Strawn, E., Basir, Z., Wang, Y., Halverson, G., Montgomery, K. and Kajdacsy-Balla, A. (2004). Genomic alterations in the endometrium may be a proximate cause for endometriosis, *Eur J Obstet Gynecol Reprod Biol* **116**: 89–99.

Jong, K., Marchiori, E., Meijer, G., Van Der Vaart, A. and Ylstra, B. (2004). Breakpoint identification and smoothing of array comparative genomic hybridization data, *Bioinformatics* **20**: 3636–3637.

Kallioniemi, A., Kallioniemi, O. P., Sudar, D., Rutovitz, D., Gray, J. W., Waldman, F. and Pinkel, D. (1992). Comparative genomic hybridization for molecular cytogenetic analysis of solid tumors, *Science* **258**: 818–821.

Kirchhoff, M., Gerdes, T., Maahr, J., Rose, H., Bentz, M., Dohner, H. and Lundsteen, C. (1999). Deletions below 10 megabasepairs are detected in comparative genomic hybridization by standard reference intervals, *Genes, Chromosomes and Cancer* **25**: 410–413.

Luo, Z. and Wahba, G. (1997). Hybrid adaptive splines, *Journal of the American Statistical Association* **92**: 107–116.

Mantripragada, K. K., Buckley, P. G., de Stahl, T. D. and Dumanski, J. P. (2004). Genomic microarrays in the spotlight, *Trends in Genetics* **20**: 87–94.

Picard, F., Robin, S., Lavielle, M., Vaisse, C. and Daudin, J. J. (2005). A statistical approach for array CGH data analysis, *BMC Bioinformatics* **6**: Art. No. 27, Feb.

Pinkel, D., Segraves, R., Sudar, D., Clark, S., Poole, I., Kowbel, D., Collins, C., Kuo, W. L., Chen, C., Zhai, Y., Dairkee, S. H., Ljung, B. M., Gray, J. W. and Albertson, D. G. (1998). High resolution analysis of DNA copy number variation using comparative genomic hybridization to microarrays, *Nat. Genet.* **20**: 207–211.

Pollack, J. R., Perou, C. M., Alizadeh, A. A., Eisen, M. B., Pergamenschikov, A., Williams, C. F., Jeffrey, S. S., Botstein, D. and Brown, P. O. (1999). Genome-wide analysis of DNA copy-number changes using cDNA microarrays, *Nat Genet* **23**: 41–46.

Rice, J. A. (1984). Bandwidth choice for nonparametric regression, *Annals of Statistics* **12**: 1215–1230.

Snijders, A. M., Nowak, N., Segraves, R. Blackwood, S., Brown, N., Conroy, J., Hamilton, G., Hindle, A. K., Huey, B., Kimura, K., Law, S., Myambo, K., Palmer, J., Ylstra, B., Yue, J. P., Gray, J. W., Jain, A. N., Pinkel, D. and Albertson, D. G. (2001). Assembly of microarrays for genome-wide measurement of DNA copy number, *Nature Genetics* **29**: 263–264.

Solinas-Toldo, S., Lampel, S., Stilgenbauer, S., Nickolenko, J., Benner, A., Dohner, H., Cremer, T. and Lichter, P. (1997). Matrix-based comparative genomic hybridization: biochips to screen for genomic imbalances, *Genes, Chromosomes and Cancer* **20**: 399–407.

Tong, T. and Wang, Y. (2005). Estimating residual variance in nonparametric regression using least squares, to appear in *Biometrika*.

Veltman, J., Schoenmakers, E. F. P. M., Eussen, B. H., Janssen, I., Merkx, G., van Cleef, B., van Ravenswaaij, C. M., Brunner, H. G., Smeets, D. and van Kessel, A. G. (2002). High-throughput analysis of subtelomeric chromosome rearrangements by use of array-based comparative genomic hybridization, *Am J Hum Genet.* **70**: 1269–1276.

Wang, P., Kim, Y., Pollack, J., Narasimhan, B. and Tibshirani, R. (2005). A method for calling gains and losses in array CGH data, *Biostatistics* **6**: 45–58.

Wang, Y. and Guo, S. W. (2004). Statistical methods for detecting genomic alterations through array-based comparative genomic hybridization (CGH), *Frontiers in Bioscience* **9**: 540–549.

Wang, Y. and Wahba, G. (1995). Bootstrap confidence intervals for smoothing splines and their comparison to Bayesian confidence intervals, *J. Statist. Comput. Simul.* **51**: 263–279.

Wessendorf, S., Fritz, B., Wrobel, G., Nessling, M., Lampel, S., Goettel, D., Kuepper, M., Joos, S., Hopman, T., Kokocinski, F., Dohner, H., Bentz, M., Schwaenen, C. and Licher, P. (2002). Automated screening for genomic imbalances using matrix-based comparative genomic hybridization, *Lab Invest* **82**: 47–60.

Yano, S., Matsuyama, H., Matsuda, K., Matsumoto, H., Yoshihiro, S. and Naito, K. (2004). Accuracy of an array comparative genomic hybridization (CGH) technique in detecting DNA copy number aberrations: comparison with conventional CGH and loss of heterozygosity analysis in prostate cancer, *Cancer Genet Cytogenet* **150**: 122–127.

Ye, J. M. (1998). On measuring and correcting the effects of data mining and model selection, *Journal of the American Statistical Association* **93**: 120–131.

In: Trends in Genome Research
Editor: Clyde R. Williams, pp. 155-172
ISBN 1-60021-027-9

Chapter 6

Molecular Characterisation of Human Common Fragile Site *FRA6E*, a Large Genomic Region Spanning 9 Mb

Antonella Russo[a*], *Francesco Acquati*[b], *Massimiliano Rampin*[a], *Laura Monti*[b], *Elisa Palumbo*[a], *Romina Graziotto*[a] *and Roberto Taramelli*[b]

[a] Dipartimento di Biologia, Università degli Studi di Padova, Via U. Bassi 58b, 35131 Padova, Italy;

[b] Dipartimento di Biotecnologie e Scienze Molecolari, Università degli Studi dell'Insubria, Via J.H. Dunant 3, 21110 Varese, Italy.

Abstract

Common fragile sites of the human genome are suggested to be potentially involved in cancer development; *FRA6E* (6q26), one of the most frequently expressed common fragile sites in humans, is located in a region frequently found rearranged in cancer. We have mapped *FRA6E* by FISH analysis with YAC, BAC and PAC genomic clones, and have characterized the fragility of the region by sequence analysis. Recent published data indicated that the location of *FRA6E* is about 2.5 Mb beyond the telomeric side of the region considered in the present study. Taken together, our data and previously reported data indicate that *FRA6E* spans approximately 9 Mb, corresponding to a chromosomal region located at 6q25.3-6q26. It has been recently suggested that unusual structural features, detected as high flexibility motives by sequence analysis, are overrepresented within fragile sites, and that this organization can be relevant for the intrinsic fragility of these regions. We have carried out a search for fragility motives within the genomic sequence corresponding to *FRA6E*, confirming the significance of unusual structural organization of chromosome sequences with respect to the location of common fragile sites. A number of expressed genes map at *FRA6E*, which can be relevant for cancer. RT-PCR analysis revealed that some of them are down-regulated in

[*] E-mail address: russo@bio.unipd.it, phone: +39 049 8276279, fax: +39 049 8276280, (Corresponding author: Antonella Russo, Dipartimento di Biologia, Università degli Studi di Padova, Via U. Bassi 58b, 35131 Padova, Italy)

melanoma tumors. The results outlined in this study underline the need for a deep investigation of the fragility regions of the human genome, which are probably wider than previously thought.

Introduction

Fragile sites are non-random chromosomal regions prone to breakage, which under specific culture conditions are expressed as decondensations, gaps or breaks. Rare fragile sites are observed in less than 5% of the human population, segregate as mendelian traits and can be associated with pathological phenotypes [Richards, 2001; Arlt *et al.*, 2003]; common fragile sites represent a normal feature of chromosomes, even though their expression is detectable only in a subset of cells [Richards, 2001; Arlt *et al.*, 2003]. The number of common fragile sites characterised at the molecular level is rapidly increasing [Arlt *et al.*, 2003; Popescu, 2003], five of them being characterised in the last two years: *FRA2G* [Limongi *et al.*, 2003], *FRA4F* [Rozier *et al.*, 2004], *FRA6E* [Denison *et al.*, 2003a], *FRA7E* [Zlotorynski *et al.*, 2003], *FRA9E* [Callahan *et al.*, 2003]. However, the molecular basis for instability of common fragile sites is still not understood. Sequence analysis suggests high flexibility and low stability structure in common fragile sites, due to overrepresentation of AT- and TA-dinucleotide repeats [Arlt *et al.*, 2003; Zlotorynski *et al.*, 2003]. This feature has been proposed as a possible common molecular basis for the fragility of rare and common fragile sites [Zlotorynski *et al.*, 2003]. Recently, it has been provided as evidence for a role of several signal transduction factors (ATR, BRCA, SMC, FA) in common fragile site induction [Casper et al., 2002; Arlt et al., 2004; Musio et al., 2005; Howlett et al., 2005]..

One innovative concept concerning the molecular organization of common fragile sites is the huge extension of these regions. For example *FRA3B,* originally reported to cover about 500 kb, was found subsequently to extend 4 Mb [Becker *et al.*, 2002]. *FRA16D* and *FRA6F* have been reported to span more than 1 Mb [Krummel *et al.*, 2000; Morelli *et al.*, 2002]; *FRA9E* accounts for almost 10 Mb [Callahan *et al.*, 2003], and *FRA4F* is a sequence of 7 Mb [Rozier *et al.*, 2004]; the still incomplete characterisation of *FRA7E* suggests that the fragility region is at least 4.5 Mb [Zlotorynski *et al.*, 2003]. Furthermore, in these fragile sequences the breakage events can occur at variable locations, and separate hotspots for fragility can be detected within them [Morelli *et al.*, 2002; Callahan *et al.*, 2003, Rozier *et al.*, 2004].

It is still controversial whether common fragile sites must be considered a risk factor for human health [Richards, 2001; Popescu, 2003]. Yunis and Soreng first proposed a possible involvement of fragile sites in carcinogenesis, as they correspond to chromosome breakpoints specifically observed in cancer [Yunis and Soreng, 1984]. Recently, common fragile sites have been reported to be highly sensitive to mutagens and carcinogens, to represent preferential sites for translocations and deletions, for gene amplification and insertion of viral sequences [see Popescu, 2003 for a review]. Furthermore, loss of heterozygosity (LOH), chromosomal deletions or altered expression of gene sequences occur for several tumours in regions including common fragile sites [Richards, 2001; Popescu, 2003, Ishii and Furukawa, 2004, Finnis et al., 2005]. *FRA3B* contains the tumour suppressor gene *FHIT* [Huebner *et al.*, 2001; Roz *et al.*, 2002]. The candidate tumour suppressor gene *WWOX* has been identified in correspondence of *FRA16D* [reviewed by Ludes-Meyers *et al.*, 2003], and functional evidence for the presence of a tumour suppressor gene has been reported in 7q31.3, the same location of *FRA7G* [Tatarelli *et al.*, 2000; Zenklusen *et al.*, 2000]. *PARK2* has been mapped into fragile site *FRA6E,* and oncosoppressive function has been suggested for this gene [Cesari *et al.*, 2003; Denison *et al.*, 2003a; Denison *et al.*, 2003b].

FRA6E was mapped at 6q25.3-q26 by conventional cytogenetics [Yunis and Soreng, 1984; Kahkonen *et al.*, 1988]. A recently published study reported the molecular mapping of *FRA6E* [Denison *et al.*, 2003a]; its extension, according to the recent release from the human genome sequencing, corresponds to a region of 3.3 Mb. Cytogenetic and LOH data indicate that 6q is frequently and preferentially deleted in several cancers; one major susceptibility region is located in 6q25-6q27 [Cooke *et al.*, 1996; Fujii *et al.*, 1996; Colitti *et al.*, 1998; Hauptschein *et al.*, 1998; Rodriguez *et al.*, 2000]. This region is the subject of intense study by our group, aimed at characterizing genes involved in cancer by positional cloning approaches [Acquati *et al.*, 1994; Magnaghi *et al.*, 1994; Tibiletti *et al.*, 1996; Tibiletti *et al.*, 2000; Acquati *et al.*, 2001].

We have also mapped *FRA6E* and our results indicate that *FRA6E* is not limited to the above mentioned size but extends its fragility region for about 9 Mb; we report here that this huge region includes a number of cancer related genes, some of which are down regulated in melanoma tumors. In addition, sequence analysis of *FRA6E* confirms the significance of an unusual structural organization of chromosome sequences with respect to the location of common fragile sites.

The results coming from this study underline the need for a more in depth investigation of fragility regions of the human genome, which are probably much greater than previously thought.

Materials and Methods

Selection of Genomic Clones

Genomic clones (YAC, BAC, PAC clones) mapping in 6q25.3-q26 were selected after screening the databases available at: NCBI, the National Center for Biotechnology Information (http://www.ncbi.nlm.nih.gov/); the Sanger Institute (http://www.sanger.ac.uk/); the Whithead Institute for Biomedical Research (http://wi.mit.edu/); the selection started for YAC clones positives for DNA markers *D6S441, D6S473* and *D6S442* since they are included in a region frequently involved in LOH events in cancer. Further selections of BAC and PAC clones were done according to the indications obtained by FISH experiments. DNA from genomic clones was obtained by standard procedure.

FISH Mapping of FRA6E

Chromosome preparations from human lymphocytes were obtained by whole blood culture (subject A), or after Ficoll-paque isolation of mononucleated cells by freshly collected buffy coats (anonimously provided by the Blood Hospital Center of Padova; subjects B-D). Lymphocytes were PHA-stimulated and cultured 72 h before harvesting. *FRA6E* expression was achieved by treating the cultures with aphidicolin (APC; 0.2 μM, Sigma) in the last 24 h of growth. Colcemid (0.1 μg/ml) was added one hour before harvest to accumulate cells at metaphase; chromosome preparations were obtained by a standard protocol.

To investigate the expression of *FRA6E* in the human lymphoblastoid cell line H691, obtained by immortalisation of peripheral B-lymphocytes from subject A, exponentially growing cells were exposed for 24 h to 0.2 μM APC. Colcemid arrest of metaphases and chromosome preparations were done as for primary lymphocytes. H691 cells have a normal diploid chromosome set and duplication time of about 24 h.

Probes were labelled by nick translation in the presence of digoxigenin-11dUTP (Roche Molecular Biochemicals), precipitated with a 50-fold excess of human Cot1 DNA and salmon sperm DNA, and resuspended in the hybridization mix (50% formamide, 10% dextran sulphate, 2xSSC). Slides were aged few days at room temperature before FISH; pretreated with 200 μg/ml RNase, and denatured by 4 min incubation in 70% formamide, 2xSCC at 70° C. Probe was denatured for 10 min at 70°C and incubated at 37°C for 60-90 min before hybridization, to achieve the preannealing of repetitive sequences present in the probe with Cot1 DNA. 100-150 ng of labelled probe were hybridised overnight at 37°C with the chromosome preparation. Detection and amplification of the probe signal was carried out after low stringency washes by using the "Fluorescent Antibody Dig Detection Set" kit (Roche Molecular Biochemicals) following the manufacturer's instructions. Slides were counterstained with DAPI and analysed under a Zeiss Axioskop fluorescence microscope. The position of each clone with respect to *FRA6E* was assessed by scoring an informative number of metaphases with the expressed fragment. Clones were considered to belong to *FRA6E* if they were observed to hybridize in different metaphases either proximally (centromerically) and distally (telomerically) to the expressed chromosome fragments, or to give a bipartite hybridization signal in correspondence of the break (A minimum of 15 metaphases with expressed fragment was considered significant to calculate percentages). A genomic clone giving a 100% proximal or distal hybridization pattern would be considered to be outside the fragile site; the significance of this result requires a largest sample size to be analysed, therefore for those clones supposed to be at the boundaries of the fragile site the total number of observations was increased accordingly. Digitalised images of each scored metaphase were collected by using a Leica DMR fluorescence microscope equipped with a high resolution photocamera (Leica DC 300F).

Computational Analysis of DNA Flexibility

DNA flexibility was evaluated by using the *TwistFlex* software, freely available at http://www.jail.cs.huji.ac.il/~netab/index.html [Zlotorynsky *et al.*, 2003]. The analysis was carried out by considering the sequence of chromosome 6 (NCBI, build 34.3) from 155.7 Mb to 163.7, at 500 kb-intervals. The region comprises the genomic sequence investigated by FISH in this study, the sequence characterised by Denison *et al.* [2003a], and the 2.5 Mb sequence interposed between. Twistflex returns a number of parameters concerning base composition and presence of dinucleotide arrays. Flexibility peaks are defined by sequence conditions predicting twist angles higher that 13.7°. Clusters of flexibility are defined by the occurrence of at least three peaks within 5 kb. The crucial parameteres influencing the flexibility properties of the sequence under analysis are the content of AT and the presence of

AT dinucleotides. More details can be found at the web address given above or in Zlotorynsky *et al.*, 2003.

Sequence Analysis

The following databases were used to verify the sequence composition and the presence of known genes in the region under study: the databases available at NCBI, the National Center for Biotechnology Information (http://www.ncbi.nlm.nih.gov/); the Ensemble Genome Browser at Sanger Institute (http://www.ensembl.org/); the Human Genome browser at UCSC (http://genome.ucsc.edu/).

RT-PCR Analysis for FRA6E Candidate Genes

Candidate genes mapping within the core fragility region defined in this study were sought by consulting the NCBI, Ensemble and UCSC databases. Among these genes, those having a potential role in cancer pathogenesis based on the database annotation were selected for expression analysis. The mRNA sequence for each of these genes was used to design a couple of oligonucleotides for RT-PCR analysis by means of the Basilisk algorithm. The primer's sequences are as follows:

NOX3: forward: 5'-GGATCGGAGTCACTCCCTTCGCTG-3'; reverse: 5'- ATGAACACCTCTGGGGTCAGCTGA-3'.
ARID1B: forward:5'-CTTACACGGAAAGCATCTGC-3'; reverse: 5'- CACAGATGACAGATGCAACC -3'.
ZDHHC14: forward:5'-GACCGTGAAACTTAAATACTGTTT-3'; reverse:5'- AGTCCTCATGCAGGGAGTC-3'.
WTAP: forward:5'-TCTGAAGAAAAACTAAAGCAACAAC-3'; reverse:5'- ACTTATTACCATTCCCTGGAGA-3'.
VIL2: forward: 5'- CCCCTGAGACTGCCGTG-3' ; reverse: 5'-CTCCTCCTGTGCCCGCTT-3'.
TULP4: forward:5'-GCGAGGAGTGGTTGGGGT-3'; reverse:5'- CACGAACATTGTAGAACTTGAC-3'.
β-ACTIN: forward:5'-CCAAGGCCAACCGCGAGAAGATGAC-3'; reverse:5'- AGGGTACATGGTGGTGCCGCCAGAC-3'.

RT-PCR reactions were carried out in a 12,5 μl final volume with 100 ng of total RNA from either snap-frozen tumor samples or cultured tumor cell lines, using the *C. Therm* One-Step RT-PCR Kit (Roche Molecular Biochemicals) following the manufacturer instructions. RT-PCR conditions were as follows: reverse transcription: 60° C for 30 min; PCR amplification: 94° C for 5 min, followed by 28 cycles of 94° C for 30 sec, 45-54° C for 30 sec and 72° C for 1 min, with a final extension step of 72° C for 7 min. The RT-PCR reactions were loaded on a 1% agarose gel and PCR product were visualized under UV light after ethidium bromide staining.

Ovarian and breast cancer cell lines were kindly provided by Dr. M. Negrini (Dipartimento di Medicina Sperimentale e Diagnostica, Università di Ferrara, Italy). Ovarian tumor samples were provided by Dr. M.G. Daidone (Istituto Nazionale Tumori- Milano, Italy.). Melanoma cell lines and tumour samples were kindly provided by Dr. M. Rodolfo (Istituto Nazionale Tumori - Milano, Italy).

Results

FISH Mapping of FRA6E with YAC, BAC and PAC Clones

In a preliminary search for genomic clones spanning *FRA6E,* YAC clones were used as probes in FISH experiments carried out on APC-treated human primary lymphocytes. The selected clones belonged to contig WC6.15 (mega-YAC CEPH library), and represented the genomic region located at 6q25-q26 which appears frequently involved in LOH events (in particular, including the DNA markers *D6S441* and *D6S44,* Figure 1). Among the clones assayed, some showed the peculiar pattern expected in correspondence of a fragility region (proximal, bipartite and distal hybridization signals with respect to the expressed chromosome fragment): YAC 785_a_4 (estimated length 1160 kb), YAC 823_b_11 (estimated length 1700 kb), and YAC 897_f_2, whose estimated size is 290 kb. The details of this preliminary analysis can be found in Table 1.

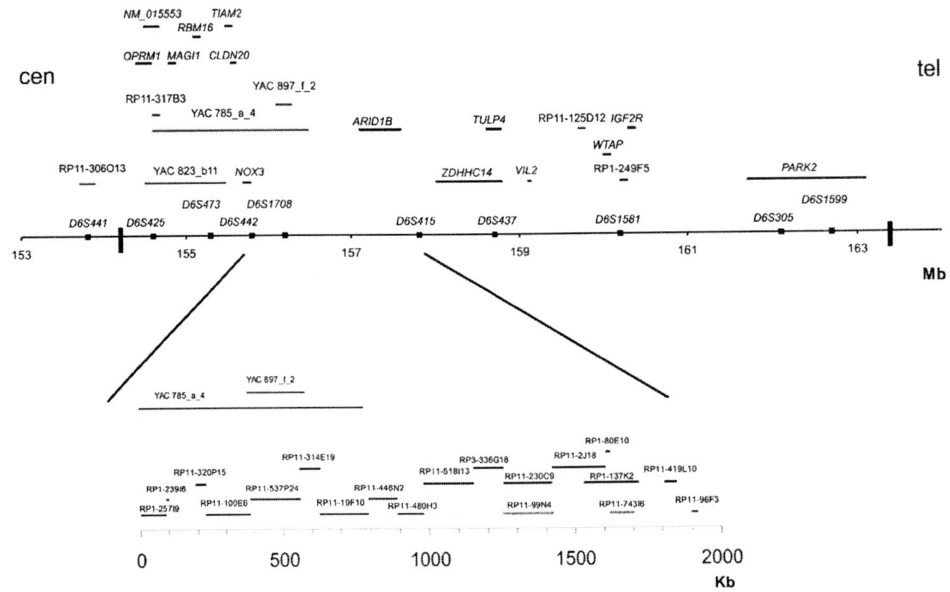

Figure 1. Physical map of *FRA6E,* showing the genomic clones used in this study, the relevant known genes, and other relevant clones located in the region. The 1.85 Mb region, investigated in details by a contig of overlapping genomic clones, is represented in a larger scale at the bottom. The position of YAC clones, as well as that of BAC clones RP11-99N4 and RP11-743I6, is based on their DNA marker content. The remaining genomic clones are fully sequenced and placed on the map accordingly. The position of a number of DNA markers is also shown on the axis. The solid vertical lines on the axis indicate the approximate boundaries of *FRA6E.*

On the basis of the above data, a panel of BAC and PAC clones was selected to refine the molecular mapping of *FRA6E.* FISH experiments were carried out on APC-treated human primary lymphocytes (Table 1), or by using an immortalised lymphoblastoid cell line (H691) derived from the donor considered for FISH experiments with YAC probes (Table 1). The latter results are reported in Table 2.

Table 1. FISH mapping of *FRA6E* on APC-treated human primary lymphocytes. The selected YAC and BAC probes hybridize in the 153.7-159.8 Mb region of chromosome 6. For each probe the frequencies of proximal, bipartite or distal hybridization signals with respect to the break are indicated.

Probe	Genomic location	Donor	Position of hybridization						Total breaks scored
			Proximal		Bipartite		Distal		
			N	%	N	%	N	%	N
RP11-306O13	153.7-153.9	B	37	100.0	0		0		37
RP11-317B3	154.6-154.7	B	12	75.0	1	6.3	3	18.7	16
y823_b_11	154.5-155.5	A	8		0		1		9
y785_a_4	154.6-156.5	A	2		0		4		6
y897_f_2	156.1-156.3	A	11	61.1	1	5.6	6	33.3	18
RP11-320P15	155.9-156.0	C	8	50.0	3	18.7	5	31.3	16
RP11-743I6	157.3-157.5	D	11	68.8	0		5	31.3	16
RP11-419L10	157.5-157.6	D	4	26.7	7	46.7	4	26.7	15
RP11-96F3	157.6-157.6	C	24	36.4	13	19.7	29	43.9	66
RP11-125D12	159.7-159.8	B	4		0		3		7

Table 2. FISH mapping of *FRA6E* on APC-treated H691 cells. The selected PAC and BAC probes hybridize in the 153.7-159.8 Mb region of chromosome 6. For each probe the frequencies of proximal, bipartite or distal hybridization signals with respect to the break are indicated.

Probe	Genomic location	Position of hybridization						Total breaks scored
		Proximal		Bipartite		Distal		
		N	%	N	%	N	%	N
RP11-320P15	155.9-156.0	8	33.3	5	20.8	11	45.8	24
RP11-100E6	156.0-156.1	9	37.5	3	12.5	12	50.0	24
RP11-537P24	1561-156.3	6	42.9	0		8	57.1	14
RP11-19F10	156.3-156.5	3	11.1	7	25.9	17	63.0	27
RP11-230C9	157.0-157.1	2	9.5	2	9.5	17	81.0	21
RP11-99N4	157.0-157.1	2	10.0	8	40.0	10	50.0	20
RP11-2J18	157.1-157.3	3	13.6	4	18.2	15	68.2	22
RP1-80E10	157.3-157.3	4	19.0	4	19.0	13	61.9	21
RP11-743I6	157.3-157.5	0		11	25.6	32	74.4	43
RP11-419L10	157.5-157.6	0		6	30.0	14	70.0	20
RP11-96F3	157.6-157.6	5	8.5	6	10.2	48	81.4	59
RP11-125D12	159.7-159.8	10		5		45		60

Two BAC clones were selected to define the location of the centromeric boundary of *FRA6E*: clone RP11-317B3, which is positive for marker *D6S425,* overlaps the most centromeric portions of YACs 823_b_11 and 785_a_4 (Figure 1 and Table 1). On a total of 16 metaphases expressing *FRA6E,* this clone was found to hybridize mainly (75%) in proximal position with respect to the break, but bipartite (6.3%) and distal (18.7%) signals were also observed (Table 1). This indicates that the genomic sequence corresponding to clone RP11-317B3 is still inside the fragile site. In contrast, the most centromeric clone tested, RP11-306O13, produced the hybridisation pattern expected for a sequence located upstream the fragility region: 100% proximal hybridisation signals on 37 APC-expressed breaks. We can therefore consider that the centromeric boundary of *FRA6E* is located between markers *D6S441* and *D6S425.*

With one exception, the additional clones selected for the analysis span about 1.85 Mb at the telomeric boundary of band q25.3 (Figure 1, bottom); all of them showed the hybridisation pattern expected in correspondence of a fragile site, as proximal, distal and bipartite fluorescent signals were observed, with variable percentages, with respect to the breaks (Tables 1-2). The remaining BAC clone (RP11-125D12) was selected in consideration of the results published by Denison *et al.* [2003a], who have mapped *FRA6E* to a genomic region of 3.3. Mb located 2.5 Mb downstream to clone RP11-96F3, still giving in the present study bipartite signals (Tables 1-2). Therefore it was crucial to understand if the fragility region characterised by us could extend as a continuum toward the whole 3.3 Mb region characterised by Denison *et al.* [2003a]. Clone RP11-125D12 maps only 300 kb upstream to the suggested centromeric boundary of *FRA6E* [Denison *et al.* 2003a] (Figure 1, top), but in our FISH experiments this clone produced the typical hybridisation pattern expected within a fragile site (Tables 1-2), thus supporting the existence of a unique fragile site at 6q25.3-q26.

Figure 2 shows representative pictures of FISH.

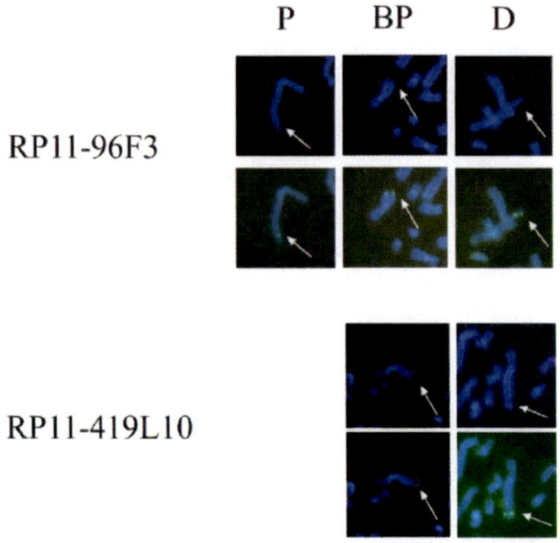

Figure 2. Representative hybridisation patterns across *FRA6E,* as observed in APC-treated metaphases from human lymphocytes (top, clone RP11-96F3) or from H691 lymphoblastoid cells (bottom, clone RP11-419L10). For each picture the DAPI staining (blue), and the merged image showing FITC (yellow) visualization of the hybridised probe are shown; arrows indicate the expressed break. P = proximal hybridisation; BP = bipartite hybridisation ; D= distal hybridisation.

Sequence Analysis

Several genes are located in the rather large genomic region encompassed by *FRA6E.* Their location is shown in Figure 1, while other relevant information is summarised in Table 3. The gene density is particularly low in the 1.85 region studied in more details by FISH analysis, which includes only two genes, *NOX3* and *ARID1B* (Figure 1).

Table 3. Genes mapping in the region characterised in the present study

Gene symbol	Ensemble Gene ID	Position (Mb)[§]	Known or putative function
OPRM1	ENSG00000112038	154.4	Mu-type opioid receptor
NM_015553	ENSG00000074706	154.5	phosphoinositide-binding protein PIP3-E
MAGI1	ENSG00000153721	154.8	membrane- associated guanylate kinase interacting protein-like 1
RBM16	ENSG00000180821	155.1	putative RNA-binding protein 16
TIAM2 (T-cell lymphoma invasion and metastasis 2)	ENSG00000146426	155.5	guanyl-nucleotide exchange factor, involved in the intracellular signaling cascade
Claudin-20	ENSG00000171217	155.6	integral membrane protein component of tight junction (TJ) strands
NOX3	ENSG00000074771	155.7	NAPDH oxidase participating in reactive oxigen generation
ARIDB1	ENSG00000049618	157.1	DNA-binding protein with chromatin remodelling function
ZDHHC14	ENSG00000175048	157.7	putative transcription factor
TULP4	ENSG00000130338	158.6	putative transcription factor
VIL2 (ezrin)	ENSG00000092820	159.1	cytovillin with membrane-cytoskeleton linking functions
WTAP	ENSG00000146457	160.1	ubiquitously expressed nuclear protein, which associates to tumor suppressor protein WT1.

[§]according to build 34.3 of the chromosome 6 sequence

Flexibility Analysis of FRA6E

Search for flexibility features of the region studied in the present work was done by using the *TwistFlex* software, freely available at http://www.jail.cs.huji.ac.il/~netab/index.html [Zlotorynsky *et al.*, 2003]. The analysis was carried out for the 1.85 Mb region representing the core region of fragility, and extended toward the region described by Denison *et al.* [2003a], including the 2.5 Mb sequence in between. As described in Materials and Methods, the AT content and the percentage of AT dinucleotides are the crucial variables describing the flexibility of a given sequence. Along the whole region examined, these values were comparable to the whole genome estimates; in particular the AT content was found about 60%, and the average percentage of AT dinucleotides was 7.60. The *TwistFlex* software indicated the presence of several peaks of flexibility in the region analysed, all of them characterised by high AT content ranging from 73 to 78%; in the peaks of flexibility the percentage of AT dinucleotides was 19.7-25.5, therefore 2-2.5 times higher than the average value observed in the whole sequence. Furthermore, percentages of TA dinucleotides were 17.6-25.5 in the flexible peaks, while the same percentage was on the average 6.46 along the whole sequence. The peak length ranged from 100 to more than 70,000 bp. Clusters of flexibility peaks are defined by the presence of at least three peaks in 5 kb. In the interval between 155.7-157.6 Mb, corresponding to the region characterised by FISH in the present study, 6.5 fragility clusters per Mb were observed (Table 4); a comparable result was obtained for the 3.3 Mb sequence region investigated by Denison *et al.* [2003a], in which 6.9 clusters/Mb were observed (Table 4). The intermediate 2.5 Mb region appeared less flexible with respect to the adjacent ones, with only 3.6 cluster per Mb detected (Table 4); however the value obtained is slightly higher than the reported threshold for flexibility [Zlotorynsky *et al.* 2003].

Table 4. Flexibility properties of *FRA6E*

Region	Coordinates	Clusters of flexibility detected at 500 kb intervals (min-max)	Clusters of flexibility detected at 500 kb intervals (mean±SE)	Clusters/Mb
Present study	155.7-157.7Mb	2-4	3.25±0.479	6.5
Intermediate region	157.7-160.2 Mb	0-3	1.80±0.490	3.6
Denison *et al.* (2003a)	160.2-163.7 Mb	2-5	3.43±0.369	6.9

Expression Analysis of Genes within FRA6E

The 1.85 Mb fragility region, which is the core region of fragility, was found to contain two genes: *NOX3* and *ARID1B* (Figure 1). The very restricted expression pattern in normal adult tissues of *NOX3* precluded a thoroughly analysis of this gene in tumor and cell lines. By contrast, *ARID1B* turned out to be expressed in normal ovarian surface epithelium (HOSE), melanocytes and normal breast tissue; therefore, we have investigated its expression pattern by semi-quantitative RT-PCR in a panel of ovarian, breast and melanoma-derived cell lines or primary tumors. As shown in Figure 3 (panels a-b), no change in the expression of *ARID1B* was observed in a panel of 7 primary ovarian tumor samples and 11 ovarian tumor cell lines when compared to the normal counterpart. The lack of amplification from the SG10G cell line was not unexpected, since this cell line has been shown to lack chromosome 6 (RT and AR, unpublished data). Similarly, we found no evidence of *ARID1B* down-regulation in a panel of five breast cancer cell lines (data not shown). By contrast, three out of six samples (50%) derived from primary melanomas or melanoma-derived cell lines showed a clear down-regulation of *ARID1B* expression when compared to the expression level observed in primary melanocytes (Figure 3, panel c). LOH analysis of the corresponding genomic region failed to detect genomic losses as possible causes of the *ARID1B* gene down regulation (data not shown).

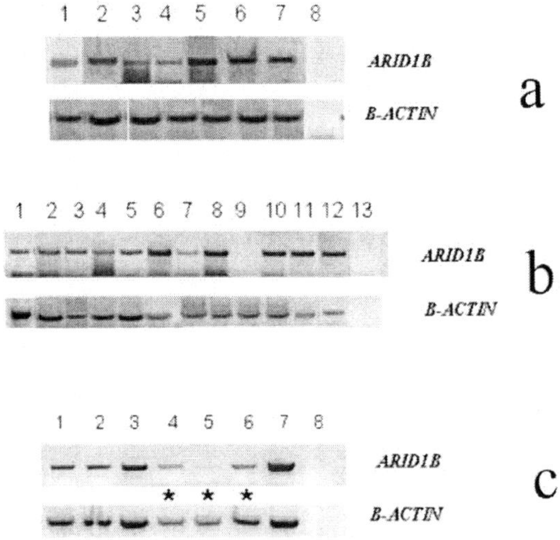

Figure 3. *ARID1B* expression analysis in primary ovarian cancer samples, ovarian cancer cell lines and melanoma-derived cell lines. Expression of *ARID1B* was assessed by RT-PCR on total RNA samples extracted from primary ovarian cancer samples (panel a), ovarian cancer cell lines (panel b) or melanoma cell lines (panel c) as described in Materials and Methods. Panel a lanes: 1-7: seven independent primary ovarian cancer samples; lane 8: negative control. Panel b lanes: 1: normal ovarian surface epithelium; 2: 12780KOV; 3: HEY 4; 4: IGROV 1; 5: INTOV 1; 6: INTOV 2; 7: IOSE 64; 8: IOSE 80; 9: SG10G; 10: SKOV 3; 11: OAW 42; 12: OV166; 13: negative control. Panel c lanes: 1: normal melanocytes; 2: SK MEL 28; 3, 5, 6 and 7: four independent melanoma-derived cell lines; 4: primary melanoma tumor sample; 8: negative control. The asterisks highlight the three melanoma samples displaying *ARID1B* down-regulation.

We have further investigated the expression profile of three additional genes that are located in the 2.5 Mb genomic region located more telomerically from the one we have characterized. The genes in the centromere to telomere order are *TULP4*, *VIL2* and *WTAP* (Figure 1) and they were chosen for expression analysis because of their biological/biochemical function, which is compatible with a role in cancer development. A fourth gene mapping within the above mentioned region, *ZDHHC14* (Figure 1), was also evaluated as a candidate gene, but it turned out not to be expressed by RT-PCR analysis in normal ovarian surface epithelium (HOSE), melanocytes and normal breast tissue, therefore it was discarded for further analysis.

Semiquantitative RT-PCR was performed for *TULP4*, *VIL2* and *WTAP* in the same panel of tumor and tumor-derived cell lines described above. No expression changes were detected for *VIL2* and *WTAP* (data not shown). The *TULP4* gene was not expressed in normal breast tissue and was very weakly expressed in normal ovarian surface epithelium, whereas it produced a strong RT-PCR product in melanocytes, therefore the expression analysis for this gene was restricted to the latter tissue. From this analysis, three out of six melanoma-derived samples (those that also showed a reduction of *ARID1* expression) displayed a decreased expression level for such gene when compared to normal melanocytes (Figure 4). Again LOH analysis of the corresponding genomic region did not detect any genomic rearrangement (data not shown).

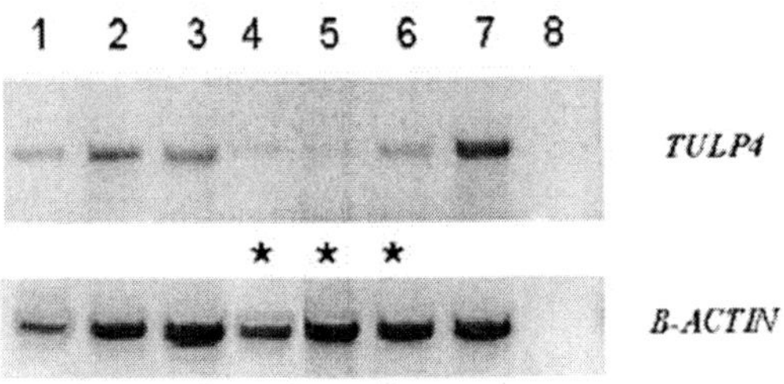

Figure 4. *TULP4* expression analysis in melanoma-derived cell lines. Expression of *TULP4* was assessed by RT-PCR on total RNA samples extracted from the same panel of melanoma cell lines used for *ARID1B* expression analysis. Lane 1: normal melanocytes; lane 2: SK MEL 28; lanes 3, 5, 6 and 7: four independent melanoma-derived cell lines; lane 4: primary melanoma tumor sample; lane 8: negative control. The asterisks highlight the three melanoma samples displaying *ARID1B* down-regulation.

Conclusion

We have reported evidence for the huge extension of common fragile site *FRA6E*, which appears three times bigger than previously suggested [Denison *et al.*, 2003a]. This conclusion is not unprecedented, as recently demonstrated for *FRA3B,* which turned out to be much wider than the previous characterization (more than 4 Mb instead of the previously defined 500 kb); indeed such fragile site contains four additional genes other than the 1.5 Mb *FHIT* gene [Becker *et al.*, 2002].

The proximal molecular boundary of *FRA6E* should be located between 153.9-154.6 Mb (NCBI build 34.3), while the distal boundary is close to position 163.5 Mb, according to previously published data [Denison *et al.*, 2003a]. Interestingly, although conventionally located at 6q26 [Kahkonen *et al.*, 1988], *FRA6E* has been already mapped at 6q25.3 by high resolution banding [Yunis and Soreng, 1984].

Recent experimental evidence support the fact that common fragile sites are largest than expected, and that these regions have a complex organization, with more than one single core of fragility. For example, Morelli *et al.* [2002] described for *FRA6F* a bipartite structure for the fragile site, with two 200 kb separate hot spots of fragility. In the wide region corresponding to *FRA9E*, the majority of clones used for FISH analysis showed equal proportions of proximal and distal hybridization [Callahan *et al.*, 2003], a result which suggests a plateau of fragility throughout the sequence, instead of a core. Also in our study many clones throughout the 1.85 Mb of DNA sequence gave comparable frequencies of proximal and distal hybridization signals, although a trend can be envisaged with distal hybridisation signals increasing from the centromeric to the telomeric limit of the region under scrutiny (Tables 1-2). Additional indication for a complex organization of *FRA6E* derives from the flexibility analysis of the whole 9 Mb sequence corresponding to *FRA6E*, supporting the existence of two regions of maximum flexibility, separated by a more stable sequence. Furthemore these results represent a further confirmation that flexibility motives, which have unusual structural features but are overrepresented within fragile sites, can be relevant for the intrinsic fragility of these regions [Zlotorynski *et al.*, 2003].

In our experiments, an higher proportion of distal signals was observed with H691 cells than with primary lymphocytes, and by comparing primary cells from different subjects it appears that the boundary of common fragile site *FRA6E* could be differently positioned in different individuals; the same result has been reported by Callahan *et al.* [2003] concerning *FRA9E*. In the light of the already known interindividual variability of expression of common fragile sites, the possibility that the boundaries of the fragile region may be detected at variable positions in different subjects is not unexpected; on the contrary, this effect may, in part, account for the discrepant observations described in the present and in the other published study [Denison *et al.*, 2003a].

In summary, common fragile sites may be composed by several juxtaposed fragility regions of variable expression. This observation underlines the need for more extensive cytogenetic analysis in order to fully understand the structural, and most importantly, the biological features of common fragile sites.

It is well known that 6q25-q26 is preferentially rearranged in cancer, as appears from the the analysis of a consistent high number of different tumours [Knuutila *et al.*, 1999; Mitelman, the "Recurrent Chromosome Aberrations in Cancer Database", http://cgap.nci.nih.gov/Chromosomes/Mitelman). A minimal region of overlapping deletions in 6q26-27 was found after detecting 6q deletion in almost one half of tumours analysed by CGH [Knuutila *et al.*, 1999; Knuutila *et al.*, 2000]. Furthermore, deletion of 6q24-qter was found as the sole chromosome anomaly in two cases of endometrial cancer [Tibiletti *et al.*, 1997].

A careful analysis of the published LOH data (summarised in Figure 5) demonstrates that DNA markers located in *FRA6E*, included those previously mapped with less accuracy, are often involved in LOH events. It is particularly interesting to note that marker *D6S442*, mapping at position 155.78 Mb i.e. in correspondence of the *NOX3* genomic sequences, has frequently been reported to be deleted in different tumours [Fujii *et al.*, 1996; Theile *et al.*, 1996]. Other markers analysed in LOH studies and mapping in *FRA6E* are *D6S473* at 155.28 Mb, *D6S415* at 157.7 Mb, *IGFR2R* at 160.3 Mb and *SOD2,* actually at 160.0 Mb but formerly supposed to be located proximally (6q25.2). All together several different studies indicated that a minimal region of deletions in tumours contains these DNA markers [de Souza *et al.*, 1995a; Queimado *et al.*, 1995; Cooke *et al.*, 1996; Fujii *et al.*, 1996; Theile *et al.*, 1996; Queimado *et al.*, 1998; Rodriguez *et al.*, 2000].

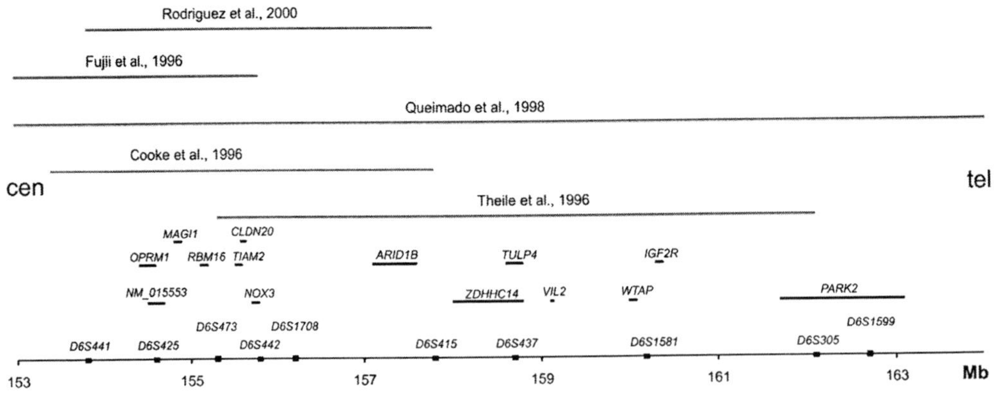

Figure 5. Critical regions of LOH (thick gray lines) involving *FRA6E*. The relevant known genes and DNA markers are also shown in the map.

A gene survey of the *FRA6E* core region and the one just telomeric to it revealed several interesting candidates for a role in cancer development and progression (Table 3). *NOX3* is a NAPDH oxidase participating in reactive oxigen generation [Cheng *et al.*, 2001]; a link between accumulation of reactive oxigen species and cell transformation is well known, therefore the presence of this gene in a chromosomal region prone to rearrangements is worth noting. *ARID1B* has been demonstrated to be a subunit of the human complex SWI/SNF which is an ATP-dependent chromatin remodelling complex [Hurlstone *et al.*, 2002; Inoue *et al.*, 2002], participating to transcriptional activation by hormone receptors including estrogen [Inoue *et al.*, 2002] and adrogen receptors [Marshall *et al.*, 2003]. The role of hormone receptors in regulating cell growth as well as the relation of receptor-mediated signalling dysfunction and cancerogenesis, are all well known. Some of the genes located in the 2.5 Mb region interposed between the sequence characterised in the present paper and that studied by Denison *et al.* (2003a] are also worth reporting when considering common fragile sites causally associated with cancer: *ZDHHC14*, encoding for a protein containing a zinc finger domain [Table 3); Ezrin, encoded by the gene *VIL2* [Table 3), which is overexpressed in several epithelial tumours [Böhling *et al.*, 1996; Ohtani *et al.*, 2002; Pang *et al.*, 2004] and appears involved in the metastatic processes [Elliot *et al.*, 2004; Khanna *et al.*, 2004]. Other relevant genes are WTAP, supposed to cooperate as splicing factor with WT1 (Table 3) and the putative transcription factor TULP4 (Table 3).

Expression analysis in primary tumours and tumour derived cell lines was carried out in this study for the four (*ARID1B, TULP4*, *VIL2* and *WTAP)* of the above genes, which were expressed in the normal tissues selected for the analysis (ovarian and breast tissues, melanocytes). *ARID1B* and *TULP4*, gave interesting results, showing a reduced expression in three melanoma tumors which retained (no LOH could be detected) the corresponding genomic region. In spite of the low number of tumor sample analysed, these data point to *ARID1B* and *TULP4* as a putative targets for down-regulation in the context of melanoma development.

The 3.3 Mb region characterised by Denison *et al.* [2003a] contains 8 genes, and among these worth noting are: the putative tumor-suppressor gene *IGF2R* [de Souza *et al.*, 1995b] at its centromeric boundary; whereas the huge *PARK2* gene, which is also proposed to be a tumour suppressor gene [Cesari *et al.*, 2003; Denison *et al.*, 2003a; Denison *et al.*, 2003b], is located at the telomeric end. 4 out the 5 genes expressed in normal epithelium of the ovary, showed reduced or absent expression in ovarian cancer cell lines and primary ovarian tumours [Denison *et al.* 2003a]. Alternative transcripts of *PARK2,* normally absent in non tumoral cells, can be found in cancer cell lines and primary tumours, a phenomenon which has been reported also for other two tumour-suppressor genes located in other fragile sites, namely *FHIT* and *WWOX* [Huebner and Croce 2001; Ludes-Meyers *et al.*, 2003].

Because so many genes with a proved or supposed role in the cancerogenesis process are present in the very large sequence corresponding to *FRA6E,* and because of the intrinsic instability of the region in which they are located, the integrity of their function should be deeply investigated in different tumors.

Acknowledgments

We are grateful to Maria Grazia Tibiletti (Laboratorio di Anatomia Patologica, Ospedale di Circolo, Varese for helpful technical assistance and discussion during the preliminary FISH experiments with YACs.

RT was supported by grants from Cofin 2003, FIRB 2003 and CARIPLO 2003. LM is a recipient of a fellowship from Amici dell'Università dell'Insubria.

References

Acquati, F; Malgaretti, N; Hauptschein, R; Rao, P; Gaidano, G; Taramelli R. A 2-Mb YAC contig linking the plasminogen-apoprotein(a) gene family to the insulin-like growth factor 2 receptor (*IGF2R*) gene on the telomeric region of chromosome 6 (6q26-q27). *Genomics*, 1994, 22, 664-666.

Acquati, F; Morelli, C; Cinquetti, R; Bianchi, MG; Porrini, D; Varesco, L; Gismondi, V; Rocchetti, R; Talevi, S; Possati, L; Magnanini, C; Tibiletti, MG; Bernasconi, B; Daidone, MG; Shridhar, V; Smith, DI; Negrini, M; Barbanti-Brodano, G; Taramelli, R. Cloning and characterization of a senescence inducing and class II tumor suppressor gene in ovarian carcinoma at chromosome region 6q27. *Oncogene*, 2001, 20, 980-988.

Arlt, MF; Casper, AM; Glover TW. Common fragile sites. *Cytogenet Genome Res*, 2003, 100, 92-100.

Arlt, MF; Xu, B; Durkin, SG; Casper, AM; Kastan, MB; Glover, TW. BRCA1 is required for common-fragile.site stability via ist G2/M checkpoint function. *Mol Cell Biol*, 2004, 24, 6701-6709.

Becker, NA; Thorland, EC; Denison, SR; Phillips, LA; Smith DI. Evidence that instability within the FRA3B region extends four megabases. *Oncogene*, 2002, 21, 8713-8722.

Bohling, T; Turunen, O; Jaaskelainen, J; Carpen, O; Sainio, M; Wahlstrom, T; Vaheri, A; Haltia, M. Ezrin expression in stromal cells of capillary hemangioblastoma. An immunohistochemical survey of brain tumors. *Am J Pathol*, 1996, 148, 367–373.

Callahan, G; Denison, SR; Phillips, LA; Shridhar, V; Smith, DI.Characterization of the common fragile site *FRA9E* and its potential role in ovarian cancer. *Oncogene*, 2003, 22, 590-601.

Casper, AM; Nghiem, P; Arlt, MF; Glover, TW. ATR regulates fragile site stability. *Cell*, 2002, 111, 779-789.

Cesari, R; Martin, ES; Calin, GA; Pentimalli, F; Bichi, R; McAdams, H; Trapasso, F; Drusco, A; Shimizu, M; Masciullo, V; D'Andrilli, G: Scambia, G; Picchio, MC; Alder, H; Godwin, AK; Croce CM. Parkin, a gene implicated in autosomal recessive juvenile parkinsonism, is a candidate tumor suppressor gene on chromosome 6q25-q27. *Proc Natl Acad Sci USA*, 2003, 100, 5956-5961.

Cheng, G; Cao, Z; Xu, X; van Meir, EG; Lambeth, JD. Homologs of gp91*phox*: cloning and tissue expression of Nox3, Nox4, and Nox5. *Gene*, 2001, 269, 131-140.

Colitti, CV; Rodabaugh, KJ; Welch, WR; Berkowitz, RS; Mok SC. A novel 4 cM minimal deletion unit on chromosome 6q25.1-q25.2 associated with high grade invasive epithelial ovarian carcinomas. *Oncogene*, 1998, 16, 555-559.

Cooke, IE; Shelling, AN; Le Meuth, VG; Charnock, ML; Ganesan, TS. Allele loss on chromosome arm 6q and fine mapping of the region at 6q27 in epithelial ovarian cancer. *Genes Chrom Cancer,* 1996, 15, 223-233.

De Souza, AT; Hankins, GR; Washington, MK; Fine, RL; Orton, TC; Jirtle, RL. Frequent loss of heterozygosity on 6q at the mannose 6-phosphate/insulin-like growth factor II receptor locus in human hepatocellular tumors. *Oncogene*, 1995a 10, 1725-1729.

De Souza, AT; Hankins, GR; Washington, MK; Orton, TC; Jirtle RL. M6P/IGF2R gene is mutated in human hepatocellular carcinomas with loss of heterozygosity. *Nature Genet.*, 1995b, 11, 447-449.

Denison, SR; Callahan, G; Becke,r NA; Phillips, LA; Smith, DI. Characterization of *FRA6E* and its potential role in autosomal recessive juvenile parkinsonism and ovarian cancer. *Genes Chrom Cancer*, 2003a, 38, 40-52.

Denison, SR; Callahan, G; Becker, NA; Phillips, LA; Smith, DI. Alterations in the common fragile site gene Parkin in ovarian and other cancers. Oncogene, 2003b, 22, 8370-8378.

Elliott, BE; Qiao, H; Louvard, D; Arpin, M. Co-operative effect of c-Src and ezrin in deregulation of cell-cell contacts and scattering of mammary carcinoma cells. *J Cell Biochem*, 2004, 92, 16-28

Finnis, M; Dayan, S ; Hobson, L. ; Chenevix-Trench, G; Friend, K; Ried, K; Venter, D; Woollatt, E; Baker, E; Richards, RI. Common fragile site *FRA16D* mutation in cancer cells. *Hum Mol Genet*, 2005, 14, 1341-1349

Fujii, H; Zhou, W; Gabrielson, E; Detection of frequent allelic loss of 6q23-q25.2 in microdissected human breast cancer tissues. *Genes Chrom Cancer*, 1996, 16, 35-39.

Hauptschein, RS; Gamberi, B; Rao, PH; Frigeri, F; Scotto, L; Venkatraj, VS; Gaidano, G; Rutner, T; Edwards, YH; Chaganti, RS; Dalla-Favera, R. Cloning and mapping of human chromosome 6q26-q27 deleted in B-cell non-Hodgkin lymphoma and multiple tumor types. *Genomics*, 1998, 50, 170-186.

Howlett, NG; Taniguchi, T; Durkin, S; D'Andrea, A; Glover, TW. The Fanconi anemia pathway is required for the DNA replication stress response and for the regulation of common fragile site stability. *Hum Mol Genet*, 2005, 14, 693-701.

Huebner, K; Croce, CM. FRA3B and other common fragile sites: the weakest links. *Nature Rev Cancer,* 2001, 1, 214-221.

Hurlstone, AF; Olave, IA; Barker, N; van Noort, M; Clevers, H. Cloning and characterization of hELD/OSA1, a novel BRG1 interacting protein. *Biochem. J*, 2002, 364, 255-264.

Inoue, H; Furukawa, T; Giannakopoulos, S; Zhou, S; King, DS; Tanese N. Largest subunits of the human SWI/SNF chromatin-remodeling complex promote transcriptional activation by steroid hormone receptors. *J Biol Chem*, 2002, 277, 41674-41685.

Ishii, H; Furokawa, Y. Alterations of common fragile sites in hematopoietic malignancies. *Int J Hematol*, 2004, 79, 238-242.

Kahkonen, M. Population cytogenetics of folate-sensitive fragile sites. I. Common fragile sites. *Hum Genet*, 1988, 80, 344-348.

Khanna, C; Wan, X; Bose, S; Cassaday, R; Olomu, O; Mendoza, A; Yeung, C; Gorlick, R; Hewitt, SM; Helman, LJ. The membrane-cytoskeleton linker ezrin is necessary for osteosarcoma metastasis. *Nature Med*, 2004, 10, 182-186.

Knuutila, S; Aalto, Y; Autio, K; Bjorkqvist, AM; El-Rifai, W; Hemmer, S; Huhta, T; Kettunen, E; Kiuru-Kuhlefelt, S; Larramendy, ML; Lushnikova, T; Monni, O; Pere, H; Tapper, J; Tarkkanen, M; Varis, A; Wasenius, VM; Wolf, M; Zhu, Y, DNA copy number losses in human neoplasms. *Am J Pathol*, 1999, 155, 683-694.

Knuutila, S; Autio, K; Aalto, Y. Online access to CGH data of DNA sequence copy number changes. *Am J Pathol*, 2000, 157, 689.

Krummel, KA; Roberts, LR; Kawakami, M; Glover, TW; Smith DI The characterization of the common fragile site FRA16D and its involvement in multiple myeloma translocations. *Genomics*, 2000, 69, 37-46.

Limongi, MZ; Pelliccia, F; Rocchi, A. Characterization of the human common fragile site FRA2G. Genomics, 2003, 81, 93-97.

Ludes-Meyers, JH; Bednarek, AK; Popescu, NC; Bedford, M; Aldaz, CM. WWOX, the common chromosomal fragile site, FRA16D, cancer gene. *Cytogenet Genome Res*, 2003.,100, 101-110.

Magnaghi, P; Citterio, E; Malgaretti, N; Acquati, F; Ottolenghi, S; Taramelli, R. Molecular characterisation of the human apo(a)-plasminogen gene family clustered on the telomeric region of chromosome 6 (6q26-27). *Hum Mol Genet*, 1994, 3, 437-442.

Marshall, TW; Link, KA; Petre-Draviam, CE; Knudsen KE. Differential requirement of SWI/SNF for androgen receptor activity. *J Biol Chem*, 2003, 278, 30605-30613.

Morelli, C; Karayianni, E; Magnanini, C; Mungall, AJ; Thorland, E; Negrini, M; Smith, DI; Barbanti-Brodano, G. Cloning and characterization of the common fragile site FRA6F harboring a replicative senescence gene and frequently deleted in human tumors. *Oncogene*, 2002, 21,7266-7276.

Musio, A; Montagna, C; Mariani, T; Tilenni, M; Focarelli, ML; Brait, L; Indino, E; Benedetti, PA; Chessa, L; Albertini, A; Ried, T; Vezzoni, P. SMC involvement in fragile site expression. *Hum Mol Genet* , 2005, 14, 525-533.

Ohtani, K; Sakamoto, H; Rutherford, T; Chen, Z; Kikuchi, A; Yamamoto, T; Satoh, K; Naftolin. F. Ezrin, a membrane-cytoskeletal linking protein, is highly expressed in atypical endometrial hyperplasia and uterine endometrioid adenocarcinoma. *Cancer Lett*, 2002, 179, 79–86.

Pang, ST; Fang, X; Valdman, A; Norstedt, G; Pousette, A; Egevad, L; Ekman, P. Expression of ezrin in prostatic intraepithelial neoplasia. *Urology*, 2004, 63, 609-612.

Popescu, NC. Genetic alterations in cancer as a result of breakage at fragile sites. *Cancer Lett.* 2003, 192,1-17.

Queimado, L; Seruca, R; Costa-Pereira, A; Castedo, S. Identification of two distinct regions of deletion at 6q in gastric carcinoma. *Genes Chrom Cancer*, 1995 14, 28-34.

Queimado, L; Reis, A; Fonseca, I; Martins, C; Lovett, M; Soares, J; Parreira, L. A refined localization of two deleted regions in chromosome 6q associated with salivary gland carcinomas. *Oncogene*, 1998, 16, 83-88.

Richards, RI. Fragile and unstable chromosomes in cancer: causes and consequences. *Trends Genet,* 2001, 17, 339-345.

Rodriguez, C; Causse, A; Ursule, E; Theillet, C. At least five regions of imbalance on 6q in breast tumors, combining losses and gains. *Genes Chrom Cance*, 2000, 27, 76-84.

Roz, L; Gramegna, M; Ishii, H; Croce, CM; Sozzi, G. Restoration of fragile histidine triad (FHIT) expression induces apoptosis and suppresses tumorigenicity in lung and cervical cancer cell lines. *Proc Natl Acad Sci USA,* 2000, 99, 3615-3620.

Rozier, L; El-Achkar, E; Apiou, F; Debatisse, M. Characterization of a conserved aphidicolin-sensitive common fragile site at human 4q22 and mouse C1: possible association with an inherited disease and cancer. *Oncogene*, 2004, 23, 6872-6880.

Tatarelli, C; Linnenbach, A; Mimori, K; Croce, CM. Characterization of the human TESTIN gene localized in the FRA7G region at 7q31.2. *Genomics*, 2000, 68, 1-12.

Theile, M; Seitz, S; Arnold, W; Jandrig, B; Frege, R; Schlag, PM; Haensch, W; Guski, H; Winzer, KJ; Barrett, JC; Scherneck, S. A defined chromosome 6q fragment (at D6S310) harbors a putative tumor suppressor gene for breast cancer. *Oncogene*, 1996, 13, 677-685.

Tibiletti, MG; Bernasconi, B; Furlan, D; Riva, C; Trubia, M; Buraggi, G; Franchi, M; Bolis, P; Mariani, A; Frigerio, L; Capella, C; Taramelli, R Early involvement of 6q in surface epithelial ovarian tumors. *Cancer Res*, 1996, 56, 4493-4498.

Tibiletti, MG; Bernasconi, B; Taborelli, M; Furlan, D; Fabbri, A; Franchi, M; Taramelli, R; Trubia, M; Capella, C. Involvement of chromosome 6 in endometrial cancer. *Br J Cancer*, 1997, 75, 1831-1835.

Tibiletti, MG; Sessa, F; Bernasconi, B; Cerutti, R; Broggi, B; Furlan, D; Acquati, F; Bianchi, M; Russo, A; Capella, C; Taramelli, R. A large 6q deletion is a common cytogenetic alteration in fibroadenomas, pre-malignant lesions, and carcinomas of the breast. *Clinical Cancer Res,* 2000, 6, 1422-1431.

Yunis, JJ; Soreng, AL. Constitutive fragile sites and cancer. Science, 1984, 226, 1199-1204.

Zenklusen, JC; Hodges, LC; LaCava, M; Green, ED; Conti, CJ. Definitive functional evidence for a tumor suppressor gene on human chromosome 7q31.1 neighboring the FRA7G site. *Oncogene*, 2000, 19, 1729-1733.

Zlotorynski, E; Rahat, A; Skaug, J; Ben-Porat, N; Ozeri, E; Hershberg, R; Levi, A; Scherer, SW; Margalit, H; Kerem, B. Molecular basis for expression of common and rare fragile sites. *Mol Cell Biol*, 2003, 23, 7143-7151.

In: Trends in Genome Research
Editor: Clyde R. Williams, pp. 173-205
ISBN 1-60021-027-9

Chapter 7

Human DNA Standard Reference Materials Developed by the National Institute of Standards and Technology[1, 2]

Barbara C. Levin, Kristy L. Richie, Margaret C. Kline, Janette W. Redman and Diane K. Hancock
Biotechnology Division, National Institute of Standards and Technology, Gaithersburg, MD 20899-8311

Abstract

The National Institute of Standards and Technology (NIST), formerly called the National Bureau of Standards (NBS), has developed over 1300 Standard Reference Materials (SRMs). The Office of Standard Reference Materials defines and describes a SRM as a:

"well-characterized material produced in quantity to improve measurement science. It is certified for specific chemical or physical properties, and is issued by NIST with a certificate that reports the results of the characterization and indicates the intended use of the material. A SRM is prepared and used for the following three purposes: 1.To help develop accurate methods of analysis; 2. To calibrate measurement systems used to facilitate exchange of goods, institute quality control, determine performance characteristics, or measure a property at the state-of-the-art limit; and 3. To assure the long-term adequacy and integrity of measurement quality assurance programs" (http://patapsco.nist.gov/srmcatalog/about/Definitions.htm).

[1]This chapter is a contribution of the US National Institute of Standards and Technology (NIST) and is not subject to copyright. Certain commercial equipment, instruments, materials, or companies are identified in this chapter to specify the experimental procedure. Such identification does not imply recommendation or endorsement by NIST, nor does it imply that the materials or equipment identified are the best available for this purpose.

[2] Correspondence should be addressed to: Dr. Barbara C. Levin, 100 Bureau Drive, Stop 8311, National Institute of Standards and Technology, Gaithersburg, Maryland 20899-8311. Telephone: (301) 975-6682, FAX: (301) 330-3447; email: barbara.levin@nist.gov

To provide quality assurance in the analysis of human DNA, five Standard Reference Materials - SRM 2390, SRM 2391b, SRM 2392, SRM 2392-I, and SRM 2395 have been developed by NIST and are currently available. Two additional DNA SRMs (# 2394 and # 2399[3]) have been developed and released since the writing of this chapter. Three of these SRMs - the DNA Profiling Standard 2390, the Polymerase Chain Reaction (PCR)-based DNA Profiling Standard 2391b, and the Human Y-Chromosome DNA Profiling Standard 2395 - are intended for use in forensic and paternity identifications, for instructional law enforcement, or non-clinical research purposes. They are not intended for any human/animal clinical diagnostic use. The DNA SRMs, 2392 and 2392-I, are for standardization and quality control when amplifying and sequencing the entire or any segment of human mitochondrial DNA (16,569 base pairs) for forensic identification, disease diagnosis or mutation detection. SRM 2394 is called the Heteroplasmy mtDNA Standard and will permit investigators to determine the limit of their heteroplasmic mutation detection techniques and hopefully, will be useful in promoting the development of new and more sensitive mutation detection methods. Orders and requests for information concerning these SRMs should be directed to: The National Institute of Standards and Technology, Standard Reference Materials Program, 100 Bureau Drive, Mail Stop 2322, Gaithersburg, MD 20899-2322, Telephone: (301) 975-6776, FAX: (301) 948-3730 E-mail: srminfo@nist.gov Web sites: www.nist.gov/srm, http://ts.nist.gov/ts/htdocs/230/232/232.htm.

SRM 2390 – RFLP DNA Profiling Standard

Standard Reference Material 2390 is designed to standardize the methodology used to detect Restriction Fragment Length Polymorphisms (RFLP) using the *Hae* III restriction enzyme. This procedure examines the variable numbers of tandem repeats (VNTR) in highly polymorphic human loci (1,2,3,4). The use of RFLP depends on the presence of a polymorphism which can vary in length. In this case, the *Hae* III restriction cleavage sites flank the tandem repeat sequences of the following commonly probed genetic loci: D1S7, D2S44, D4S139, D5S110, D10S28, and D17S79 and the less commonly probed loci: D7S467, D7Z2, D8S358, D14S13, D17S26, and DYZ1. Different length DNA fragments are generated depending on the number of tandem repeats in an individual. SRM 2390 was originally certified in 1992 and was technically revised in 2001 to update the allelic band sizes based on the latest state-of-the-art forensic practices. While the allelic band sizes are ideally determined by the actual number of tandem repeats, the reported sizes depend on the methodology used to measure them (5). In 1991, the Federal Bureau of Investigation (FBI), the Royal Canadian Mounted Police (RCMP) and many state and local laboratories were using *Hae* III in their RFLP procedures for forensic and paternity testing (6,7). The restriction enzyme *Hae* III was the enzyme of choice because: 1. It is an extremely hardy enzyme, 2. It recognizes a four base sequence (GGCC), 3. It produces relatively small size fragments, and 4. The smaller fragment sizes have better resolution than those obtained with other enzymes (e.g., *Pst* I, *Hinf* I, *Alu* I) (7). In addition, the presence of DNA methylation does not interfere with the enzymatic activity of *Hae* III to recognize or cleave its restriction site.

The DNA Profiling SRM 2390 contains DNA from two sources 1. The cell line, K562 (Life Technologies, Inc., Rockville, MD), which was derived from a female with chronic myelogenous leukemia and 2. TAW (Analytical Genetic Testing Center, Inc., Denver, CO), an apparently healthy male. This SRM provides quality control for the following procedures:

[3]SRM 2399 provides quality control to clinical laboratories that test human samples for Fragile X and that need to determine the accurate number of CGG trinucleotide repeats.

1. Extracting the DNA from the cell pellet, 2. Quantifying the extracted DNA, 3. Determining the restriction enzyme cutting efficiency, 4. Separating the DNA electrophoretically, 5. Blotting the separated DNA onto a nylon membrane using an alkaline transfer solution, 6. Hybridizing the sample DNA to radioactively-labeled DNA probes, 7. Exposing the membrane to X-ray film, and 8. Imaging the developed autoradiogram with a computerized imaging system to determine band sizes. The cells and DNA are provided as 1. A cell pellet containing approximately 3 x 10^6 cells, 2. Extracted genomic DNA and 3. *Hae* III digested DNA. In addition, the SRM contains a DNA molecular size standard for sizing the allele fragments (DNA Analysis Marker System, Gibco BRL Products, Life Technologies, Gaithersburg, MD); a set of quantitative DNA standards consisting of six tubes containing DNA in concentrations from 6 ng to 250 ng; and a visualization marker set based on adenovirus DNA which is cut with restriction enzymes to produce twelve bands ranging from 594 to 35,937 base pairs. The visualization marker is used to assess the DNA separation on the electrophoretic gel. Agarose pretested for compatibility with all the DNA components is also included.

SRM 2390 has 20 components and is packaged in three boxes (containing a total of 19 components) plus a separate container for the agarose. Components #1-5 comprise the DNA Analysis Marker System (Life Technologies, Inc.) for Southern blotting applications using ^{32}P- labeled probes. Components #6-11 plus the loading buffer #19 enable the user to evaluate the quality and quantity of the extracted DNA. Component #18 is an adenovirus DNA visible ladder containing a mixture of digested and undigested adenovirus DNA with fragments ranging from 594 to 35,937 bp. Components 12-17 are the cells and extracted DNA, both *Hae* III treated and untreated from both the female (K562) and male (TAW) sources. These materials and other components of the SRM were obtained from Life Technologies, Inc., Rockville, MD and from Analytical Genetic Testing Center, Inc., Denver, CO.

Interlaboratory Evaluation of SRM 2390

Twenty laboratories participated in an Interlaboratory Evaluation of the 2001 revised SRM 2390 (Table 1) and the data from these laboratories were used to produce the certified allelic band sizes shown in Table 2 and informational band sizes shown in Table 3. Table 2 lists the certified values (expected allelic band sizes and sizing uncertainty) for band size measurements of the cell pellet and extracted K562 and TAW DNA at the six commonly probed genetic loci mentioned above. Table 3 provides informational values for K562 and TAW DNA band sizes at the six less commonly probed loci itemized above. The chromosome location of these various loci as well as those in SRM 2391b are given in Table 4.

All laboratories received the above components, instructions, and a questionnaire. All laboratories used the basic FBI protocol (8) or modifications thereof for RFLP sizing. This protocol consists of the following steps: 1. Extracting DNA from the cell pellet; 2. Quantifying the amount of DNA extracted using the set of quantitative controls supplied with the SRM; 3. Cutting the DNA with a *Hae* III restriction enzyme; 4. Testing the restriction process by gel electrophoresis; 5. Running all electrophoresis on an analytical gel with tris-acetate buffer in the presence of ethidium bromide and appropriate viral DNA markers for assessing proper separation; 6. Blotting the separated DNA onto a nylon membrane using an alkaline transfer solution; 7. Hybridizing the sample DNA to radioactively - labeled DNA probes; 8. Exposing the membrane to X-ray film; and 9. Imaging the developed autoradiogram with a computerized imaging system to determine band sizes. Some of the laboratories participating in the interlaboratory evaluation used probes that were fluorescently labeled rather than radioactively labeled.

In summary, NIST has prepared a standard reference material SRM 2390 to provide quality control and quality assurance to forensic laboratories that are still using RFLP for human identification. Most laboratories are currently using short tandem repeats (STRs) rather than RFLP. The PCR method with STRs is much shorter (days versus weeks with radioactive probes); it requires smaller samples of DNA (1 ng vs. 50-500 ng); the condition of the DNA is less important (may be low molecular weight vs. intact high molecular weight); and finally, the PCR approach may be done on a robot that can process high throughput volumes. There are also some PCR disadvantages, which include that the presence of some inhibiting factors in the sample will prevent the amplification and the primers may fail if the primer site contains a mutation. Therefore, some laboratories are still conducting RFLP analysis and can use SRM 2390 in several different ways depending on their quality assurance needs. Components of this SRM are designed to provide assurance that each step of the protocol is functioning properly, but they can also be used for trouble shooting, for calibrating equipment, and for testing the efficacy of new lots of reagents.

Table 1. Participants in the Interlaboratory Recertification of SRM 2390 in 2001

LABORATORY	LOCATION
Arizona Department of Public Safety Crime Laboratory	Phoenix, AZ
Broward County Sheriff's Office, Crime Laboratory	Ft. Lauderdale, FL
Connecticut Forensic Science Laboratory	Meriden, CT
Illinois State Police, Forensic Science Center	Chicago, IL
Illinois State Police, Springfield Forensic Science Lab.	Springfield, IL
Indianapolis-Marion County Forensic Services Agency	Indianapolis, IN
Kentucky State Police Crime Laboratory	Frankfort, KY
LabCorp, Forensic Identity Testing	RTP, NC
Maryland State Police Crime Laboratory	Pikesville, MD
Metro-Dade Police Crime Laboratory	Miami, FL
Minnesota Dept. of Public Safety Bureau of Criminal Apprehension	St. Paul, MN
New York State Police Forensic Investigation Center	Albany, NY
North Carolina State Bureau of Investigation Crime Lab.	Raleigh, NC
Orange County Sheriff's Coroner Dept. DNA Lab.	Santa Ana, CA
Pennsylvania State Police DNA Laboratory	Greensburg, PA
South Carolina Law Enforcement Division DNA Lab.	Columbia, SC
Vermont Forensic Lab., Department of Public Safety	Waterbury, VT
Washington State Patrol Crime Laboratory	Seattle, WA
Washoe County Sheriff's Office Crime Laboratory	Reno, NV
Wisconsin State Crime Laboratory	Milwaukee, WI

Table 2. Certified Values for Band Sizes of SRM 2390 in 2001

DNA Locus [n][a]	DNA Source K562 Band 1	K562 Band 2	TAW Band 1	TAW Band 2
D1S7 [n=20]	4585[b] ± 29.9[c]	4237 ± 23.6	7773 ± 63.2	6886 ± 41.3
D2S44 [n=20]	2905 ± 19.5	1788 ± 14.3	3711 ± 23.2	1288 ± 8.7
D4S139 [n=20]	6474 ± 49.2	3440 ± 22.2	10854 ± 117	8185 ± 64.7
D5S110 [n=17]	3700 ± 23.2	2926 ± 17.4	3343 ± 20.4	1444 ± 11.5
D10S28 [n=19]	1754 ± 11.4	1180 ± 9.7	3935 ± 24.5	1788 ± 10.2
D17S79 [n=15]	1979 ± 14.8	1514 ± 11.1	1753 ± 11.2	1515 ± 11.7

a. Number of data sets received for this locus.
b. Mean number of base pairs calculated from the means of the three preparations (cell, genomic and *Hae* III digested) from all the laboratories.
c. The uncertainty which is the half-width of a 95%/95% statistical tolerance interval for each band. A 95%/95% statistical tolerance interval provides 95% confidence that it contains at least 95% of the relevant population. For each band, this refers to the population of individual results for any of the three preparations, obtained by a population of laboratories similar to those in this interlaboratory study (9).

Table 3. Informational Values for Additional Loci Examined for SRM 2390 in 2001

DNA Locus [n][a]	DNA Source K562 Band 1	K562 Band 2	TAW Band 1	TAW Band 2
D7S467 [n=5]	4677[b]	3217	4496	4339
D7Z2[c] [n=1]	2736		2747	
D8S358 [n=1]	5878	1303	3417	2383
D14S13[d] [n=2]	1642		1579	
D17S26 [n=1]	4823	1358	5514	4852
DYZ1[e] [n=1]			3571	

a. Number of laboratories that submitted data for this specific locus.
b. Mean (in base pairs) of values submitted by all the laboratories that tested these probes.
c. Human-specific monomorphic locus having a known sequence length of 2731 bp.
d. Both K562 and TAW are apparent homozygotes at this locus.
e. Y chromosome locus

Table 4. The chromosome location of the RFLP, STR, and PCR-based markers used in SRM 2390, SRM 2391b, or CODIS.

Chromosome Location	SRM 2390 RFLP Markers	SRM 2391b STR Markers	SRM 2391b CODIS STR Markers	SRM 2391b PCR Markers
1	D1S7	F13B		D1S80
2	D2S44	TPOX D2S1338	TPOX	
3		D3S1358	D3S1358	
4	D4S139	FGA	FGA	
5	D5S110	CSF1PO D5S818	CSF1PO D5S818	
6		F13A1 SE33		DQα
7	D7S467 D7Z2	D7S820	D7S820	
8	D8S358	LPL D8S1179	D8S1179	
9				
10	D10S28			
11		TH01	TH01	
12		vWA	vWA	
13		D13S317	D13S317	
14	D14S13			
15		FES/FPS Penta E		
16		D16S539	D16S539	
17	D17S26			
18		D18S51	D18S51	
19		D19S433		
20				
21		D21S11 Penta D	D21S11	
22				
X				Amelogenin [a]
Y				Amelogenin [a]

[a] Amelogenin is used for gender typing. The X-chromosome gene has 106 base pairs; whereas, the Y-chromosome has 112 base pairs. Therefore, a female (2 X-chromosomes) will have one peak and a male (1 X-chromosome and 1 Y-chromosome) will have two peaks.

Table 5. Laboratories Participating in the Interlaboratory Testing for SRM 2391 in 1995

LABORATORY	LOCATION
Alabama Department of Forensic Sciences	Birmingham, AL
Armed Forces DNA Identification Laboratory	Rockville, MD
Broward Sheriff's Crime Laboratory	Fort Lauderdale, FL
California Department of Justice NA Laboratory	Berkeley, CA
Chicago Police Crime laboratory	Chicago, IL
Commonwealth of Virginia Division of Forensic Sciences	Richmond, VA
Connecticut Dept. of Public Safety Forensic Science Lab.	Meriden, CT
Directions des Expertises Judiciaries	Montreal, Quebec, Canada
Dubai Police Headquarters C.I.D. Criminal Laboratory	Dubai, United Arab Emirates
FBI Forensic Science Research & Training Center	Quantico, VA
Forensic Science Associates	Richmond, CA
Georgia Bureau of Investigation Div. of Forensic Sciences	Decatur, GA
Illinois State Police Crime Laboratory	Springfield, IL
Kentucky State Police	Frankfort, KY
Metro-Dade Police Department	Miami, FL
Michigan State Police DNA Laboratory	East Lansing, MI
Minnesota Forensic Science Laboratory	St. Paul, MN
Office of the Chief Medical Examiner	New York, NY
Orange County Sheriff, Coroner Dept. Forensic Science Services	Santa Ana, CA
Roche Biomedical Laboratories, Inc.	Research Triangle Park, NC
Royal Canadian Mounted Police Central Forensic Laboratory	Ottawa, Ontario, Canada
U. CA Berkeley School of Public Health, Forensic Science Group.	Berkeley, CA
U. North Texas, Health Science Center of Fort Worth	Fort Worth, TX

SRM 2391b - PCR and STR DNA Profiling Standard

DNA SRM 2391, a PCR-based DNA Profiling Standard, was first issued in 1995 to provide standardization and quality control for forensic identification and paternity testing procedures. As in SRM 2390, it is intended to provide quality assurance for genetic testing, instructional law enforcement, and non-clinical research. It is not intended for use in human or animal clinical diagnostics. SRM 2391 was originally certified for use with the genetic locus D1S80 (pMCT118) (10) and specific primers (11).

The procedures used in the development of SRM 2391 at NIST were based on those of the FBI (PCR-Based Typing Protocols, FBI Laboratory, Quantico, VA, 12/12/94). These procedures consisted of: 1. Extraction of DNA from cells spotted on special filter paper; 2. Amplification of the DNA at the D1S80 locus (11); 3. Separation of the amplified alleles by electrophoresis of the DNA in a gel system that generates good resolution of the allelic ladder; 4. Detection in the gel by silver staining or fluorescent dye followed by image analysis.

The original SRM 2391 contained human cells from two cell culture lines from which DNA could be extracted; genomic DNA from those two cell lines plus eight other individuals; and PCR-amplified DNA from the two cell lines plus four of the eight individuals. A D1S80 allelic ladder for characterization of amplified DNA and a DNA size marker to assure proper electrophoretic separations were also included. SRM 2391 was composed of two boxes (A and B) containing a total of 20 components. The genomic DNA components were from Roche Molecular Systems, Inc., Alameda, CA and the cells, genomic and amplified DNA from cell lines GM 09947A and GM 09948 were obtained from Life Technologies, Inc., Gaithersburg, MD. They were qualified and licensed for forensic use from the National Institute of General Medical Science (NIGMS) repository in Camden, NJ.

Table 6. Certified Values for SRM 2391[a]

DNA SOURCE	COMPONENT NUMBER	D1S80 ALLELES
Genomic 1	3	28, 31
Genomic 2	4	18, 24
Genomic 3	5	18, 18
Genomic 4	6	21, 24
Genomic 5	7	17, 28
Genomic 6	8	24, 37
Genomic 7	9	24, 28
Genomic 8	10	17, 21
Genomic GM 09947A	11	18, 31
Genomic GM 09948	12	18, 25
Amplified 1	13	28, 31
Amplified 2	14	18, 18
Amplified 3	15	24, 37
Amplified 4	16	17, 21
Amplified GM 09947A	17	18, 31
Amplified GM 09948	18	18, 25
Cells GM 09947A	19	18, 31
Cells GM 09948	20	18, 25

a. The certified values represent the pooled results from analyses performed at two laboratories plus NIST.

Interlaboratory Evaluation of SRM 2391

Prior to certification, various components of SRM 2391 were tested by 20 laboratories (Table 5). Table 6 shows the certified values for the D1S80 alleles determined by three laboratories including NIST. Table 7 shows informational values determined for AmpliType™ HLA-DQα, AmpliType™ PM, TH01, F13A01, vWA, and FES/FPS. AmpliType HLA-DQα was an amplification and typing kit produced by Cetus and was used in the qualitative detection and identification of the human leukocyte antigen (HLA) DQα alleles found on chromosome 6. The kit allowed one to amplify a 239 or 242 bp fragment from the HLA-DQα locus. The typing was performed by hybridization of the amplified DNA to probe strips and permitted visual detection of the probes that were complementary to the unknown DNA sample. AmpliType™ PM PCR Amplification and Typing Kit allowed the typing of 6 polymorphic loci using a reverse dot format. TH01, F13A01, vWA, and FES/FPS are STR loci. See Table 4 for the chromosomal location of these markers.

Recertification of SRM 2391

Since the issuance of SRM 2391 in 1995, this SRM has been recertified as 2391a in 1998 and as SRM 2391b in 2002. Each ensuing version placed more emphasis on the use of Short Tandem Repeat (STR) loci for human identity rather than D1S80. The initial certificate for SRM 2391 had limited information on only four STR loci, TH01, F13A01, vWA and FES/FPS. The forensic community requested that SRM 2391 include STR information for all the DNA samples and that the STR information include the FBI's 13 CODIS (COmbined DNA Index System) core STR loci (Table 4). The CODIS core loci are CSF1PO, D3S1358, D5S818, D7S820, D8S1179, D13S317, D16S539, D18S51, D21S11, FGA, TH01, TPOX, and vWA. In addition, STR loci F13A01, F13B, FES/FPS, LPL, Penta D, Penta E, D2S1338, D19S433, and SE 33 were certified for SRM 2391b as well as D1S80, AmpliType ® HLA-DQA1, AmpliType ® PM, and Amelogenin. Therefore, a total of 26 loci were analyzed for the recertification of SRM 2391 as SRM 2391b (Tables 4, 8-10).

There are a number of advantages using PCR methods with STR loci over RFLP as mentioned above. The more STR loci that one examines, the greater the power of discrimination and much work has been done on multiplexing the STR loci, so multiple loci can be examined at the same time.

The laboratories that participated in an interlaboratory evaluation of SRM 2391b were: NIST, Gaithersburg, MD; Pennsylvania State Police DNA Laboratory, Greensburg, PA; Oregon State Police Forensic Laboratory, Portland, OR; Promega Corp., Madison, WI; and Applied Biosystems, Foster City, CA. The values in Tables 8-10 are the pooled results from all the laboratories that participated in the interlaboratory evaluation. The amplification kits that were used at NIST to genotype the various STR loci are shown in Table 11.

Twelve components are included in each SRM 2391b unit. Components #1 through #10 each contain 20 μL of genomic DNA at a concentration of approximately 1 ng/μL. Vials #1 through 8 contain Genomic DNA 1 through Genomic DNA 8, respectively. Vial #9 contains Genomic DNA from GM09947A and Vial #10 contains Genomic DNA from GM09948. Components #11 and #12 consist of GM09947A cells and GM09948 cells at a concentration of 2 x 10^5 on a 7 mm Scleicher & Schull 903 ™ filter paper circle 1, respectively.

In summary, SRM 2391b is designed to provide quality assurance to laboratories that each step of the PCR methodology to examine STR loci is operating correctly and within the proper limits. The examination of multiple STR loci increases the power of discrimination between individuals. The recent improvement in the ability to multiplex and examine many STR loci simultaneously also enhances the utility of this method.

Table 7. Other Information Values for SRM 2391

DNA Source	Component #	AmpliType HLA-DQα	AmpliType PM (polymarker)	TH01	F13A01	vWA	FES/FPS
Genomic 1	3	2, 4	AA, AB, AA, AA, CC	6, 7	6, 7	N/A	N/A
Genomic 2	4	1.1, 3	AB, BB, AB, AB, AC	8, 9.3	7, 7	N/A	N/A
Genomic 3	5	1.3, 4	BB, AA, BB, BB, AA	9.3, 9.3	3.2, 4	N/A	N/A
Genomic 4	6	4, 4	AB, AA, AB, AA, AB	7, 9	5, 6	N/A	N/A
Genomic 5	7	4, 4	BB, AA, BC, AA, BC	7, 7	5, 7	N/A	N/A
Genomic 6	8	4, 4	AB, AB, AB, AB, AC	9, 9.3	3.2, 5	N/A	N/A
Genomic 7	9	1.2, 4	BB, BB, CC, AB, BB	6, 7	5, 8	N/A	N/A
Genomic 8	10	1.2, 2	BB, BB, AC, AA, BB	7, 8	3.2, 5	N/A	N/A
Genomic GM 09947A	11	4, 4	AA, AB, AB, AA, AC	8, 9.3	6, 16	17, 18	10, 12
Genomic GM 09948	12	1.2, 3	AB, AB, BB, AB, BC	6, 9.3	6, 6	17, 17	11, 11
GM09947A Cells	19	4, 4	AA, AB, AB, AA, AC	8, 9.3	6, 16	17, 18	10, 12
GM09948 Cells	20	1.2, 3	AB, AB, BB, AB, BC	6, 9.3	6, 6	17, 17	11, 11

Table 8. Certified Values for the FBI's CODIS 13 STR Loci

Component No.	Contents	CSF1PO	D3S1358	D5S818	D7S820	D8S1179	D13S317	D16S539	D18S51	D21S11	FGA	TH01	TPOX	vWA
1	Genomic 1	12,12	14,17	12,12	9,10	13,13	11,13	12,14	14,14	29,33.2	21,22	6,7	8,11	17,17
2	Genomic 2	11,12	15,16	12,12	9,10	11,16	8,11	12,12	10,14	29,30	20,22	8,9.3	8,10	14,16
3	Genomic 3	11,12	15,15	11,11	12,13	14,16	11,12	11,12	16,20	28,31.2	23,25	9.3,9.3	8,11	18,19
4	Genomic 4	11,12	15,17	11,11	8,10	14,14	12,12	9,10	18,18	28,30	18,22	7,9	8,9	17,17
5	Genomic 5	10.12	15,18	11,12	8,10	15,16	11,12	9,11	14,16	28,30	23,26	7,7	10,11	16,20
6	Genomic 6	10,13	14,17	12,12	8,11	10,16	12,13	12,13	18,18	28,29	21,26	9,9.3	8,8	16,18
7	Genomic 7	10,11	14,15	11,12	9,9	13,15	11,12	10,10	13,16	28,31.2	23,24	6,7	8,11	16,16
8	Genomic 8	10,12	15,18	12,13	9,10	12,14	9,13	9,11	15,18	30,31	24,28	7,8	8,12	15,17
9	Genomic GM09947A	10,12	14,15	11,11	10,11	13,13	11,11	11,12	15,19	30,30	23,24	8,9.3	8,8	17,18
10	Genomic GM09948	10,11,12	15,17	11,13	11,11	12,13	11,11	11,11	15,18	29,30	24,26	6,9.3	8,9	17,17
11	GM09947A cells	10,12	14,15	11,11	10,11	13,13	11,11	11,12	15,19	30,30	23,24	8,9.3	8,8	17,18
12	GM09948 cells	10,11 or 10,11,12[a]	15,17	11,13	11,11	12,13	11,11	11,11	15,18	29,30	24,26	6,9.3	8,9	17,17

[a]The relative intensity of the 12 allele is less than 7% of that of the dominant 10 allele.

Table 9. Certified Values for Additional STR Loci for SRM 2391b

Component	Contents	F13A01	F13B	FES/FPS	LPL	Penta D	Penta E	D2S1338	D19S433	SE33
1	Genomic 1	6,7	10,10	12,12	10,11	10,15	7,12	17,23	13,16.2	20,30.2
2	Genomic 2	7,7	8,10	10,11	10,11	9,11	7,12	17,26	14,16	23.2,28.2
3	Genomic 3	3.2,4	9,10	11,12	11,12	11,12	13,14	20,24	12,14	14.2,26.2
4	Genomic 4	5,6	6,9	10,13	10,12	8,9	5,12	17,23	11,13	22,28.2
5	Genomic 5	5,7	8,9	11,13	10,12	10,13	7,13	17,19	12.2,14	14,30.2
6	Genomic 6	3.2,5	9,10	11,11	10,12	9,12	12,14	25,25	12,14	20,21
7	Genomic 7	5,8	6,8	11,11[a]	11,12	3.2,11	12,16	17,22	13,15.2	13.2,20
8	Genomic 8	3.2,5	6,8	10,11	9,11	8,9	5,10	22,22	12.2,15	16,27.2
9	Genomic GM09947A	6,16	8,10	10,12	11,12	12,12	12,13	19,23	14,15	19,29.2
10	Genomic GM09948	6,6	8,8	11,11	10,12	8,12	11,11	23,23	13,14	23.2,26.2
11	GM09947A cells	6,16	8,10	10,12	11,12	12,12	12,13	19,23	14,15	19,29.2
12	GM09948 cells	6,6	8,8	11,11	10,12	8,12	11,11	23,23	13,14	23.2,26.2

[a] Genomic 7 has a variant allele at the FES/FEP locus. Preliminary sequence analysis indicates sequence changes on either side of the STR.

Table 10. Certified Values for AmpliType® HLA-DQA1, AmpliType® PM, and Amelogenin for SRM 2391b

DNA Source	Component Number	AmpliType® HLA-DQA1	AmpliType® PM					Amelogenin
Genomic 1	1	2,4.1	AA	AB	AA	AA	CC	XY
Genomic 2	2	1.1,3	AB	BB	AB	AB	AC	XX
Genomic 3	3	1.3,4.1	BB	AA	BB	BB	AA	XY
Genomic 4	4	4.1,4.2/4.3	AB	AA	AB	AA	AB	XX
Genomic 5	5	4.1,4.1	BB	AA	BC	AA	BC	XX
Genomic 6	6	4.1,4.1	AB	AB	AB	AB	AC	XX
Genomic 7	7	1.2,4.1	BB	BB	CC	AB	BB	XY
Genomic 8	8	1.2,2	BB	BB	AC	AA	BB	XX
Genomic GM09947A	9	4.1,4.2/4.3	AA	AB	AB	AA	AC	XX
Genomic GM09948	10	1.2,3	AB	AB	BB	AB	BC	XY
GM09947A Cells	11	4.1,4.2/4.3	AA	AB	AB	AA	AC	XX
GM09948 Cells	12	1.2,3	AB	AB	BB	AB	BC	XY

For certified values for D1S80, see table 6.

Table 11. Amplification Kits used at NIST to Genotype STR Loci for SRM 2391b

STR Locus	Applied Biosystems				Promega			
	Identi-filer	Profiler Plus	COfiler	SGM Plus	Power Plex 16	Power Plex ES	Power Plex 16 Bio	FFFL
Amelogenin	X	X	X	X	X	X	X	
CSF1PO	X		X		X		X	
D2S1338	X			X				
D3S1358	X		X	X	X	X	X	
D5S818	X	X			X		X	
D7S820	X	X	X		X		X	
D8S1179	X	X		X	X	X	X	
D13S317	X	X	X		X		X	
D16S539	X			X	X		X	
D18S51	X	X		X	X	X	X	
D19S433	X			X				
D21S11	X	X		X	X	X	X	
F13A01								X
F13B								X
FES/FPS								X
FGA	X	X		X	X	X	X	
LPL								X
PENTA D					X		X	
PENTA E					X		X	
SE33						X		
TH01	X		X	X	X	X	X	
TPOX	X		X		X		X	
vWA	X	X		X	X	X	X	

SRM 2392 and SRM 2392-I - Human Mitochondrial Amplification and Sequencing Standards

Human mitochondrial DNA (mtDNA) was completely sequenced in 1981 and found to consist of a circular double-stranded molecule containing 16,569 base pairs (12). This sequence determined by Anderson *et al.* is referred to as the Cambridge Reference Sequence (CRS) and was a consensus sequence based primarily on the results from a human placenta, partly on the sequence from HeLa cells, and in five nucleotide positions where the human results were ambiguous, the authors inserted the results from the bovine mtDNA that they had also sequenced. In 1999, Andrews *et al.* (13) rediscovered and resequenced the original placenta and found that the 1981 sequence contained a number of rare polymorphisms that were specific for that placenta plus a number of errors.

Each human cell can have a few dozen to several thousand molecules of mtDNA (14, 15). Sequence analysis of mtDNA is being used by the forensic community for human identification especially in those cases where genomic DNA is highly degraded or non-existent (16, 17). Forensic analysis to distinguish between individuals is primarily based on the considerable sequence variation found in the two hypervariable regions (HV1, HV2) located in the non-coding displacement loop (D-loop) or control region. These are the areas designated by primer sets 1, 57 and 58 (Table 12). The medical community is also using sequence analysis of mtDNA for diagnoses of diseases associated with specific mutations and deletions (18). A third area of research which is largely unexplored and which needs sequence analysis is the examination of the mutagenic effects of chemical and physical agents on mtDNA (19, 20).

Human mtDNA SRMs 2392 and 2392-I were developed at NIST to be used for quality control when amplifying and sequencing DNA for forensic identifications, medical diagnostics, or mutation detection. SRM 2392, which became available in 1999, compares the entire mtDNA sequences of two lymphoblastoid cell lines from two apparently normal individuals (CHR and 9947A[4]) (21) with the 1981 Cambridge Reference Sequence. SRM 2392 also contains the cloned DNA from the CHR HV1 region which contains a C-stretch, an area beyond which sequencing becomes very difficult. In 2003, we developed human mtDNA amplification and sequencing SRM 2392-I (22,23), which contains the DNA from cell line HL-60[5] (a promyelocytic cell line prepared from the peripheral blood leukocytes of a female with acute promyelocytic leukemia). The sequencing results from SRM 2392-I are compared with both the 1981 and 1999 Cambridge Reference Sequences and the sequences obtained for SRM 2392. The information on the entire mtDNA sequences (but not the DNA) from GM03798[6] (a normal human lymphoblast cell line) and GM10742A[6] [a cell line from an individual with Leber Hereditary Optic Neuropathy (LHON)] are provided for information and comparison purposes. Both human mtDNA SRMs 2392 and 2392-I complement one another and provide additional DNA templates for quality assurance when amplifying and sequencing unknown specimens.

Fifty-eight unique primer sets were designed to allow any area or the entire mtDNA (16,569 base pairs) to be amplified and sequenced using the same conditions. The sequences of these primers shown in Table 12 are the same as those used for SRM 2392 (21) with the exception of the reverse primer of set 51. The original reverse primer of set 51 was designed to bind to the CRS sequence. Andrews *et al.* (13) in their reevaluation of the placenta originally used to sequence human mtDNA in 1981 (12) found a C, not a G, at np 14368. Therefore, the reverse primer was redesigned.

With one exception, none of the differences in the coding region of the three normal templates (CHR, 9947A, GM03798) correspond to published mutations associated with specific diseases; although some of these differences did result in amino acid changes when compared with the Cambridge Reference Sequence (12, 13). However, HL-60 did have four mutations that corresponded with mutations that have been associated with the disease Leber Hereditary Optic Neuropathy (LHON), which causes blindness in young adults (18). Due to this finding, we also sequenced the entire mtDNA of a cell line (GM10742A) derived from a person diagnosed with LHON to determine how many mutations these two cell lines would have in common. Two of the four LHON associated mutations were in both cell lines. GM10742A had an additional two LHON mutations. All the differences from the CRS (both

[4] Life Technologies, Inc., Gaithersburg, MD. This cell line is also used in SRM 2391b.

[5] DNA was prepared by the Professional Services Department of American Type Culture Collection (ATCC, Manassas, VA).

[6] NIGMS Human Genetic Mutant Cell Repository, Coriell Institute for Medical Research, 401 Haddon Ave., Camden, NJ.

1981 and 1999) from all five templates that were sequenced are shown in Figure 1 and Table 13. This table also indicates if the mutation produces an amino acid change in the resultant protein. Since we have no information on the identity of HL-60, we do not know if that individual also developed LHON.

SRM 2392 was revalidated at NIST in 2003 and the expiration date was extended to 2008.

Interlaboratory Evaluation of SRM 2392 and 2392-I

An interlaboratory evaluation of the amplification, sequencing, and data analysis of the CHR template for SRM 2392 was conducted by The Bode Technology Group, Inc., Sterling, VA; IIT Research Institute, Newington, VA; and Lark Technologies, Inc., Houston, TX plus NIST. Another interlaboratory evaluation of the amplification, sequencing, and data analysis of HL-60 for SRM 2392-I was conducted by the FBI Laboratory, FBI Academy, Quantico, VA; Armed Forces DNA Identification Laboratory (AFDIL), Armed Forces Institute of Pathology, Rockville, MD; and the Georgia Bureau of Investigation (GBI), Decatur, GA plus NIST. Corroboration of the SRM results provides quality assurance that any unknown mtDNA is also being amplified and sequenced correctly.

For SRM 2392, each participant of the interlaboratory evaluation was provided:

1. Two tubes of DNA from the CHR cell culture line, one contained extracted DNA ready for PCR amplification of the entire mtDNA, and the other contained the cloned DNA ready for cycle sequencing of the HV1 region (this DNA did *not* need to be PCR amplified).
2. Fifty-eight sets of primers labeled with either F# (forward primer) or R# (reverse primer). Forward and reverse primers with the same number were paired and numbered from the 5' end. Primers were diluted to 10 μmol/L and ready for use. Also sent was the -21M13 primer to do the sequencing of the cloned HV1 region of the CHR DNA.
3. A copy of the protocol used at NIST to amplify and sequence the DNA. The participants in the interlaboratory evaluation, however, were free to use any protocol with which they were familiar and
4. A form table to record the results. This table provided the number of the Primer Set, the region that each Primer Set amplified, and the length of the amplified region. The laboratory was asked to fill in the differences found when they compared the sequence that they determined for the CHR template with that of the Cambridge Reference Sequence (12).

All of the laboratories examining CHR essentially followed the NIST protocol. Any changes to the protocol are listed in the section on Materials and Methods in reference 21. Each laboratory was instructed to amplify and sequence the 58 areas designated by the 58 primer sets and also to sequence the cloned DNA for the HV1 region. Labs 1, 2 and 3 found essentially the same polymorphisms. Laboratory 4 had less experience with sequencing mtDNA and did find differences that the other laboratories did not observe. This interlaboratory evaluation was considered successful in that most of the laboratories found the same results. The differences noted by Laboratory 4 confirm and emphasize the need for a standard reference material for sequencing mtDNA. If Laboratory 4 had the NIST mtDNA SRM 2392 and had run it simultaneously with their unknown sample, they would have realized that they were finding an undue number of differences and could have reexamined their procedures to try to determine the reason for these differences.

For SRM 2392-I, each participant in the interlaboratory evaluation was asked to amplify and sequence the entire mtDNA of HL-60. NIST provided: 1. A tube of DNA containing the extracted DNA ready for PCR amplification, 2. The 58 sets of primers labeled with either F# (forward primer) or R# (reverse primer), 3. A table to record the results, and 4. Any other supplies that were needed and requested by the participants. They were allowed to use any protocol for amplification or sequencing that they wished, but were requested to provide a copy of that protocol to NIST. NIST also requested copies of the electropherograms to enable us to resolve any discrepancies; although, as it turned out, all four laboratories obtained identical results. The differences in the methodologies used by the laboratories participating in the interlaboratory evaluation of HL-60 are described in references 22 and 23.

Table 12. Primer Sets Used for the Amplification and Sequencing of mtDNA in SRMs 2392 and 2392-I

Primer Set Number	Nucleotide Positions of Forward and Reverse Primers	Primer Sequence
1	F15	CACCCTATTAACCACTCACG
(HV2)	R484	TGAGATTAGTAGTATGGGAG
2	F361	ACAAAGAACCCTAACACCAGC
	R921	ACTTGGGTTAATCGTGTGACC
3	F756	CATCAAGCACGCAGCAATG
	R1425	AATCCACCTTCGACCCTTAAG
4	F873	GGTTGGTCAATTTCGTGCCAG
	R1425	AATCCACCTTCGACCCTTAAG
5	F1234	CTCACCACCTCTTGCTCAGC
	R1769	GCCAGGTTTCAATTTCTATCG
6	F1587	TGCACTTGGACGAACCAGAG
	R2216	TGTTGAGCTTGAACGCTTTC
7	F1657	CTTGACCGCTCTGAGCTAAAC
	R2216	TGTTGAGCTTGAACGCTTTC
8	F1993	AAACCTACCGAGCCTGGTG
	R2216	TGTTGAGCTTGAACGCTTTC
9	F2105	GAGGAACAGCTCTTTGGACAC
	R2660	AGAGACAGCTGAACCCTCGTG
10	F2417	CACTGTCAACCCAACACAGG
	R3006	ATGTCCTGATCCAACATCGAG
11	F2834	CCCAACCTCCGAGCAGTACATG
	R3557	AGAAGAGCGATGGTGAGAGC
12	F2972	ATAGGGTTTACGACCTCGATG
	R3557	AGAAGAGCGATGGTGAGAGC
13	F3234	AGATGGCAGAGCCCGGTAATC
	R3557	AGAAGAGCGATGGTGAGAGC

Table 12. Continued

Primer Set Number	Nucleotide Positions of Forward and Reverse Primers	Primer Sequence
14	F3441	ACTACAACCCTTCGCTGACG
	R3940	TGAAGCCTGAGACTAGTTCGG
15	F3635	GCCTAGCCGTTTACTCAATCC
	R4162	TGAGTTGGTCGTAGCGGAATC
16	F3931	TCAGGCTTCAACATCGAATACG
	R4728	TTATGGTTCATTGTCCGGAGAG
17	F4183	TTTCTACCACTCACCCTAGCATTAC
	R4728	TTATGGTTCATTGTCCGGAGAG
18	F4392	CCCATCCTAAAGTAAGGTCAGC
	R4983	GGTTTAATCCACCTCAACTGCC
19	F4447	TTGGTTATACCCTTCCCGTAC
	R4982	GTTTAATCCACCTCAACTGCC
20	F4797	CCCTTTCACTTCTGAGTCCCAG
	R5553	AGGGCTTTGAAGGCTCTTG
21	F4976	ATTAAACCAGACCCAGCTACG
	R5553	AGGGCTTTGAAGGCTCTTG
22	F5318	CACCATCACCCTCCTTAACC
	R5882	GCTGAGTGAAGCATTGGACTG
23	F5700	TAAGCACCCTAATCAACTGGC
	R6262	GCCTCCACTATAGCAGATGCG
24	F5999	TCTAAGCCTCCTTATTCGAGC
	R6526	ATAGTGATGCCAGCAGCTAGG
25	F6242	CGCATCTGCTATAGTGGAGG
	R6526	ATAGTGATGCCAGCAGCTAGG
26	F6426	GCCATAACCCAATACCAAACG
	R7030	TGGGCTACAACGTAGTACGTG
27	F6744	GGCTTCCTAGGGTTTATCGTG
	R7255	TTTCATGTGGTGTATGCATCG
28	F7075	GAGGCTTCATTCACTGATTTCC
	R7792	GGGCAGGATAGTTCAGACGG
29	F7215	CGACGTTACTCGGACTACCC
	R7792	GGGCAGGATAGTTCAGACGG
30	F7645	TATCACCTTTCATGATCACGC
	R8215	GACGATGGGCATGAAACTG
31	F7901	TGAACCTACGAGTACACCGACTAC
	R8311	AAGTTAGCTTTACAGTGGGCTCTAG
32	F8164	CGGTCAATGCTCTGAAATCTGTG
	R8669	CATTGTTGGGTGGTGATTAGTCG
33	F8539	CTGTTCGCTTCATTCATTGCC
	R9059	GTGGCGCTTCCAATTAGGTG
34	F8903	CCCACTTCTTACCACAAGGC
	R9403	GTGCTTTCTCGTGTTACATCG
35	F9309	TTTCACTTCCACTCCATAACGC
	R9848	GAAAGTTGAGCCAATAATGACG
36	F9449	CGGGATAATCCTATTTATTACCTCAG
	R9995	AGAGTAAGACCCTCATCAATAGATGG
37	F9754	AGTCTCCCTTCACCATTTCCG
	R10275	AAAGGAGGGCAATTTCTAGATC

Table 12. Continued

Primer Set Number	Nucleotide Positions of Forward and Reverse Primers	Primer Sequence
38	F10127	ACTACCACAACTCAACGGCTAC
	R10556	GGAGGATATGAGGTGTGAGCG
39	F10386	GGATTAGACTGAACCGAATTGG
	R11166	CATCGGGTGATGATAGCCAAG
40	F10704	GTCTCAATCTCCAACACATATGG
	R11267	TGTTGTGAGTGTAAATTAGTGCG
41	F11001	AACGCCACTTATCCAGTGAACC
	R11600	CTGTTTGTCGTAGGCAGATGG
42	F11403	GACTCCCTAAAGCCCATGTCG
	R11927	TTGATCAGGAGAACGTGGTTAC
43	F11760	ACGAACGCACTCACAGTCG
	R12189	AAGCCTCTGTTGTCAGATTCAC
44	F11901	TGCTAGTAACCACGTTCTGGTG
	R12876	GATATCGCCGATACGGTTG
45	F12357	AACCACCCTAACCCTGACTTCC
	R12876	GATATCGCCGATACGGTTG
46	F12601	TTCATCCCTGTAGCATTGTTCG
	R13123	AGCGGATGAGTAAGAAGATTCC
47	F12793	TTGCTCATCAGTTGATGATACG
	R13343	TTGAAGAAGGCGTGGGTACAG
48	F13188	CACTCTGTTCGCAGCAGTATG
	R13611	TCGAGTGCTATAGGCGCTTGTC
49	F13518	CATCATCGAAACCGCAAAC
	R13935	TGTGATGCTAGGGTAGAATCCG
50	F13715	GAAGCCTATTCGCAGGATTTC
	R14118	TGGGAAGAAGAAAGAGAGGAAG
51[a]	F13899	TTTCTCCAACATACTCGGATTC
	R14388	TTAGCGATGGAGGTAGGATTCG (old primer)
	R14388	TTAGCGATGGAGGTAGGATTGG (new primer)
52	F14189	ACAAACAATGGTCAACCAGTAAC
	R14926	TGAGGCGTCTGGTGAGTAGTGC
53	F14470	TCCAAAGACAACCATCATTCC
	R14996	CGTGAAGGTAGCGGATGATTC
54	F14909	TACTCACCAGACGCCTCAACCG
	R15396	TTATCGGAATGGGAGGTGATTC
55	F15260	AGTCCCACCCTCACACGATTC
	R15774	ACTGGTTGTCCTCCGATTCAGG
56	F15574	CGCCTACACAATTCTCCGATC
	R16084	CGGTTGTTGATGGGTGAGTC
57 (HV1)	F15971	TTAACTCCACCATTAGCACC
	R16451	GCGAGGAGAGTAGCACTCTTG
58	F16097	TACATTACTGCCAGCCACCATG
	R336	TTAAGTGCTGTGGCCAGAAG
-21M13	F	TGTAAAACGACGGCCAGT

[a] During the development of SRM 2392-I, reverse primer 51 was changed. When sequencing this area of human mtDNA, one should use the new reverse primer 51.

Differences Between SRM 2392 and SRM 2392-I Templates, GM03798, GM10742A, and the Cambridge Reference Sequence

The Cambridge Reference Sequence (CRS) for human mtDNA was first published in 1981 and revised in 1999 (12, 13). All investigators, who subsequently examined human mtDNA, have used the numbering system of the CRS and have compared their sequence findings to that sequence. The CRS DNA, however, is not available for use as a positive control during actual experiments; whereas, NIST SRM 2392 and 2392-I are available. Table 13 shows the mtDNA differences compared to the CRS that were found at NIST with all five templates - CHR, 9947A, GM03798, HL-60 and GM10742A. Compared to the 1981 CRS, CHR mtDNA had 13 differences in the non-coding regions and 33 differences in the coding regions, 9947A mtDNA had 9 differences in the non-coding regions and 23 differences in the coding regions, HL-60 had 11 differences in the non-coding regions and 33 differences in the coding regions. GM03798 and GM 10742A, whose data are included for comparison and information, had 4 and 12 differences in the non-coding regions, respectively and 19 and 14 differences in the coding regions, respectively. All of these differences are shown in Figure 1 along with many of the LHON disease mutation sites that have been noted in the literature (18). With one exception, none of the base pair changes found in the coding regions of the three normal templates sequenced at NIST correlate with any of the changes found associated with LHON or other published disease states.

Table 13. Certified Human mtDNA Sequence Differences from the Cambridge Reference Sequence (CRS) Found in the Two Templates (CHR and 9947A) in NIST SRM 2392, One Template (HL-60) in NIST SRM 2392-I and in GM03798 and GM10742A.

Comparison with the Cambridge Reference Sequence (CRS)								
CRS		Template	Template	Template	Template	Template	Amino acid change	Region
# [a]	Base[b] 1981/1999	CHR[d]	9947A[d]	HL-60	GM03798	GM10742A		
73	A	G	-	G	-	G		HV2
93	A	-	G	-	-	-		HV2
150	C	-	-	T	-	-		HV2
152	T	-	-	C	-	-		HV2
185	G	-	-	-	-	A		HV2
195	T	C	C	-	-	-		HV2
204	T	C	-	-	-	-		HV2
207	G	A	-	-	-	-		HV2
214	A	-	G	-	-	-		HV2
228	G	-	-	-	-	A		HV2
263*R	A	G	G	G	G	G		HV2
295	C	-	-	T	-	T		HV2
303-309	-	C (ins)	CC (ins)	-	-	-		HV2
311-315*R	-	C (ins)	C (ins)	C (ins)	C (ins)	C (ins)		HV2
462	C	-	-	-	-	T		HV2
482	T	-	-	-	-	C		HV2
489	T	-	-	C	-	C		HV2
709	G	A	-	-	A	-		12sRNA
750 *R	A	G	G	G	G	G		12sRNA
1438*R	A	G	G	G	G	G		12sRNA
1719	G	A	-	-	-	-		16sRNA
2706	A	G	-	G	-	G		16sRNA
2841	T	-	-	-	-	A		16sRNA
3010	G	-	-	-	A	A		16sRNA
3106-3107*E	C/del	del C	del C	del C	del C	del C		16sRNA
3394	T	-	-	-	-	C	Tyr → His	ND1 LHON

Table 13. Continued

Comparison with the Cambridge Reference Sequence (CRS)								
CRS		Template CHR[d]	Template 9947A[d]	Template HL-60	Template GM03798	Template GM10742A	Amino acid change	Region
# [a]	Base[b] 1981/1999							
3423*E	G/T	T	T	T	T	T	Silent	ND1
4135	T	-	C	-	-	-	Tyr → His	ND1
4216	T	-	-	C	-	C	Tyr → His	ND1 LHON
4769*R	A	G	G	G	G	G	Silent	ND2
4985*E	G/A	A	A	A	A	A	Silent	ND2
5186	A	G	-	-	-	-	Silent	ND2
5228	C	-	-	G	-	-	Silent	ND2
5633	C	-	-	T	-	-		tRNA Ala
6221	T	C	-	-	-	-	Silent	COI
6371	C	T	-	-	-	-	Silent	COI
6791	A	G	-	-	-	-	Silent	COI
6849[h]	A	G(0.3A)[h]	-	-	-	-	Thr → Ala[h]	COI
7028	C	T	-	T	-	T	Silent	COI
7476	C	-	-	T	-	-		tRNA Ser
7645	T	-	C	-	-	-	Silent	COII
7861	T	-	C	-	-	-	Silent	COII
8020	G	-	-	-	-	A	Silent	COII
8448	T	-	C	-	-	-	Met → Thr	ATPase 8
8503	T	C	-	-	-	-	Silent	ATPase 8
8860*R	A	G	G	G	G	nd	Thr → Ala	ATPase6
9315	T	-	C	-	-	-	Phe → Leu	COIII
9559*E	G/C	C	C	C	C	C	Arg → Pro	COIII
10172	G	-	-	A	-	-	Silent	ND3
10398	A	-	-	G	-	G	Thr → Ala	ND3
11251	A	-	-	G	-	G	Silent	ND4
11287	T	-	-	-	-	C	Silent	ND4

Table 13. Continued

Comparison with the Cambridge Reference Sequence (CRS)								
CRS		Template CHR[d]	Template 9947A[d]	Template HL-60	Template GM03798	Template GM10742A	Amino acid change	Region
# [a]	Base[b] 1981/1999							
11335*E	T/C	C	C	C	C	C	Silent	ND4
11719	G	A	-	A	-	A	Silent	ND4
11778	G	-	-	-	-	A	Arg → His	ND4 LHON
11878	T	C	-	-	-	-	Silent	ND4
12071[het]	T	-	-	C/T[het]	-	-	Phe→Leu[het]	ND4
12612	A	G	-	G	-	G	Silent	ND5
12705	C	T	-	-	-	-	Silent	ND5
13572	T	-	C	-	-	-	Silent	ND5
13702*E	G/C	C	C	C	C	C	Gly → Arg	ND5
13708	G	A	-	A	-	A	Ala → Thr	ND5 LHON
13759	G	-	A	-	-	-	Ala → Thr	ND5
13966	A	G	-	-	-	-	Thr → Ala	ND5
14199*E	G/T	T	T	T	T	T	Pro → Thr	ND6
14272*E	G/C	C	C	C	C	C	Phe → Leu	ND6
14365*E	G/C	C	C	C	C	C	Silent	ND6
14368*E	G/C	C	C	C	C	C	Phe → Leu	ND6
14470	T	C	-	-	-	-	Silent	ND6
14569	G	-	-	A	-	-	Silent	ND6
14766*E	T/C	T	C	T	C	T	Ile → Thr	ND6
14798	T	-	-	-	-	C	Phe → Leu	CYT B
15257	G	-	-	A	-	-	Asp→ Asn	CYT B LHON
15326*R	A	G	G	G	G	G	Thr → Ala	CYT B
15452	C	-	-	A	-	A	Leu → Ile	CYT B
15646	C	-	-	-	T	-	Silent	CYT B
15812	G	-	-	A	-	-		CYT B LHON
16069	C	-	-	T	-	T	Val → Met	HV1
16126	T	-	-	-	-	C		HV1

Table 13. Continued

Comparison with the Cambridge Reference Sequence (CRS)								
CRS		Template CHR[d]	Template 9947A[d]	Template HL-60	Template GM03798	Template GM10742A	Amino acid change	Region
# [a]	Base[b] 1981/1999							
16183	A	C	-	-	-	-		HV1
16184-93	-	C (ins)	-	-	-	-		HV1
16189	T	C	-	-	-	-		HV1
16193	C	-	-	T	-	-		HV1
16223	C	T	-	-	-	-		HV1
16278	C	T	-	T	-	-		HV1
16292	C	-	-	-	-	T		HV1
16311	T	-	C	-	-	-		HV1
16357	T	-	-	-	C	-		
16362	T	-	-	C	-	-		HV1
16519	T	C	C	-	C	nd		HV1

a : Numbers correspond to Cambridge Reference Sequence (12).
b: Base found in 1981 (12)/ Base found in 1999 (13).
d: SRM 2392 (21, 23).
e: SRM 2392-I (22, 23).
- : Base pair same as in 1981 Cambridge Reference Sequence (12).
h : Possible heteroplasmic site. This heteroplasmy seen in the mtDNA from the first CHR cell culture line is not seen in the mtDNA from the second CHR cell culture line. The second CHR cell culture line agrees with the CRS at np 6849. It is DNA from the second CHR cell culture line that is supplied in NIST SRM 2392.
*R: Rare polymorphisms in Cambridge Reference Sequence discovered by reanalysis of original placenta (13).
*E: Error in Cambridge Reference Sequence discovered by reanalysis of original placenta (13).
del: Deletion
ins: Insertion
het: Heteroplasmy found in HL-60 at np 12071.
HV1: Non-coding region found from 16024 and 16569.
HV2: Non-coding region found from 1 and 576.

CHR DNA: Sequence based on two amplifications and cycle sequencing procedures with DNA from the first cell culture line and at least one amplification and cycle sequencing procedure with DNA from the second cell culture line.
9947A DNA: Sequence based on two amplifications and cycle sequencing procedures.
HL-60 DNA: Sequence based on two amplifications and cycle sequencing procedures in both the forward and reverse directions for a total of 4 sequences
ATPase 6: ATP synthase 6
ATPase 8: ATP synthase 8
CYTB: Cytochrome B
COI: Cytochrome C Oxidase I
COII: Cytochrome C Oxidase II
COIII: Cytochrome C Oxidase III
ND1: NADH dehydrogenase 1
ND2: NADH dehydrogenase 2
ND3: NADH dehydrogenase 3
ND4: NADH dehydrogenase 4
ND5: NADH dehydrogenase 5
ND6: NADH dehydrogenase 6

In summary, the mtDNA genome of HL-60, a promyelocytic leukemia cell line, has been completely sequenced by four laboratories and is now available as NIST SRM 2392-I to the forensic and medical communities. NIST human mtDNA SRM 2392 also continues to be available and includes the DNA from two apparently healthy individuals. Both SRM 2392 and 2392-I contain all the information (e.g., the sequences of 58 unique primer sets) needed to use these SRMs as positive controls for the amplification and sequencing of any DNA. Compared to the templates in SRM 2392, the HL-60 mtDNA in SRM 2392-I has two tRNA differences and more polymorphisms resulting in amino acid changes. Four of these HL-60 mtDNA polymorphisms have been associated with Leber Hereditary Optic Neuropathy (LHON), one as an intermediate mutation and three as secondary mutations. The mtDNA from cell line GM10742A from an individual with LHON was also completely sequenced for comparison and contained some of the same LHON mutations. The combination of these particular LHON associated mutations is also found in phylogenetic haplogroup J and its subset, J_2, and may only be indicative that HL-60 belongs to haplogroup J, one of nine haplogroups that characterize Caucasian individuals of European descent or may mean that haplogroup J is more prone to LHON. Both these mtDNA SRMs will provide enhanced quality control in forensic identification, medical diagnosis, and single nucleotide polymorphism (SNP) detection to the scientific and medical communities when they sequence human mtDNA.

SRM 2395 – Human Y-Chromosome DNA Profiling Standard

SRM 2395 is the Human Y-Chromosome DNA Profiling Standard and is designed to provide quality control to scientists conducting genetic tests involving the polymerase chain reaction (PCR), to law enforcement agents using it as an instructional aid, and to researchers engaging in non-clinical studies that involve the human Y-chromosome. It is not intended for any human or animal clinical diagnostic use. The Y-chromosome is a paternally-transmitted chromosome inherited by males only and is the factor that determines the gender of an individual's offspring. Females have two X chromosomes (one from each parent), while males have one X (from their mother) and one Y (from their father). Therefore, Y-chromosome short tandem repeat (STR) loci are useful in forensic cases such as sexual assaults to distinguish between the DNA of the male assailant and the female victim. These STRs can also be used in paternity testing, identity verification, evolutionary studies to determine population origins, and male lineage genealogy studies (e.g., to determine if the descendants of Sally Hemmings also descended from Thomas Jefferson or other males from the same paternal lineage). Thus, two additional uses of Y-chromosome SRM 2395 are to serve as positive controls in paternity determinations and in identifications of male perpetrators in rape cases. By obtaining the certified results with SRM 2395, the investigators will have the quality assurance that their results with their unknown samples are correct.

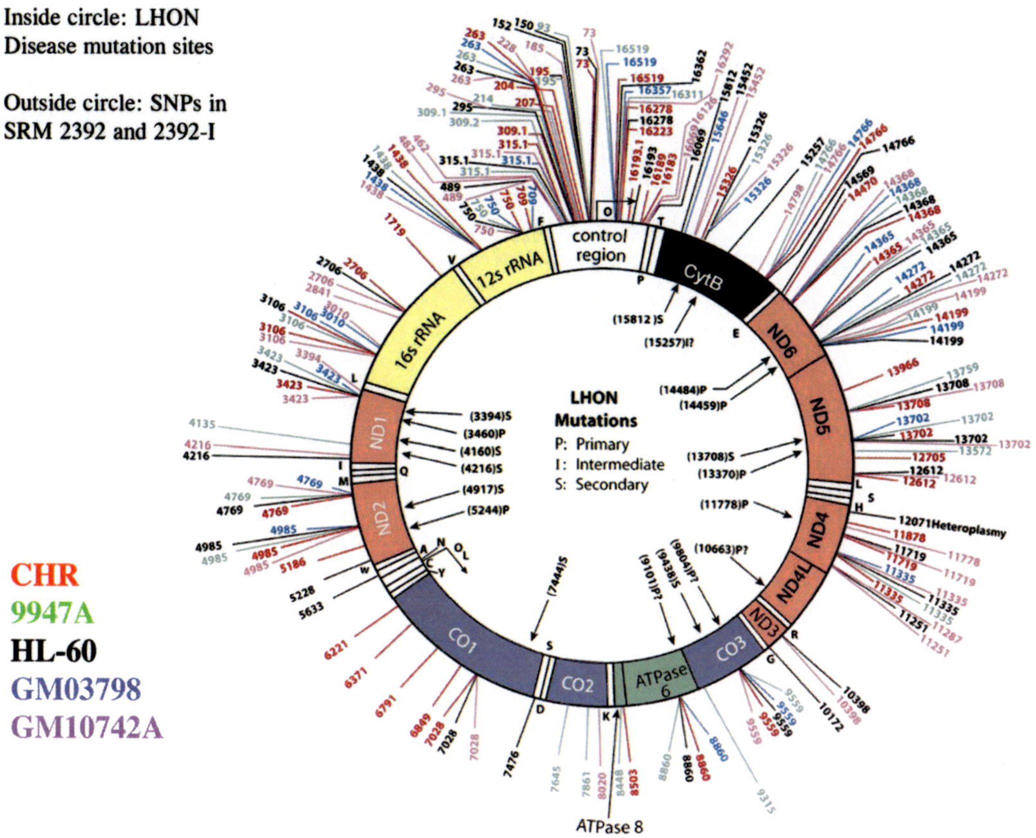

Figure 1. Schematic of Human mtDNA Showing Single Nucleotide Differences from Cambridge Reference Sequence found in SRM 2392, SRM 2392-I, and DNA templates from cell lines GM03798 and GM10742A.

SRM 2395 is composed of well-characterized human genomic DNA from five males and one female (negative control) and consists of the following specific genetic STR loci that have been certified by sequencing of the various alleles: DYS19, DYS385 a/b, DYS388, DYS389 I/II, DYS390, DYS391, DYS392, DYS393, DYS426, DYS435, DYS436, DYS437, DYS438, DYS439, DYS447, DYS448, DYS460, DYS461, DYS462, and Y-GATA-H4 (Tables 14, 15) (24 – 35). Table 16 provides informational values for five additional Y STR loci (nine allele calls) that have been typed, but not yet sequenced: DYS450, DYS456, DYS458 DYS464 a/b/c/d, and YCAII a/b. Additional information on each Y chromosome marker can be found at a NIST-sponsored database on the Internet at http://www.cstl.nist.gov/biotech/strbase and the positions of these STR markers along the Y chromosome are shown in Figure 2. Table 17 contains a summary of the sequence information for the 22 sequenced Y STR loci.

For this SRM, genomic DNA components were extracted from whole blood obtained from Millennium Biotech, Inc., Ft. Lauderdale, FL. NIST used four commercial kits to obtain typing results: The ReliaGene Y-PLEX ™ 6 kit (30) was used to type DYS19, DYS389II, DYS390, DYS391, DYS393, and DYS385 a/b; ReliaGene Y-PLEX ™ 5 was used to type DYS389I/II, DYS392, DYS438, and DYS439; the Promega PowerPlex®Y prototype kit was used to type DYS19, DYS385 a/b, DYS389I/II, DYS390, DYS391, DYS392, DYS393, DYS437, DYS438, and DYS439; and the OligoTrail 20 plex prototype kit was used to type DYS19, DYS 385a/b, DYS389I/II, DYS 390, DYS391, DYS392, DYS393, YCAIIa/b, and DYS388. Three NIST multiplex assays [NIST 20 plex (27), NIST 11 plex (32,33) and NIST 10 plex (29)] were also used to examine the various Y STR markers.

Six components, labeled A through F, are included in each SRM unit and each component contains 50 µL of genomic DNA at a concentration of approximately 2 ng/µL. Components A through E are male genomic DNA 1 through 5, respectively. Component F is female genomic DNA, which serves as a negative control for Y-chromosome specific assays.

Interlaboratory Evaluation of SRM 2395

The STR values for this SRM represent the pooled results from analyses performed at NIST, ReliaGene Technologies, Inc. (New Orleans, LA), OligoTrail LLC (Evanston, IL), and the Forensic Laboratory for DNA Research at Leiden University Medical Center (Leiden, The Netherlands). Sequencing of all (except DYS462) STR markers was performed at NIST. DYS462 was sequenced at Leiden University, who also confirmed the sequences of DYS19, DYS388, DYS389 I/II, DYS390, DYS391, DYS392, DYS393, DYS460, and DYS461.

In summary, the attributes of the Y-chromosome SRM 2395 can be compared to those of the mitochondrial DNA SRMs 2392 and 2392-I in that the Y-chromosome is inherited through the paternal lineage and the mtDNA is inherited through the maternal lineage. Thus, they both can be used to detect evolutionary backgrounds. However, they differ in that the Y-chromosome STR markers are only found in the male population; whereas, all individuals (males and females) have mtDNA that they have inherited from their mothers. If multiple loci are examined, the Y-chromosome STRs can be used to discriminate between individual males. The mtDNA will be similar among maternally-related family members whose DNA can be used to verify identification of missing children, unknown soldier remains, and criminal cases in which blood is found at the scene, but the suspect is not available. The mtDNA SRM can also be used to trace the inheritance of mitochondrial diseases and help in the diagnosis of diseases that have be correlated with mtDNA mutations. The Y-chromosome SRM 2395 will be especially helpful in distinguishing between the male and female DNA in sexual assault cases and in paternity disputes. All of the DNA SRMs that have been developed at NIST will serve to provide quality control and quality assurance that laboratories are testing their unknown samples correctly and obtaining accurate results.

Table 14. Certified values for the European minimal haplotype and U.S. core Y-STR loci.

Component ID	Gender Name	DYS19	DYS389I	DYS389II	DYS390	DYS391	DYS392	DYS393	DYS385 a/b	DYS438	DYS439
A	Male 1	14	13	29	25	11	13	13	12-15	12	12
B	Male 2	14	13	28[a]	23	11	11	12	14-17	9	12
C	Male 3	16	14	32	21[b]	12	11	13	17-20	11	11
D	Male 4	15	12	28[a]	22	10	11	14	14-15	11	11
E	Male 5	17	14	31	24	10	12	14	13-15	10	11
F	Female	-	-	-	-	-	-	-	-	-	-

[a] In DYS389II, components B and D both contain a total number of repeats equal to 28, but can be distinguished since B has 5-10-3-10 and D has 5-11-3-9 of the TCTG-TCTA-TCTG-TCTA repeats, respectively (see Table 17).

[b] At the DYS390 locus, component C has a variant allele. Size-based analytical systems should type this sample as a 21 repeat allele although sequence information reveals a T-to-A polymorphism internal to the repeat.

Table 15. Certified values for other commonly used Y-STR markers

Component ID	Name	DYS 388	DYS 426	DYS 435	DYS 436	DYS 437	DYS 447	DYS 448	DYS 460	DYS 461	DYS 462	H4
A	Male 1	12	12	12	12	15	24	19[b]	11	12	11	12[c]
B	Male 2	15	11	11	12	14	25[a]	21[b]	10	13	11	12[c]
C	Male 3	12	11	11	12	14	25[a]	21[b]	9	13	12	12[c]
D	Male 4	12	11	11	12	16	23	21[b]	11	11	13	12[c]
E	Male 5	13	11	11	12	14	26	20[b]	11	12	12	11[c]
F	Female	-	-	-	-	-	-	-	-	-	-	-

[a] In DYS447, components B and C both have a total of 25 repeats. However, B contains 9-1-8-1-6, while C has 7-1-8-1-8 of the following [TAATA]-[TAAAA]-[TAATA]-[TAAAA]-[TAATA] repeats, repectively (see Table 17).

[b] Three different nomenclatures have been published for DYS448 (32). The one listed here follows Redd *et al.* (28).

[c] The H4 nomenclature follows Butler *et al.* (27).

Table 16. Informational values for additional Y-STR loci.

Component ID	Name	DYS 450	DYS 456	DYS 458	DYS464 a/b/c/d expanded	DYS464 a/b/c/d conservative	YCAII a/b
A	Male 1	10	15	16	14-15-15-17	14-15-17	19-23
B	Male 2	10	15	15	12-13-13-17	12-13-17	19-22
C	Male 3	8	15	17	13-16-16-18	13-16-18	19-19
D	Male 4	9	15	16	13-13-14-14	13-14	20-20
E	Male 5	10	15	16	11-14-14-15	11-14-15	19-21
F	Female	--	--	--	--	--	--

Table 17. Repeat sequences of Y-chromosome STRs

STR Loci	STR sequence
DYS19	$[TAGA]_X$ tagg $[TAGA]_Y$
DYS388	$[ATT]_X$
DYS391	$[TCTA]_X$
DYS392	$[TAT]_X$
DYS393	$[AGAT]_X$
DYS426	$[GTT]_X$
DYS435	$[TGGA]_X$
DYS436	$[GTT]_X$
DYS438	$[TTTTC]_X$
DYS439	$[GATA]_X$
DYS460	$[ATAG]_X$
DYS461	$[TAGA]_X$CAGA
DYS462	$[TATG]_X$
DYS385a	$[GAAA]_X$
DYS385b	$[GAAA]_X$
GATA-H4	$[TAGA]_X$
DYS3891	$[TCTG]_X[TCTA]_Y$
DYS38911	$[TCTG]_X[TCTA]_Y \ldots [TCTG]_{X'}[TCTA]_{Y'}$
DYS390	$[TCTG]_X[TCTA]_Y[TCTG]_{X'}[TCTA]_{Y'}$*
DYS447	$[TAATA]_X [TAAAA][TAATA]_Y[TAAAA][TAATA]_{X'}$
DYS448	$[AGAGAT]_X N_{42}[AGAGAT]_Y$
DYS437	$[TCTA]_X[TCTG]_Y[TCTA]_{X'}$

X + Y + X` + Y` = Total number of repeat units in each loci. For details, see SRM 2395 certificate of analysis and Table 4 at http://patapsco.nist.gov/srmcatalog/certificates/2395.pdf

* In male genomic DNA 3, one TCTA changed to ACTA. See Table 4 in the certificate of analysis.

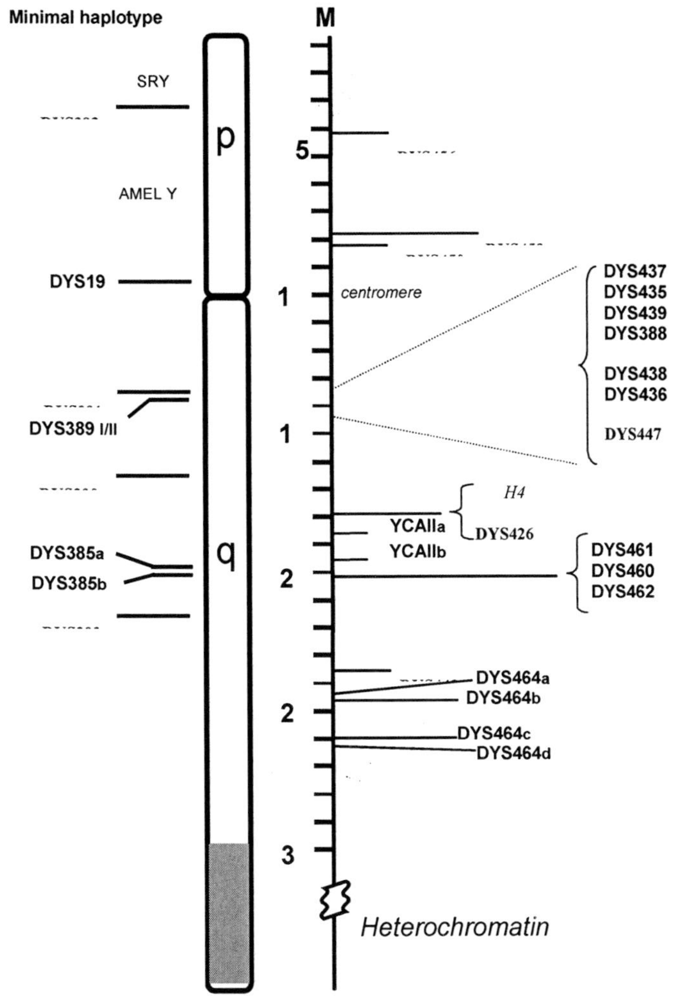

Figure 2. Y-STR Marker Positions for Loci in SRM 2395

Acknowledgments

All of the analytical determinations and technical measurements leading to the certification of SRMs 2390, 2391, 2392, 2392-I, and 2395 were performed in the NIST Biotechnology Division of the Chemical Science and Technology Laboratory at the National Institute of Standards and Technology. The technical and support aspects involved in the preparation, certification and issuance of these SRMs were coordinated through the Standard Reference Materials Program by J. C. Colbert, C. S. Davis, and B. S. MacDonald.

For SRM 2390, the technical aspects of this recertification were conducted by D. J. Reeder, formerly of the NIST Biotechnology Division. Material stability studies and coordination of the interlaboratory study were conducted by K. L. Richie of the NIST Biotechnology Division. Data analysis was performed by D.L. Duewer of the NIST Analytical Chemistry Division. Statistical consultation was provided by H-K Liu of the NIST Statistical Engineering Division.

For SRM 2391b, the analytical determinations and technical measurements leading to the certification of this SRM were performed by M. C. Kline and J. W. Redman of the NIST Biotechnology Division. The overall direction of the technical measurement leading to the certification was under the chairmanship of J. M. Butler of the NIST Biotechnology Division. The DNA, amplified and genomic, was obtained from Roche Molecular Systems, Inc., Alameda, CA. The cell lines - GM09947A and GM09948 - were obtained from Marligen Biosciences, Inc., Ijamsville, MD.

For SRM 2392, the analytical determinations and technical measurements leading to the certification of this SRM were performed by B. C. Levin, H. Cheng, L. Tully, M. P. Jones and D. J. Reeder. The leader of the NIST DNA Technologies Group in the Biotechnology Division, D. J. Reeder, provided overall direction leading to the certification. DNA from GM09947A was obtained from Life Technologies, Inc. Funding was received from the National Institute of Justice through the NIST Office of Law Enforcement Standards and the Advanced Technology Program at NIST. P. Reddy provided help and advice on the cloning of the HV1 region.

For SRM 2392-I, the analytical determination, technical measurements and analysis of data for the certification of this SRM were performed by D. K. Hancock, K. L. Richie, K. A. Holland (on sabbatical from Gettysburg College, Gettysburg, PA), and B. C. Levin of the NIST DNA Technologies Group, Biotechnology Division, Chemical Science and Technology Laboratory. The overall direction and coordination of the technical measurements leading to the certification was performed by B. C. Levin of the NIST DNA Technologies Group, Biotechnology Division, Chemical Science and Technology Laboratory. This research was supported by Interagency Agreement number 1999-IJ-R-094 from the National Institute of Justice.

For SRM 2395, the overall direction and coordination of the technical activities leading to certification were under the chairmanship of Margaret C. Kline and John M. Butler of the NIST Biotechnology Division. Analytical determination and technical measurements leading to the certification of this SRM were performed by J.M. Butler, R. Schoske, P.M. Vallone, M.C. Kline, and J.W. Redman of the NIST Biotechnology Division. This research was supported by Interagency Agreement number 1999-IJ-R-094 from the National Institute of Justice.

For SRMs 2394 and 2399, which were developed and released following the submission of this chapter, more information can be obtained from The National Institute of Standards and Technology, Standard Reference Materials Program, 100 Bureau Drive, Mail Stop 2322, Gaithersburg, MD 20899-2322, Telephone: (301) 975-6776, FAX: (301) 948-3730

E-mail: srminfo@nist.gov

Web sites: www.nist.gov/srm, http://ts.nist.gov/ts/htdocs/230/232/232.htm.

References

[1] Reeder, D.J., NIST Standards Development for RFLP DNA Profiling. *Proceedings of the Second International Symposium on Human Identification, Promega Corporation*, p. 245-261 (1991).

[2] National Institute of Standards and Technology, "Certificate of Analysis, *Standard Reference Material* **2390**, DNA Profiling Standard," Standard Reference Materials

Program, NIST, Gaithersburg, MD (1992, 2001). (http://patapsco.nist.gov/srmcatalog/certificates/2390.pdf)

[3] Reeder, D.J., Kline, M.C., and Richie, K.L., An Overview of Reference Materials Prepared for Standardization of DNA Typing Procedures. Fresenius' *J. Anal. Chem.* **352**:246-249 (1995).

[4] Levin, B.C., Cheng, H., Kline, M.C., Redman, J.W., and Richie, K.L., A Review of the DNA Standard Reference Materials Developed by the National Institute of Standards and Technology. Fresenius' *J. Anal. Chem.* **370**:213-219 (2001).

[5] Duewer, D.L., Currie, L.A., Reeder, D.J., Leigh, S.D., Liu, H-K., and Mudd, J.L., Interlaboratory Comparison of Autoradiographic DNA Profiling Measurements. 4. Protocol Effects, *Anal. Chem.*, **69**:1882-1892, (1997).

[6] Eisenberg, A.J., Gibson, P., Nandi, S., and Wang, L., The Development and Implementation of a Hae III Based RFLP System for Parentage Testing in Texas. *Proceedings from the Second International Symposium on Human Identification*, Promega Corporation, p. 163-180 (1991).

[7] Budowle, B., The RFLP Technique. *Crime Laboratory Digest* **15**:97-98 (1988).

[8] Budowle, B. and Baechtel, F.S. Modifications to Improve the Effectiveness of Restriction Fragment Length Polymorphism Typing, Applied Theories. *Electrophoresis* **1**: 181-187 (1990).

[9] Hahn, G.J. and Meeker, W.Q. *Statistical Intervals: a Guide for Practitioners*. John Wiley, New York, NY (1991).

[10] Nakamura, Y., Carlson, M., Krapcho, V., and White, R., Isolation and Mapping of a polymorphic DNA Sequence (pMCT118) on Chromosome 1p (D1S80). *Nucleic Acids Res.* **16**: 9364 (1988).

[11] Kasai, K., Nakamura, Y., and White, R., Amplification of a Variable Number of Tandem repeats (VNTR) Locus (pMCT118) by the Polymerase Chain Reaction (PCR) and its Application to Forensic Science. *J. For. Sci.* **35**: 1196-1200 (1990).

[12] Anderson, S., Bankier, A. T., Barrell, B. G., deBrujin, M. H. L., Coulson, A. R., Drouin, J., Eperon, I. C., Nierlich, D. P., Roe, B. A., Sanger, F., Schreier, P. H., Smith, A. J. H., Staden, R., and Young, I. G., Sequence and Organization of the Human Mitochondrial Genome. *Nature* **290**: 457-465 (1981).

[13] Andrews, R.M., Kubacka, I., Chinnery, P.F., Lightowlers, R.N., Turnbull, D.M., Howell, N. (1999). Reanalysis and revision of the Cambridge Reference Sequence for human mitochondrial DNA. *Nature Genetics* **23**:147 (1999).

[14] Bogenhagen, D., and Clayton, D. A., The Number of Mitochondrial Deoxyribonucleic Acid Genomes in Mouse L and Human HeLa Cells. *J. Biol. Chem.* **249**: 7991-7995 (1974).

[15] King, M. P., and Attardi, G., Human Cells Lacking MtDNA: Repopulation with Exogenous Mitochondria by Complementation. *Science* **246**: 500-503 (1989).

[16] Holland, M. M., Fisher, D. L., Mitchell, L. G., Rodriquez, W. C., Canik, J. J., Merril, C. R., and Weedn, V. W., Mitochondrial DNA Sequence Analysis of Human Skeletal Remains: Identification of Remains from the Vietnam War. *J. Forensic Sciences* **38**: 542-553. (1993).

[17] Holland, M. M., Fisher, D. L., Roby, R. K., Ruderman, J., Bryson, C., and Weedn, V. W., Mitochondrial DNA Sequence Analysis of Human Remains. *Crime Laboratory Digest* **22**: 109-115 (1995).

[18] Wallace, D. C., Mitochondrial Genetics: a Paradigm for Aging and Degenerative Diseases. *Science* **256**: 628-632 (1992).

[19] Grossman, L. I., Mitochondrial Mutations and Human Disease. *Env. & Mol. Mutag.* **25**: (supplement 26) 30-37 (1995).

[20] Ballinger, S. W., Bouder, T. G., Davis, G. S., Judice, S. A., Nicklas, J. A., and Albertini, R. J., Mitochondrial Genome Damage Associated with Cigarette Smoking. *Cancer Research* **56**: 5692-5697 (1996).

[21] Levin, B.C., Cheng, H., and Reeder, D.J., A Human Mitochondrial DNA Standard Reference Material for Quality Control in Forensic Identification, Medical Diagnosis, and Mutation Detection. *Genomics* **55**: 135-146 (1999).

[22] Levin, B.C., Holland, K.A., Hancock, D.K., Coble, M., Parsons, T.J., Kienker, L.J., Williams, D.W., Jones, MP, and Richie, K.L., Comparison of the Complete mtDNA Genome Sequences of Human Cell Lines - HL-60 and GM10742A - from Individuals with Pro-myelocytic Leukemia and Leber Hereditary Optic Neuropathy, Respectively, and the Inclusion of HL-60 in the NIST Human Mitochondrial DNA Standard Reference Material - SRM 2392-I. *Mitochondrion* **2**:387-400 (2003).

[23] Levin, B.C., Hancock, D.K., Holland, K.A., Cheng, H., and Richie, K.L., Human Mitochondrial DNA - *Amplification and Sequencing Standard Reference Materials* – SRM 2392 and SRM 2392-I. NIST Special Publication 260-155, National Institute of Standards and Technology, Gaithersburg, MD (2003).

[24] Jobling, M.A., Pandya, A., and Tyler-Smith, C. The Y-Chromosome in Forensic Analysis and Paternity Testing. *Int. J Legal Med.* **110:**118-124 (1997).

[25] Kayser, M. *et al.* Evaluation of Y-Chromosomal STRs: a Multicenter Study. *Int. J. Legal Med.***110**:125-133 (1997).

[26] Roewer, L. *et al.* Online Reference Database of European Y-Chromosomal Short Tandem Repeat (STR) Haplotypes. *Forensic Sci. Int.* **118**:106-113 (2001).

[27] Butler, J.M., Schoske, R., Vallone, P.M., Kline, M.C., Redd, A.J., and Hammer, M.F. A Novel Multiplex for Simultaneous Amplification of 20 Y-Chromosome STR Markers. *Forensic Sci. Int.***129:**10-24 (2002).

[28] Redd, A.J., Agellon, A.B., Kearney, V.A., Contreras, V.A., Karafet, T., Park, H., de Knijff, P., Butler, J. M., and Hammer, M. F. Forensic Value of 14 Novel STRs on the Human Y-Chromosome. *Forensic Sci. Int.***130:** 97-111 (2002).

[29] Schoske, R., Vallone, P.M., Ruitberg, C.M., and Butler, J.M. Multiplex PCR Design Strategy Used for the Simultaneous Amplification of 10 Y-Chromosome Short Tandem Repeat (STR) Loci. *Anal. Bioanal. Chem.***375:**333-343 (2003).

[30] Sinha, S. et al. Development and Validation of a Multiplexed Y-Chromosome STR Genotyping System, Y-PLEX. 6, for Forensic Casework. *J. Forensic Sci.* **48:**93-103 (2003).

[31] Butler, J.M. Recent Developments in Y-STR and Y-SNP Analysis. *Forensic Sci. Rev.* (in press, 2003).

[32] Schoske, R. The Design, *Optimization and Testing of Y-Chromosome Short Tandem Repeat Megaplexes*; Ph.D. Dissertation, American University (2003).

[33] Schoske, R., Vallone, P.M., Kline, M.C., Redman, J.W., and Butler, J.M. High-Throughput Y-STR Typing of U.S. *Populations With 27 Regions of the Y-Chromosome Using Two Multiplex PCR Assays.* submitted (2003).

[34] Vallone, P.M., and Butler, J.M. Y-SNP Typing Using Allele-Specific Hybridization and Primer Extension. submitted (2003).

[35] Y Chromosome Consortium. A Nomenclature System for the Tree of Human Y-Chromosomal Binary Haplogroups. *Genome Res.***7**:339-348 (2002).

In: Trends in Genome Research
Editor: Clyde R. Williams, pp. 207-223
ISBN 1-60021-027-9

Chapter 8

Bioinformatics Software and Databases for Proteomics

Mauno Vihinen[*]
Institute of Medical Technology, FI-33014 University of Tampere, Finland, and Research Unit, Tampere University Hospital, FI-33520 Finland

Abstract

The completion of numerous genome projects is changing the focus of research to the gene products, most often proteins. Proteomics approaches can be divided into four clearly distinct classes based on studied systems and produced data. Proteomics and other data intensive techniques rely on bioinformatics to organize, analyze, store and distribute large data sets. The major trends and bioinformatics services of the four subcategories of proteomics, i.e. expression proteomics, interaction proteomics, functional proteomics, and structural proteomics are discussed. Numerous references and links are provided to validated proteomics databases and programs. Since many of the bioinformatics routines in proteomics can be run in Internet mainly Internet-based systems are described, especially those that are freely available.

Introduction

The completion of numerous genome projects is changing the focus of research to the gene products, most often proteins. Functional genomics aims to identify the functions, abundance, reactions, interactions, localization, and structures of gene products. Proteomics has been defined as a field which reveals the identities, abundances, biochemical and cellular functions, interactions, and structures of all proteins in an organism, organ, or organelle, and their variation during time, space, and physiological state.

[*] E-mail address: mauno.vihinen@uta.fi, tel. +358-3-3551 7735, fax +358-3-3551 7710 (Correspondence to Professor Mauno Vihinen, Institute of Medical Technology, FI-33014 University of Tampere, Finland)

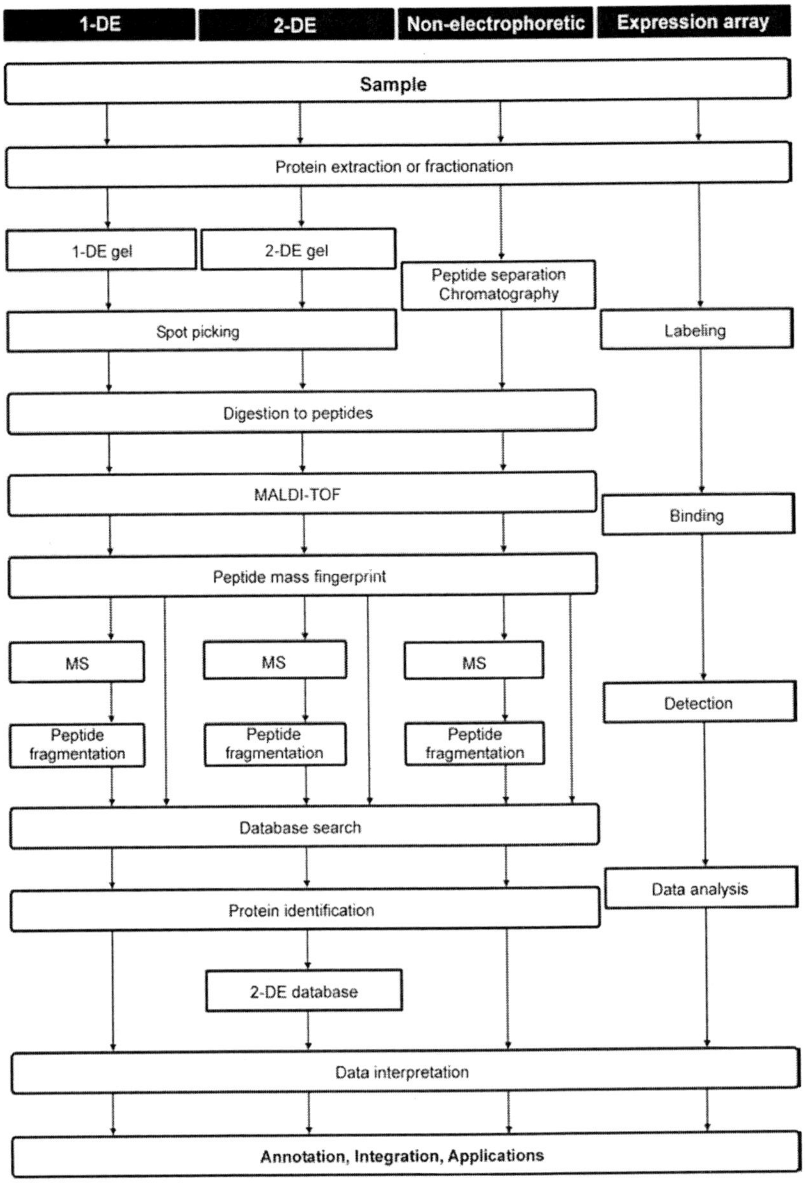

Figure 1. Schematic overview of proteomics methods. One-dimensional gel electrophoresis can be used to investigate e.g. protein complexes, while 2-DE technique has the widest application range. Non-electrophoretic methods are run in liquid phase, requiring a multistep separation before protein identification. Several array technologies have been developed. In a typical expression array samples are labeled in the same way as in cDNA or oligonucleotide microarrays. After running a gel, a spot of interesting complexes or proteins in 1-DE or 2-DE method, respectively, are picked and digested with proteases to generate characteristic peptides for each individual protein. Peptide mass fingerprint is obtained with mass spectrometry and peptide fragmentation can be used for sequencing in tandem-MS instruments. Peptide mass fingerprints and sequence information are compared to information in databases to identify the proteins. Images of 2-DE gels can be annotated and distributed in Internet as databases. By combining and integrating information from various sources for the identified proteins it is possible to describe changes in proteomes in detail and to correlate the expression patterns to cellular processes.

Proteomics approaches can be divided into four clearly distinct classes based on studied systems and produced data. Expression proteomics studies protein production. Differential proteome analysis, i.e. comparison of different samples, forms the basis of this approach. Interaction proteomics, also known as cell-map proteomics, reveals interactions of proteins and their subcellular localization. In functional proteomics the effects of functional inactivation or perturbation are studied. Structural proteomics, which has also been called structural genomics, is defined as large-scale three-dimensional structure analysis.

Proteomics started with the introduction of two-dimensional gel electrophoresis (2-DE) technology (Figure 1). Recently several new techniques have been developed including methods for protein identification, protein arrays, localization methods, two-hybrid method, and phage display technology. Together all these methods produce vast amounts of data. Proteomics and other data intensive techniques rely on bioinformatics to organize, analyze, store and distribute large data sets (Wojcik and Schäcther, 2000, Vihinen, 2001, Dowsey *et al.*, 2003, Vihinen, 2004).

New rivals for 2-DE technology have recently emerged from several new techniques. Protein arrays or chips are prepared by attaching suitable baits onto a solid support (Cutler, 2003). Antibodies are the most common bait molecules and there are already commercial antibody arrays available. In the future microfluidics-based arrays (lab-on-a-chip) may become common. Other new improvements include liquid chromatography mass spectrometry (LC-MS) approach, especially with isotope coded affinity tags (ICAT) (Gygi *et al.*, 1999a). LC-MS methods are run directly from liquid samples thereby avoiding the labor intensive 2-DE, which has limited dynamic range. At the moment, these methods are best suited for the analysis of subproteomes or complexes. 2-DE technique is likely remain in wide use also in the future because of many of its benefits. The gels provide an overall view on the whole data, and post-translational modifications (Mann and Jensen, 2003) such as phosphorylation and glycosylation can be investigated as well as the proportions of different splice variants. The new methods cannot be utilized for such studies, but, however, they are more amenable for automation.

MS is the most commonly used method for protein identification (Figure 1). Gel running, spot picking and MS analysis can be automated with robotics making high-throughput proteomics feasible. Proteins are identified from MS data by comparing peptide mass fingerprints to those in databases. Further accuracy can be obtained with tandem MS, in which the downstream instrument is used for sequencing a few residues from the N-terminus of peptides.

Gel matching forms the basis for 2-DE data analysis. Plenty of proteomics data can be found from Internet and literature. To make this data easily accessible for the proteomics community, systematic formats should be used. Proteomics Standards Initiative (PSI) (Table 1), which is a workgroup for Human Proteome Organization (HUPO), develops standards for mass spectrometry, protein-protein interaction data as well as general proteomics formats. These standards are based on XML (eXtensible Markup Language) schemas. XML facilitates easy exchange of the data between different programs and allows also distribution to different devices. A format and a standard have been published for interaction information (Hermajakob *et al.*, 2004a) and there is also a PSI-MS schema for spectra data. HUP-ML is a project for general proteomics data representation, exchange and distribution. Details of experiments can be collected and stored with LIMS (laboratory information management system) packages.

Various bioinformatics programs, databases and services needed in different steps during proteome analysis projects are discussed here. Since many of the bioinformatics routines in proteomics can be run in Internet, mainly Internet-based systems are described, especially those that are freely available. Majority of the discussion is related to the 2-DE technique, because the new methods are still under development and there are not many dedicated bioinformatics resources for them.

Protein Identification

Protein identification from spots on 2-DE gels is one of the first analysis steps. MS of the protein spots and their unique digestion fingerprints with MALDI/TOF (Matrix-Assisted Laser Desorption/Ionisation/Time-of-Flight) or ESI (Electrospray Ionization) MS is the standard method. Proteins can be further characterized by sequence tagging with tandem mass spectrometry (MS-MS).

For protein identification, sequence databases are searched for proteins with similar fingerprints. The more accurate and complete the sequence databases, the more reliable identifications can be obtained. Genome sequencing projects have remarkably increased the fidelity of the identification, because the complete genome for an organism allows the prediction of all fingerprint patterns. However, alternative splicing of genes and post-translational modifications of proteins are still poorly known for most genes/proteins and therefore there are still problems in identification in some cases.

Protein spots from gels can be directly used for mass spectrometric analyses. Whole proteins cannot be analyzed with MS. Therefore proteins are cleaved with proteases to peptides of characteristic molecular weights. Fingerprints that consist of pI, Mr, peptide masses, sequence tags or amino acid composition can be used for protein identification.

ExPASy server of the Swiss Institute of Bioinformatics (SIB) provides the largest selection of Internet tools and links for proteomics. Manually annotated sequence databases such as SwissProt or LocusLink contain more reliable functional annotations than automatically generated entries. The Human Proteomics Initiative (HPI) of SIB and the European Bioinformatics Institute (EBI) is an effort to automatically annotate, describe and distribute highly curated information concerning human protein sequences (O'Donovan *et al.*, 2001).

Dozens of web-accessible MS tools can be grouped to services for protein molecular weight calculation and protein sequence tags, for peptide mass fingerprinting, for fingerprinting with sequence tag information, and other tools e.g. for amino acid composition, isoelectric points, post-translational modifications and digestion information (Table 2). For a detailed grouping see (Vihinen, 2001). The launch of several of these routines simultaneously is possible with CombSearch and ProteinProspector.

The performance of some of the major peptide mass fingerprinting (Mascot and MS-Fit) and MS/MS peptide sequence information programs (ProFound and SEQUEST) has been evaluated with real data. ProFound and SEQUEST identified more proteins correctly, however the results were far from complete and combined use of methods for the same task might give better results (Chamrad *et al.*, 2004).

Table 1. General Proteomics links

Human Proteomics Organization	http://www.hupo.org/
Proteomics Standard Initiative	http://psidev.sourceforge.net/
PSI Molecular Interaction standard	http://psidev.sf.net/mi/xml/doc/user/
PSI-MS Format	http://psidev.sourceforge.net/ms/index.html
HUP-ML	http://www1.biz.biglobe.ne.jp/~jhupo/HUP-ML/hup-ml.htm
ExPASy	http://www.expasy.ch
SwissProt	http://www.expasy.org/sprot/
EntrezGene	http://www.ncbi.nlm.nih.gov/entrez/query.fcgi?db=gene
HPI	http://www.expasy.org/sprot/hpi/

Table 2. Mass spectrometry programs in the Internet

AACompIdent	http://www.expasy.ch/tools/aacomp/	Amino acid composition
AACompSim	http://www.expasy.ch/tools/aacsim/	Amino acid composition
Amino Acid Information	http://prowl.rockefeller.edu/aainfo/contents.htm	Amino acid properties
CombSearch	http://www.pdg.cnb.uam.es/cursos/hola/pages/visualizacion/programas_manuales/spdbv_userguide/us.expasy.org/tools/CombSearch/index.html	Query system for several MS analysis programs
Compute pI/Mw tool	http://www.expasy.ch/tools/pi_tool.html	Computation of pI and MW
Exact Mass Calculator	http://www.sisweb.com/cgi-bin/mass11.pl	Mass calculation
FindMod	http://www.expasy.ch/tools/findmod/	Prediction of post-translational modifications
GlycoMod	http://www.expasy.ch/tools/glycomod/	Prediction of attached oligosaccharide structures
GPM	http://h112.thegpm.org/tandem/thegpm_tandem.html	Tandem MS mass fingerprinting
JPAT 2.2 API	http://www.pixelgate.net/~mjones/java/jpat/jpat2/	Query system for several MS analysis program
Mascot	http://www.matrixscience.com/search_form_select.html	Peptide fingerprint and sequence tag analysis
MassSearch	http://mendel.ethz.ch:8080/Server/ServerBooklet/MassSearchEx.html	Mass fragment search
Mass Spectrometer	http://www.sisweb.com/cgi-bin/mass8.pl	Generation of mass spectrum chart
MS-Comp	http://prospector.ucsf.edu/ucsfhtml4.0/mscomp.htm	Amino acid composition comparison
MS-Digest	http://prospector.ucsf.edu/ucsfhtml4.0/msdigest.htm	Calculation of masses of protein cleavage products
MS-Fit	http://prospector.ucsf.edu/ucsfhtml4.0/msfit.htm	Peptide mass fingerprinting
MS-Isotope	http://prospector.ucsf.edu/ucsfhtml4.0/msiso.htm	Calculation of isotope patterns

Table 2. Continued

MS-Product	http://prospector.ucsf.edu/ucsfhtml4.0/msprod.htm	Calculation of masses of protein cleavage products
MS-Seq	http://prospector.ucsf.edu/ucsfhtml4.0/msseq.htm	Peptide sequence tag analysis
MS-Tag	http://prospector.ucsf.edu/ucsfhtml4.0/mstagfd.htm	Peptide sequence tag analysis
MultiIdent	http://www.expasy.ch/tools/multiident/	Amino acid composition, mass and sequence tag analysis
PepFrag	http://prowl.rockefeller.edu/prowl/pepfragch.html	Peptide sequence tag analysis
PeptideMass	http://www.expasy.ch/tools/peptide-mass.html	Peptide mass calculation
PeptIdent	http://www.expasy.ch/tools/peptident.html	Peptide mass fingerprinting
PeptideSearch	http://www.mann.embl-heidelberg.de/GroupPages/PageLink/peptidesearchpage.html	Peptide mass and sequence analysis
ProFound	http://prowl.rockefeller.edu/profound_bin/WebProFound.exe	Peptide mass fingerprinting
PropSearch	http://abcis.cbs.cnrs.fr/propsearch/	Database search with amino acid composition
ProteinProspector	http://prospector.ucsf.edu/	Query system for several MS analysis programs
PROWL	http://prowl.rockefeller.edu/	Peptide mass and fragment ion search
TagIdent	http://www.expasy.ch/tools/tagident.html	Peptide mass and sequence analysis

Table 3. Gel comparison and 2-DE database links

Flicker	http://www.lecb.ncifcrf.gov/flicker/
2DWG	Http://www-lecb.ncifcrf.gov/2dwgDB/
WORLD-2DPAGE	Http://www.expasy.ch/ch2d/2d-index.html
2DHunt	Http://www.expasy.ch/ch2d/2DHunt
Guidelines for federated databases	Http://www.expasy.ch/ch2d/fed-rules.html
Make2D-DBII	www.expasy.ch/ch2d/make2ddb.html
ProteomeWeb	http://proteomeweb.anl.gov/
GELBANK	http://gelbank.anl.gov/

Gel Comparison

Gels have to be compared for qualitative and quantitative information regarding protein expression. After the scan further processing may be necessary to enhance the images e.g. by increasing contrast, or by subtracting the background. Since it is not possible to apply equal amounts of proteins to gels, the intensities in the images can differ and the data should be normalized. The crucial step is spot detection and quantitation. To compare gels for different samples (treated in different ways, healthy vs disease-associated samples, etc.) gel matching has to be performed. Conclusions on quantitative changes should be made with great care and optimally the images ought to be for gels and samples that have been prepared, run and stained in the same way.

For image analysis can be used some freeware programs such as Flicker (Lemkin, 1997a) (Table 3). In this area commercial programs such as PDQuest (BioRad), Melanie3 (GeneBio), and Progenesis (PerkinElmer) are clearly more advanced than public domain programs.

Gel matching has remained a tedious step in 2-DE analysis until recently. The gels are never exactly identical, because there are inhomogeneities arising from many factors such as sample preparation, staining, unequal mobility in gels, and variations of electrophoretic conditions. During the last few years novel methods for automatic gel matching have been developed. Some very expensive commercial applications are on the market. In Progenesis the spot detection, gel warping, and auto matching is fully automated and does not allow any manual intervention. The problem with fully automated systems is that they cannot be manually adjusted and optimized even if needed. On the other hand, long training is not needed to run them.

The quality and performance of commercial packages has been compared in three areas: spot detection, gel matching, and spot quantitation. Z3 was found to require less manual intervention than Melanie (Raman *et al.*, 2002), while Progenesis is better in gel matching than PDQUEST (Rosengren *et al.*, 2003).

Once matched, the gels can be analyzed both for qualitative and quantitative differences in protein expression. The identified and matched spots are the starting point for more detailed data mining. Such investigations include studies of coexpressed proteins, synthesis rates and expression levels; analysis of protein function and localization, effects of post-translational modifications and regulation; validation and identification of drug targets; diagnostics and risk analysis; search for disease markers (e.g. tumor markers) for disease conditions and progression, differential proteome analysis; and responses to treatments, agents and pathogens.

Together with nucleotide microarray analysis, proteomics indicate system-wide expression characteristics. The correlation of these two kinds of expression data is not necessarily straightforward (Anderson and Seilhamer, 1997, Gygi *et al.*, 1999b). When more proteomics data comes accessible many of the methods used for large-scale data analysis of microarray information will also be applied to proteomics.

Databases of 2-DE Information

2-DE gels contain typically at least hundreds of protein spots. A large number of gel images along with identified and annotated protein spots have been made publicly available. The gels have been generated with different methods in different conditions, and it may be difficult or even impossible to compare gels from different laboratories. Different staining procedures or even different details in staining are likely to prevent quantitative comparison over the images especially for low-expression proteins. Data from other laboratories and experiments can still be useful when utilized carefully, e.g. in tentative identification of proteins.

The 2-DE databases in Internet can be classified as general, organ/tissue-specific or cell/organism-specific registries. Powerful searches can be made from a dedicated meta-database, 2DWG (Lemkin, 1997b) (Table 3). WORLD-2DPAGE has an index of 2-DE databases and services. Another search engine is called 2DHunt. 2-DE databases can be used e.g. for the search of a protein function, expression pattern or cellular localization along with annotations.

If a laboratory wants to distribute their own gel images certain guidelines should be followed (Appel *et al.*, 1996). Federated databases can be established with the Make2D-DBII software (Mostaguir *et al.*, 2003). This program has a relational format and it facilitates integration e.g. to sequence and functional annotations.

Virtual, computational protein expression gels like in ProteomeWeb (Babnigg and Giometti, 2003) drawn based on measured or calculated pI and Mr can be useful for identification of proteins, especially those having low expression levels, with the usual caveats for post-translational modifications. For comparison to other experiments and results from other systems and methods, integration of data sources is instrumental. This is where ontologies, controlled vocabularies, and standards are needed. ProteomeWeb (Babnigg and Giometti, 2003) is an example of large-scale integration and annotation of protein expression data. This system includes information e.g. on gene annotations, chromosomal localization and gene codon usage. The same authors distribute experimental gel patterns for organisms for completed genomes (Babnigg and Giometti, 2004). GELBANK includes protein identifications in about 100 gels for human, *Methanococcus jannaschii*, *Pyrococcus furiosus*, and *Shewanella oneidensis*. Very large number of 2-DE information annotated in detail can be found at the Danish Centre for Human Genome Research. This resource is one of the largest individual sites with information for several organisms with emphasis on cell regulation in disease and health.

Interaction Proteomics

Proteins exert their functions only in contacts with other molecules. Interaction proteomics investigates the complexes and networks in which proteins are involved. Several experimental and computational methods can be used for interaction analysis. (Yeast) two-hybrid system (Uetz *et al.*, 2000) has been used to generate large data sets of interacting protein pairs. Systematic co-precipitation and MS studies have revealed very large protein complex networks (e.g. Gavin *et al.*, 2002, Ho *et al.*, 2002). With phage display a large number of interactions with peptide ligands and epitopes, single chain antibody fragments or enzyme substrates can be screened. Also cDNA libraries can be displayed on phages (Zozulya *et al.*, 1999). Expression profiles investigated by microarrays can also provide indirect interaction information (Cho *et al.*, 1998, Hughes *et al.*, 2000). Specific microarrays have been developed to screen for different types of interactions (Schweitzer *et al.*, 2003).

Lots of interaction information has been published in literature. Data mining with natural language processing (NLP) to automatically extract information from Medline abstracts or full-text articles (Hirschman *et al.*, 2002, Chiang and Yu, 2003) have been utilized in several databases.

Different interaction analysis approaches provide complementary information. Two recent large-scale comparative analyses of interaction networks in yeast obtained by several different ways indicated that only a small fraction of interactions have been detected with more than one method (von Mering *et al.*, 2002, Bader and Hogue, 2002). Use of multiple data sets is highly recommended whenever possible.

Interaction databases can be divided in two groups, those containing only experimental data and those including also - or only - inferred or predicted information. The following databases contain experimentally verified data. Interactions for yeast proteins from two-hybrid analysis are available in Yeast Protein Linkage Map (Table 4) for the Uetz *et al.* (2000) data sets along with interactions published in literature (Schwikowski *et al.*, 2000). Another yeast data source is Yeast Interacting Proteins Database (Ito *et al.*, 2001). Neither of these registries has been updated recently. Genetic interactions have been studied in large scale in yeast by utilizing deletion mutations to phenotypic characterization (Tong et al., 2004). This is one example of numerous techniques in which methods of molecular biology are utilized to derive knowledge about protein function and other properties.

PIMRider, a commercial data source, also offers four free services for academic scientists, *Helicobacter pylori, Drosophila melanogaster* interactions, human immunodeficiency virus and human protein interactions, and transforming growth factor β (TGF-β) interactions. Molecular INTeraction (MINT) contains experimentally verified protein-protein interactions of both direct and indirect relationships (Zanzoni *et al.*, 2002). Protein Quarternary Structure Database (PQS) is the best resource for interpreted subunit interactions in protein entries in PDB, whereas Nucleic Acid Database (NDB) offer the structures of all physically determined protein-nucleic acid complexes.

Inferred information along with experimental interaction data can be found at several sources. The Biomolecular Interaction Network Database (BIND) describes interactions, molecular complexes and pathways (Bader and Hogue, 2003) for proteins, nucleic acids and small molecules. The Database of Interacting Proteins (DIP) contains data of protein-protein interactions and interaction networks (Salwinski *et al.*, 2004). Human Protein Reference Database (HRPD, Peri *et al.*, 2004) contains not only interactions but also data for expression, associated diseases, post-translational modifications and subcellular localization. PPID (Protein-Protein Interaction Database) concentrates on three organims, human, rat and mouse. Systematic interaction databases are being built in an open access project IntAct (Hermjakob *et al.*, 2004b). STRING (von Mering *et al.*, 2003) has also predicted interactions altogether for more than 100 organisms.

Table 4. Links for interaction proteomics

Yeast Protein Linkage Map	http://depts.washington.edu/~sfields/yp_interactions/index.html
Yeast Interacting Proteins Database	http://itolab.cb.k.u-tokyo.ac.jp/Y2H/
PIMRider	http://pim.hybrigenics.com/pimriderext/common/
MINT	http://cbm.bio.uniroma2.it/mint/
BIND	http://www.bind.ca/Action
PQS Protein Quearternary Structure	http://pqs.ebi.ac.uk/
Nucleic Acid Database	http://ndbserver.rutgers.edu/
DIP	http://dip.doe-mbi.ucla.edu
Human Protein Reference Database	http://www.hprd.org/
Protein-Protein Interaction Database	http://www.anc.ed.ac.uk/mscs/PPID/
Search Tool for the Retrieval of Interacting Genes/Proteins	http://string.embl.de/
KEGG	http://www.genome.ad.jp/kegg
Phosphoprotein Database	http://www.phosphosite.org/Login.jsp
Biocarta	http://www.biocarta.com/genes/index.asp
Signaling Gateway	http://www.signaling-gateway.org/
Signal Transduction Knowledge Environment	http://stke.sciencemag.org/

Table 5. Functional proteomics links

TBASE	http://jaxmice.jax.org/index.html
OMIM	http://www.ncbi.nlm.nih.gov/entrez/query.fcgi?db=OMIM
Locus-specific mutation databases	http://www.hgvs.org/
RNAiDB	http://nematoda.bio.nyu.edu/
PhenoBlast	http://nematoda.bio.nyu.edu/cgi-bin/rnai3/ace/phenoblast.cgi
Saccharomyces Deletion Project	http://www-sequence.stanford.edu/group/yeast_deletion_project/deletions3.html

Table 6. Structural bioinformatics links

Protein Data Bank	http://www.rcsb.org/pdb/
Chime	http://www.umass.edu/microbio/chime/
RasTop	http://www.geneinfinity.org/rastop/
PyMol	http://pymol.sourceforge.net/
Cn3D	http://130.14.29.110/Structure/CN3D/cn3d.shtml
WebMol	http://www.cmpharm.ucsf.edu/cgi-bin/webmol.pl
MSD	http://www.ebi.ac.uk/msd/index.html
PDBsum	http://www.biochem.ucl.ac.uk/bsm/pdbsum/
STING	http://trantor.bioc.columbia.edu/SMS/STINGm/
SRS-3D	http://srs3d.ebi.ac.uk/
Biotech Validation Suite for Protein Structures	http://biotech.ebi.ac.uk:8400/
Protein Explorer	http://molvis.sdsc.edu/protexpl/frntdoor.htm
Kinemage	http://kinemage.biochem.duke.edu/
CATH	http://cathwww.biochem.ucl.ac.uk/latest/index.html
SCOP	http://scop.mrc-lmb.cam.ac.uk/scop/
DALI	http://ekhidna.biocenter.helsinki.fi/dali/start

Kyoto Encyclopedia of Genes and Genomes (KEGG) includes all kinds of molecular interactions; metabolic pathways, regulatory pathways, and molecular assemblies (Kanehisa *et al.*, 2002). Bioinformatics services for signaling molecules and pathways have been recently reviewed (Vihinen, 2003). Here we can mention a few excellent resources; Phosphoprotein Database (PPDB), which is based on 2-DE analysis of phosphorylation sites; Biocarta, a compilation of pathways; and the largest resources of this kind from Nature and Science journals, the Signaling Gateway and Signal Transduction Knowledge Environment (STKE), respectively.

Protein interaction networks have been calculated based on the expression information by applying reverse engineering based e.g. on linear system of equations (Yeung *et al.*, 2002), Bayesian (D'Haeseleer *et al.*, 2000) or Boolean networks (Friedman *et al.*, 2000).

Functional Proteomics

Protein function can be revealed by inactivating or perturbing the protein. This can be achieved at different levels. Deletions or direct mutations leading to a knockout model can be easily produced for many unicellular organisms. Mouse has been the most widely used animal model for vertebrates. TBASE (Table 5) is a large database of knockout models, especially for mouse. This resource has also descriptions of phenotypes of heterozygous and homozygous knockouts. Animal models related to human diseases can be found from OMIM (On-line Mendelian Inheritance in Man). Locus-specific mutation databases are already available for more than 500 genes.

Protein (enzyme) specific inhitors can be utilized for activity/function modulation. Antisense oligonucleotides bind to complementary mRNA and thereby prevent transcription (see Dean, 2001). RNA interference (RNAi) technique is widely used for gene silencing. Short double-stranded RNA molecules can be very effective inhibitors of gene expression. Originally described for *Caenorhabditis elegans* (Fire *et al.*, 1998) the technique has subsequently been applied to many other organisms including human (Elbashir *et al.*, 2001). RNAiDB is a dedicated database for large-scale RNAi analysis in *C. elegans* (Gunsalus *et al.*, 2004). Another tool, PhenoBlast gives ranked information about phenotypic similarities in experiments. Genomewide RNAi experiments have started to emerge (e.g. Boutros *et al.*, 2004, Nollen *et al.*, 2004).

Almost all yeast genes have already been knocked out in Saccharomyces Deletion Project. In another project double mutants are generated (Tong *et al.*, 2001). Transferred DNA (T-DNA) insertional mutagenesis was applied to produce mutations to the majority of *Arabidopsis thaliana* genes (Alonso et al., 2003). There are several other consortia for investigating the effects of deletions in other organisms.

Structural Proteomics

Proteins can be functional only in folded three-dimensional structure. Therefore structural information is crucial for understanding the function of a protein. Three-dimensional structures determined either with X-ray crystallography or nuclear magnetic resonance (NMR) spectroscopy are collected to Protein Data Bank (PDB) (Table 6). Large-scale structural proteomics (Sali *et al.*, 2003) has numerous obstacles, however it is making progress both on crystallography (Jhoti, 2001) and NMR (Rehm *et al.*, 2002) fronts.

Structures can be visualised with freely available programs like Chime, RasTop, PyMol, Cn3D, or WebMol. Several web services including Astex viewer at MSD, STING and SRS-3D, offer simultaneous views of structure and sequence, or even several aligned structures and sequences. Some programs specialize in the production of annotated animations or sequences of visualizations, designed to highlight important structural features. The two best-known programs in this category are Protein Explorer and Kinemage. PDB structures and their features are reachable via PDBsum, which lists a large number of structure-related features for each entry and provides links to other services. Information on the quality of the determined structures in many levels is provided by services available at Biotech Validation Suite for Protein Structures.

For understanding protein functions, it is essential to analyze their modes of binding to various ligands. The MSDsite service has many tools for this purpose for all ligands found in protein three-dimensional structures.

There is only a limited number of different protein structure and architectures. The exact number of folds is not known, most estimates range from about 1,000 to a few thousand folds. Protein folds are classified in CATH (Orengo *et al.*, 1997), SCOP (Andreeva *et al.*, 2004), and DALI (Holm and Sander, 1996). Already the smallest organisms have hundreds of different proteins and higher organisms have tens of thousands of genes and even much more of proteins. Thus, there is a great need for structural information, whether obtained by experimental or theoretical means.

Acknowledgements

Financial support from the National Technology Agency of Finland, and the Medical Research Fund of Tampere University Hospital.

References

Alonso, J. M., Stepanova, A. N., Leisse, T. J., Kim, C. J., Chen, H., Shinn, P., Stevensson, D. K., Zimmerman, J., Barajas, P., Cheuk, R., Gadrinab, C., Heller, C., Jeske, A., Koesema, E., Meyers, C. C., Parker, H., Prednis, L., Ansari, Y., Choy, N., Deen, H., Geralt, M., Hazari, N., Hom, E., Karnes, M., Mulholland, C., Ndubaku, R., Schmidt, I., Guzman, P., Aguilar-Henonin, L., Schmid, M., Weigel, D., Carter, D. E., Marchand, T., Risseeuw, E., Brogden, D., Zeko, A., Crosby, W. L., Berry, C. C. and Ecker, J. R. (2003) Genome-wide insertional mutagenesis of *Arabidopsis thaliana. Science* **301**, 653-657.

Anderson, L. and Seilhamer., J. (1997) A comparison of selected mRNA and protein abundances in human liver. *Electrophoresis* **18**, 533-537.

Andreeva, A., Howorth, D., Brenner, S. E., Hubbard, T. J. P., Chothia, C. and Murzin, A. G. (2004) SCOP database in 2004: refinements integrate structure and sequence family data. *Nucleic Acids Res.* **32** Database issue, D226-D229.

Appel, R. D., Bairoch, A., Sanchez, J. C., Vargas, J. R., Golaz, O., Pasquali, C. and Hochstrasser, D. F. (1996) Federated two-dimensional electrophoresis database: a simple means of publishing two-dimensional electrophoresis data. *Electrophoresis* **17**, 540-546.

Babnigg, G. and Giometti, C. S. (2003) ProteomeWeb: A Web-based interface for the display and interrogation of proteomes. *Proteomics* **3**, 584-600.

Babnigg, G. and Giometti, C. S. (2004) GELBANK: a database of annotated two-dimensional gel electrophoresis patterns of biological systems with completed genomes. *Nucleic Acids Res*. **32**, D582-D585.

Bader, G. D. and Hogue, C. W. (2002) Analyzing yeast protein-protein interaction data obtained from different sources. *Nat. Biotechnol.* **20**, 991-997.

Bader, G. D. and Hogue, C. W. (2003) An automated method for finding molecular complexes in large protein interaction networks. *BMC Bioinformatics.* **4**, 2.

Boutros, M., Kiger, A. A., Armknecht, S., Kerr, K., Hild, M., Koch, B., Haas, S. A., Heidelberg Fly Array Consortium, Paro, R., Perrimon, N. (2004) Genome-Wide RNAi analysis of growth and viability in *Drosophila* cells. *Science* **303**, 832-835.

Chamrad, D. C., Körting, G., Stühler, K., Meyer, H. E., Klose, J. and Blüggel, M. (2004) Evaluation of algorithms for protein identification from sequence databases using mass spectrometry data. *Proteomics* **4**, 619-628.

Chiang, J. H. and Yu, H. C. (2003) MeKE: discovering the functions of gene products from biomedical literature via sentence alignment. *Bioinformatics* **19**, 1417-1422.

Cho, R. J., Campbell, M. J., Winzeler, E. A., Steinmetz, L., Conway, A., Wodicka, L., Wolfsberg, T. G., Gabrielian, A. E., Landsman, D., Lockhart DJ. and Davis RW. (1998) A genome-wide transcriptional analysis of the mitotic cell cycle. *Mol. Cell* **2**,65-73.

Cutler, P. (2003) Protein arrays: The current state-of-the-art. *Proteomics* **3**, 3-18.

Dean, N. M. (2001) Functional genomics and target validation approaches using antisense oligonucleotide technology. *Curr. Opin. Biotechnol.* **12**, 622-625.

D'Haeseleer, P., Liang, S. and Somogyi, R. (2000) Genetic network inference: from co-expression clustering to reverse engineering. *Bioinformatics* **16**, 707-726.

Dowsey, A. W., Dunn, M. J. and Guang-Zong, Y. (2003) The role of bioinformatics in two-dimensional gel electrophoresis. *Proteomics* **3**, 1567-1596.

Elbashir, S. M., Harborth, J., Lendeckel, W., Yalcin, A., Weber K. and Tuschl T. (2001) Duplexes of 21-nucleotide RNAs mediate RNA interference in cultured mammalian cells. *Nature* **411**, 494-498.

Fire A., Xu S., Montgomery M. K., Kostas, S. A., Driver S. E., and Mello, C. C. (1998). Potent and specific genetic interference by double-stranded RNA in *Caenorhabditis elegans*. *Nature* **391**, 806-811.

Friedman, N., Linial, M., Nachman, I. and Pe'er, D. (2000) Using Bayesian networks to analyze expression data. *J. Comput. Biol.* **7**, 601-620.

Gavin, A. C., Bosche, M., Krause, R., Grandi, P., Marzioch, M., Bauer, A., Schultz, J., Rick, J. M., Michon, A. M., Cruciat, C. M., Remor, M., Hofert, C., Schelder, M., Brajenovic, M., Ruffner, H., Merino, A., Klein, K., Hudak, M., Dickson, D., Rudi, T., Gnau, V., Bauch, A., Bastuck, S., Huhse, B., Leutwein, C., Heurtier, M. A., Copley, R. R., Edelmann, A., Querfurth, E., Rybin, V., Drewes, G., Raida, M., Bouwmeester, T., Bork, P., Seraphin, B., Kuster, B., Neubauer, G. and Superti-Furga, G. (2002) Functional organization of the yeast proteome by systematic analysis of protein complexes. *Nature* **415**, 141-147.

Gunsalus, K. C., Yeh, W-C., MacMenamin, P. and Piano, F (2004) RNAiDB and PhenoBlast: web tools for genome-wide phenotypic mapping projects. *Nucleic Acids Res.* **32** Database issue, D406-D410.

Gygi, S. P., Rist, B., Gerber, S. A., Turecek, F., Gelb, M. H. and Aebersold, R. (1999a) Quantitative analysis of complex protein mixtures using isotope-coded affinity tags. *Nature Biotechnol.* **17**, 994-999.

Gygi, S. P., Rochon, Y., Franza, B. R. and Aebersold, R. (1999b) Correlation between protein and mRNA abundance in yeast. *Mol. Cell. Biol.* **19**, 1720-1730.

Hermjakob, H., Montecchi-Palazzi, Bader, G., Wojcik, J., Salwinski, L., Ceol, A., Moore, S., Orchard, S., Sarkans, U., von Mering, C., Roechert, B., Poux, S., Jung, E., Mersch, H., Kersey, P., Lappe, M., Lix, Y., Zeng, R., Rana, D., Nikolski, M., Husi, H., Brun, C., Shanker, K., Grant, S. G. N., Sander, C., Bork, P., Zhu, W., Pandey, A., Brazma, A., Jacq, B., Vidal, M., Sherman, D., Legrain, P., Cesareni, G., Xenarios, I., Eisenberg, D., Steipe, B., Hogue, C. and Apweiler, R. (2004a) The HUPO PSI Molecular Interaction Format - A community standard for the representation of protein interaction data. *Nature Biotechnol.* **22**, 177-183.

Hermjakob, H., Montecchi-Palazzi, L., Lewington, C., Mudali, S., Kerrien, S., Orchard, S., Vingron, M., Roechert, B., Roepstorff, P., Valencia, A., Margalit, H., Armstrong, J., Bairoch, A., Cesareni, G., Sherman, D., Apweiler, R. (2004b) IntAct - an open source molecular interaction database. *Nucleic Acids Res.* **32**: 32 Database issue, D452-D455.

Hirschman, L., Park, J. C., Tsujii, J., Wong, L. and Wu, C. H. (2002) Accomplishments and challenges in literature data mining for biology. *Bioinformatics* **18**, 1553-1561.

Ho, Y., Gruhler, A., Heilbut, A., Bader, G. D., Moore, L., Adams, S. L., Millar, A., Taylor, P., Bennett, K., Boutilier, K., Yang, L., Wolting, C., Donaldson, I., Schandorff, S., Shewnarane, J., Vo, M., Taggart, J., Goudreault, M., Muskat, B., Alfarano, C., Dewar, D., Lin, Z., Michalickova, K., Willems, A. R., Sassi, H., Nielsen, P. A., Rasmussen, K. J., Andersen, J. R., Johansen, L. E., Hansen, L. H., Jespersen, H., Podtelejnikov, A., Nielsen, E., Crawford, J., Poulsen, V., Sorensen, B. D., Matthiesen, J., Hendrickson, R. C., Gleeson, F., Pawson, T., Moran, M. F., Durocher, D., Mann, M., Hogue, C. W., Figeys, D. and Tyers, M. (2002) Systematic identification of protein complexes in *Saccharomyces cerevisiae* by mass spectrometry. *Nature* **415**, 180-183.

Holm, L. and Sander, C. (1996) Mapping the protein universe. *Science* **273**, 595-602.

Hughes, T. R., Marton, M. J., Jones, A. R., Roberts, C. R., Stoughton, R., Armour, C. D. Bennett, H. A., Coffey, E., Dai, H., He, Y. D., Kidd, M. J., King, A. M., Meyer, M. R., Slade, D., Lum, P. Y., Stepaniants, S. B., Shoemaker, D. D., Gachotte, D., Chakraburtty, K., Simon, J., Bard, M. and Friend, S. H. (2000) Functional discovery via a compendium of expression profiles. *Cell* **102**, 109-126.

Ito, T., Chiba, T., Ozawa, R., Yoshida, M., Hattori, M. and Sakaki, Y. (2001) A comprehensive two-hybrid analysis to explore the yeast protein interactome. *Proc. Natl. Acad. Sci. USA* **98**, 4569-4574.

Jhoti, H. (2001) High-troughput structural proteomics using X-rays. *Trends. Biotechnol.* **19**, 567-571.

Kanehisa, M., Goto, S., Kawashima, S., Okuno, Y., and Hattori, M. (2004) The KEGG resources for deciphering the genome. *Nucleic Acids Res.* **32** Database issue, D277-D280.

Lemkin, P. F. (1997a) Comparing two-dimensional electrophoretic gel images across the Internet. *Electrophoresis* **18**, 461-470.

Lemkin, P.F. (1997b) The 2DWG meta-database of two-dimensional electrophoretic gel images on the Internet. *Electrophoresis* **18**, 2759-2773.

Mann, M. and Jensen, O. N. (2003) Proteomic analysis of post-translational modifications. *Nature Biotechnol.* **21**, 255-261.

von Mering, C., Huynen, M., Jaeggi, D., Schmidt, S., Bork, P. and Snel, B. (2003) STRING: a database of predicted functional associations between proteins. *Nucleic Acids Res.* **31**, 258-261.

von Mering, C., Krause, R., Snel, B., Cornell, M., Oliver, S. G., Fields, S. and Bork, P. (2002) Comparative assessment of large-scale data sets of protein-protein interactions. *Nature* **417**, 399-403.

Mostaguir, K., Hoogland, C., Binz, P-A. and Appel, R. A. (2003) The Make 2D-DB II package: Conversion of federated two-dimensional gel electrophoresis databases into a relational format and interconnection of distributed databases. *Proteomics* **3**, 1441-1444.

Nollen, E. A. A., Garcia, S. M., van Haaften, G., Kim, J., Chavez, A., Morimoto, R. I. and Plasterk, R. H. A. (2004) Genome-wide RNA interference screen identifies previously undescribed regulators of polyglutamine aggretation. *Proc. Natl. Acad. Sci. USA* **101**, 6403-6408.

O'Donovan, C., Apweiler, R. and Bairoch, A. (2001) The human proteomics initiative (HPI). *Trends. Biotechnol.* **19**, 178-181

Orengo, C.A., Michie, A.D., Jones, S., Jones, D.T., Swindells, M.B., and Thornton, J.M. (1997) CATH - A hierarchic classification of protein domain structures. *Structure* **5**, 1093-1108.

Peri, S., Navarro, J. D., Kristiansen, T. Z., Amanchy, R., Surendranath, V., Muthusamy, B., Gandhi, T. K. B., Chandrika, K. N., Deshpande, N., Suresh, S., Rashmi, B. P., Shanker, K., Padma, N., Niranjan, V., Harsha, H. C., Talreja, N., Vrushabendra, B. M., Ramya, M. A., Yatish, A. J., Joy, M., Shivashankar, H. N., Kavitha, M. P., Menezes, M., Choudhury, D. R., Ghosh, N., Sarawana, R., Chandran, S., Mohan, S., Jonnalagadda, C. K., Prasad, C. K., Kumar-Sinha, C., Deshpande, K. S., and Pandey, A. (2004) Human protein reference database as a discovery resource for proteomics. *Nucleic Acids Res.* **32** Database issue, D497-D501.

Raman, B., Cheung, A. and Marten, M. R. (2002) Quantitative comparison and evaluation of two commercially available, two-dimensional electrophoresis image analysis software packages, Z3 and Melanie. *Electrophoresis* **23**, 2194-2202.

Rehm, T., Huber, R. and Holak, T. A. (2002) Application of NMR in structural proteomics: Screening for proteins amenable to structural analysis. *Structure* **10**,1613-1618.

Rosengren, A. T., Salmi, J. M., Aittokallio, T., Westerholm, J., Lahesmaa, R., Nyman, T. A. and Nevalainen, O. S. (2003) Comparison of PDQuest and Progenesis software packages in the analysis of two-dimensional electrophoresis gels. *Proteomics* **3**, 1936-1946.

Sali, A., Glaeser, R., Earnest, T. and Baumeister, W. (2003) From words to literature in structural proteomics. *Nature* **422**, 216-225.

Salwinski, L., Miller, C. S., Smith, A. J., Pettit, F. K., Bowie, J. U. and Eisenberg, D (2004) The Database of Interacting Proteins: 2004 update. *Nucleic Acids Res.* **32** Database issue D449-D451.

Schweitzer, B., Predki, P. and Snyder, M. (2003) Microarrays to characterize protein interactions on a whole-proteome scale. *Proteomics* **3**, 2190-2199.

Schwikowski, B., Uetz, P. and Fields, S. (2000) A network of protein-protein interactions in yeast. *Nature Biotech.* **18**, 1257-1261.

Taylor, C. F., Paton, N. W., Garwood, K. L., Kirby, P. D., Staed, D. A., Ying, Z., Deutsch, E. W., Selway L., Walker, J., Riba-Garcia, I., Mohammed, S., Deery, M. J., Howard, J. A., Dunkley, T., Aebersold, R., Kell, D. B., Lilley, K. S., Roepstorff, P., Yates, J. R., Brass, A., Brown, A. J. P., Cash, P., Gaskell, S. J., Hubbard, S. J. and Oliver, S. G. (2003) A systematic approach to modeling, capturing, and dissemination of proteomics experimental data. *Nature Biotechnol.* **21**, 247-254.

Tong, A. H., Evangelista, M., Parsons, A. B., Xu, H., Bader, G. D., Page, N., Robinson, M., Raghibizadeh, S., Hogue, C. W., Bussey, H., Andrews, B., Tyers, M. and Boone, C. (2001) Systematic genetic analysis with ordered arrays of yeast deletion mutants. *Science* **294**, 2364-2368.

Tong, A. H. Y., Lesage, G., Bader, G. D., Ding, H.,. Xu, H., Xin, X., Young, J., Berriz, G. F., Brost, R. L., Chang, M., Chen, Y., Cheng, X., Chua, G., Friesen, H., Goldberg, D. S., Haynes, J., Humphries, C., He, G., Hussein, S., Ke, L., Krogan, N., Li, Z., Levinson, J. N., Lu, H., Menard, P., Munyana, C., Parsons, A. B., Ryan, O., Tonikian, R., Roberts, T., Sdicu, A. M., Shapiro, J., Sheikh, B., Suter, B., Wong, S. L., Zhang, L. V., Zhu, H., Burd, C. G., Munro, S., Sander, C., Rine, J., Greenblatt, J., Peter, M., Bretscher, A., Bell, G., Roth, F. P., Brown, G. W., Andrews, B., Bussey, H. and Boone, C. (2004) Global mapping of the yeast genetic interaction network. *Science* **303**, 808-813.

Uetz, P., Giot, L., Cagney, G., Mansfield, T. A, Judson, R. S., Knight, J. R., Lockshon, D., Narayan, V., Srinivasan, M., Pochart, P., Qureshi-Emili, A., Li, Y., Godwin, B., Conover, D., Kalbfleisch, T., Vijayadamodar, G., Yang, M., Johnston, M., Fields, S. and Rothberg, J. M. (2000) A comprehensive analysis of protein-protein interactions in *Saccharomyces cerevisiae*. *Nature* **403**, 623-627.

Vihinen, M. (2001) Bioinformatics in proteomics. *Biomol. Eng.* **18**, 241-248.

Vihinen, M. (2004) Bioinformatics in proteomics. In *Handbook of Proteomic Methods*, P. M. Conn (ed), pp. 419-428, Humana Press.

Wojcik, J. and Schächter, V. (2000) Proteomic databases and software on the web. *Brief. Bioinf.* **1**, 250-259

Zanzoni, A., Montecchi-Palazzi, L., Quondam, M., Ausiello, G., Helmer-Citterich, M. and Cesareni, G. (2002) MINT: a Molecular INTeraction database. *FEBS Letters*, **513,** 135-140

Zozulya, S., Lioubin, M., Hill, R. J., Abram, C. and Gishizky, M. L. (1999) Mapping signal transduction pathways by phage display. *Nature Biotechnol.* **17**, 1193-1198.

Yeung, M. K., Tegner, J. and Collins, J. J. (2002) Reverse engineering gene networks using singular value decomposition and robust regression. *Proc. Natl. Acad. Sci. USA* **99**, 6163-6168.

Index

A

B

C

F

G

H

I

N

O

P

Q

R

S

W

X

Y

Z